Acute and Chronic Complications of Diabetes

Editors

LEONID PORETSKY
EMILIA PAULINE LIAO

ENDOCRINOLOGY AND METABOLISM CLINICS OF NORTH AMERICA

www.endo.theclinics.com

Consulting Editor
DEREK LEROITH

December 2013 • Volume 42 • Number 4

ELSEVIER

1600 John F. Kennedy Boulevard • Suite 1800 • Philadelphia, Pennsylvania, 19103-2899

http://www.theclinics.com

ENDOCRINOLOGY AND METABOLISM CLINICS OF NORTH AMERICA Volume 42, Number 4
December 2013 ISSN 0889-8529, ISBN-13: 978-0-323-26094-7

Editor: Jessica McCool
Developmental Editor: Susan Showalter

Endocrinology and Metabolism Clinics of North America (ISSN 0889-8529) is published quarterly by Elsevier Inc., 360 Park Avenue South, New York, NY 10010-1710. Months of issue are March, June, September, and December. Periodicals postage paid at New York, NY and additional mailing offices. Subscription prices are USD 330.00 per year for US individuals, USD 581.00 per year for US institutions, USD 165.00 per year for US students and residents, USD 415.00 per year for Canadian individuals, USD 718.00 per year for Canadian institutions, USD 480.00 per year for international individuals, USD 718.00 per year for international institutions, and USD 245.00 per year for international and Canadian and foreign students/residents. To receive student/resident rate, orders must be accompanied by name of affiliated institution, date of term, and the signature of program/residency coordinator on institution letterhead. Orders will be billed at individual rate until proof of status is received. Foreign air speed delivery is included in all *Clinics* subscription prices. All prices are subject to change without notice. **POSTMASTER:** Send address changes to *Endocrinology and Metabolism Clinics of North America*, Elsevier Health Sciences Division, Subscription Customer Service, 3251 Riverport Lane, Maryland Heights, MO 63043. **Customer Service: Telephone: 1-800-654-2452** (U.S. and Canada); **1-314-447-8871** (outside U.S. and Canada). **Fax: 1-314-447-8029. E-mail: journalscustomerservice-usa@elsevier.com** (for print support); **journalsonlinesupport-usa@elsevier.com** (for online support).

Reprints. For copies of 100 or more, of articles in this publication, please contact the Commercial Rights Department, Elsevier Inc., 360 Park Avenue South, New York, NY 10010-1710; phone: +1-212-633-3874; fax: +1-212-633-3820; E-mail: reprints@elsevier.com.

Endocrinology and Metabolism Clinics of North America is covered in *MEDLINE/PubMed (Index Medicus)*, *EMBASE/Excerpta Medica, Current Contents/Clinical Medicine, Current Contents/Life Sciences, Science Citation Index, ISI/BIOMED, BIOSIS,* and *Chemical Abstracts.*

Printed and bound by CPI Group (UK) Ltd, Croydon, CR0 4YY

Transferred to digital print 2012

Contributors

CONSULTING EDITOR

DEREK LEROITH, MD, PhD
Director of Research, Division of Endocrinology, Metabolism, and Bone Diseases, Department of Medicine, Mount Sinai School of Medicine, New York, New York

EDITORS

EMILIA PAULINE LIAO, MD
Assistant Professor, Department of Medicine, Albert Einstein College of Medicine, Bronx; Associate Program Director, Endocrinology, Beth Israel Medical Center, New York, New York

LEONID PORETSKY, MD
Professor, Department of Medicine, Albert Einstein College of Medicine, Bronx; Division Chief, Endocrinology, Beth Israel Medical Center, New York, New York

AUTHORS

MAZEN ALSAHLI, MD
Staff Specialist, Division of Endocrinology, Department of Medicine, Southlake Regional Health Center, Newmarket; Adjunct Professor of Medicine, Department of Medicine, Faculty of Medicine, University of Toronto, Toronto, Ontario, Canada

SUSAN M. BISSETT, MclinRes
School of Dental Sciences, Institute of Cellular Medicine, Newcastle University, Newcastle upon Tyne, United Kingdom

BRIGID S. BOLAND, MD
Gastroenterology Fellow, Division of Gastroenterology, Department of Medicine, University of California, San Diego, La Jolla, California

CAROLINA CASELLINI, MD
Research Associate, Internal Medicine, Strelitz Diabetes Center, Eastern Virginia Medical School, Norfolk, Virginia

STEVEN R. COHEN, MD, MPH
Division of Dermatology, Albert Einstein College of Medicine, Montefiore Medical Center, Bronx, New York

SARAH D. CORATHERS, MD
Assistant Professor of Pediatrics, Division of Endocrinology, Cincinnati Children's Hospital Medical Center; Assistant Professor of Internal Medicine, Division of Endocrinology, University of Cincinnati Medical Center, Cincinnati, Ohio

ANDREW DREXLER, MD
Department of Endocrinology, Gonda Diabetes Center, University of California, Los Angeles School of Medicine, Los Angeles, California

STEVEN V. EDELMAN, MD
Professor of Medicine, Division of Endocrinology and Metabolism, University of California, San Diego, La Jolla; Director, Division of Endocrinology and Metabolism, Diabetes Care Clinic, Veterans Affairs Medical Center, San Diego, California

MARIANA GARCIA-TOUZA, MD
Assistant Professor of Medicine, Diabetes and Cardiovascular Research Center; Division of Endocrinology, Diabetes and Metabolism, Department of Internal Medicine, University of Missouri Columbia School of Medicine, Columbia, Missouri

GEOFFREY GAUNAY, MD
Resident, Sol and Margaret Berger Department of Urology, Beth Israel Medical Center, New York, New York

JOHN E. GERICH, MD
Professor of Medicine, Division of Endocrinology, Department of Medicine, University of Rochester School of Medicine, Rochester, New York

GEORGE HAN, MD, PhD
Albert Einstein College of Medicine, Bronx, New York

ANKUR JINDAL, MD
Assistant Professor of Clinical Medicine, Hospital Medicine, Department of Internal Medicine; Diabetes and Cardiovascular Research Center, University of Missouri, Columbia, Missouri

NIDHI JINDAL, MD
Nephrology Fellow, Division of Nephrology and Hypertension, Department of Internal Medicine, University of Missouri Columbia School of Medicine, Columbia, Missouri

PAUL J. KIM, DPM, MS
Associate Professor, Department of Plastic Surgery, Georgetown School of Medicine, Center for Wound Healing and Hyperbaric Medicine, MedStar Georgetown University Hospital, Washington, DC

JELENA MALETKOVIC, MD
Department of Endocrinology, Gonda Diabetes Center, University of California, Los Angeles School of Medicine, Los Angeles, California

BLAIR MURPHY-CHUTORIAN, BA, MSIV
University of California, Irvine, Irvine, California

HARRIS M. NAGLER, MD
President and Chair, Sol and Margaret Berger Department of Urology, Beth Israel Medical Center, New York; Professor of Urology, Albert Einstein College of Medicine of Yeshiva University, Bronx, New York

ANINDITA NANDI, MD
Attending Physician, Division of Endocrinology and Metabolism, Beth Israel Medical Center, Albert Einstein College of Medicine, New York, New York

MARIE-LAURE NEVORET, MD
Clinical Research Coordinator, Internal Medicine, Strelitz Diabetes Center, Eastern Virginia Medical School, Norfolk, Virginia

HENRI PARSON, PhD
Director, Microvascular Biology; Assistant Professor, Internal Medicine, Strelitz Diabetes Center, Eastern Virginia Medical School, Norfolk, Virginia

SHAWN PEAVIE, DO
Fellow, Division of Endocrinology, University of Cincinnati Medical Center, Cincinnati, Ohio

LEONID PORETSKY, MD
Professor, Department of Medicine, Albert Einstein College of Medicine, Bronx; Division Chief, Endocrinology, Beth Israel Medical Center, New York, New York

PHILIP M. PRESHAW, BDS, FDSRCSEd, FDS(RestDent)RCSEd, PhD
Professor of Periodontology, School of Dental Sciences, Institute of Cellular Medicine, Newcastle University, Newcastle upon Tyne, United Kingdom

DANIEL F. ROSBERGER, MD, PhD, MPH
Clinical Assistant Professor of Ophthalmology, Weill-Cornell Medical College of Cornell University; Medical and Surgical Director, MaculaCare, PLLC, New York, New York

MARZIEH SALEHI, MD, MS
Associate Professor of Internal Medicine, Division of Endocrinology, University of Cincinnati Medical Center, Cincinnati, Ohio

JAMES R. SOWERS, MD
Professor of Medicine, and Medical Pharmacology and Physiology; Diabetes and Cardiovascular Research Center, University of Missouri; Division of Endocrinology, Diabetes and Metabolism, Department of Internal Medicine, University of Missouri Columbia School of Medicine; Department of Internal Medicine, Harry S Truman Memorial Veterans Hospital; Department of Medical Physiology and Pharmacology, University of Missouri, Columbia, Missouri

JOHN S. STEINBERG, DPM
Associate Professor, Department of Plastic Surgery, Georgetown School of Medicine, Center for Wound Healing and Hyperbaric Medicine, MedStar Georgetown University Hospital, Washington, DC

DORON S. STEMBER, MD
Faculty, Sol and Margaret Berger Department of Urology, Beth Israel Medical Center, New York; Assistant Professor, Albert Einstein College of Medicine of Yeshiva University, Bronx, New York

GARY E. STRIKER, MD
Professor, Departments of Geriatrics and Medicine, Icahn School of Medicine at Mount Sinai, New York, New York

AARON I. VINIK, MD, PhD
Professor of Medicine/Pathology/Neurobiology, Director of Research and Neuroendocrine Unit, Internal Medicine, Strelitz Diabetes Center, Eastern Virginia Medical School, Norfolk, Virginia

HELEN VLASSARA, MD
Professor of Geriatrics and Medicine, Departments of Geriatrics and Medicine, Icahn School of Medicine at Mount Sinai, New York, New York

ADAM WHALEY-CONNELL, DO, MSPH
Associate Professor of Medicine, Diabetes and Cardiovascular Research Center, University of Missouri; Division of Endocrinology, Diabetes and Metabolism, Department of Internal Medicine; Division of Nephrology and Hypertension, Department of Internal Medicine, University of Missouri Columbia School of Medicine; Associate Chief of Staff for Research and Development, Harry S Truman Memorial Veterans Hospital, Columbia, Missouri

JAMES D. WOLOSIN, MD
Chief, Division of Gastroenterology, Sharp Rees-Stealy Medical Group, San Diego, California

Contents

indicated that tight glucose control and lifestyle modification can dramatically reduce the incidence and prevalence of diabetic retinopathy. Research over the past several years has yielded a tremendous increase in our knowledge of the pathogenesis of the damage to the retina that occurs in diabetes and has facilitated our ability to intervene and control the damage. New intravitreal medical therapies supported by government- and industry-supported research are gradually replacing standard laser photocoagulation for the treatment of all forms of retinopathy.

Diabetic neuropathy (DN) is the most common and troublesome complication of diabetes mellitus, leading to the greatest morbidity and mortality and resulting in a huge economic burden for diabetes care. The clinical assessment of diabetic peripheral neuropathy and its treatment options are multifactorial. Patients with DN should be screened for autonomic neuropathy, as there is a high degree of coexistence of the two complications. A review of the clinical assessment and treatment algorithms for diabetic neuropathy, painful neuropathy, and autonomic dysfunction is provided.

In this article, the literature is reviewed regarding the role of blood pressure variability and nocturnal nondipping of blood pressure as well as the presence of diabetic kidney disease (DKD), in the absence of albuminuria, as risk predictors for progressive DKD. The importance of glycemic and blood pressure control in patients with diabetes and chronic kidney disease, and the use of oral hypoglycemic agents and antihypertensive agents in this patient cohort, are also discussed.

This review provides an overview of the vast gastrointestinal tract complications of diabetes that can occur from the mouth to the anus. The presentation, diagnosis, and management of gastrointestinal disorders, ranging from gastroparesis, celiac disease, and bacterial overgrowth to nonalcoholic fatty liver disease, are reviewed to heighten awareness. When managing care of patients with diabetes, one should keep in mind the potential gastrointestinal complications, as well as the frequent disorders that are not related to diabetes.

The diabetic foot is at high risk for complications because of its role in ambulation. Peripheral neuropathy and peripheral vascular disease can lead to chronic foot ulcers, which are at high risk for infection, in part attributable to areas of high pressure caused by lack of tolerance of the soft tissue and bone and joint deformity. If left untreated, infection and ischemia lead to tissue death, culminating in amputation. Treatment strategies include antibiosis, topical therapies, offloading, debridement, and surgery. A multidisciplinary team approach is necessary in the prevention and treatment of complications of the diabetic foot.

ENDOCRINOLOGY AND METABOLISM CLINICS OF NORTH AMERICA

RELATED INTEREST

Medical Clinics of North America, Volume 97, Issue 5 (September 2013)
The Diabetic Foot
Andrew J.M. Boulton, *Editor*
Available at: http://www.medical.theclinics.com/

Foreword

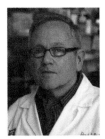

Derek LeRoith, MD, PhD
Consulting Editor

This issue on diabetic complications provides discussion of both basic pathophysiology and practical treatment for both researchers and clinicians. The next issue will focus on conditions closely associated with diabetes. Given the epidemic of obesity and type 2 diabetes, these are most timely topics for *Endocrinology and Metabolism Clinics of North America*.

Hypoglycemia is one of the major acute complications that diabetic individuals have to deal with, especially those on sulphonylureas and insulin therapy. The risk is further increased when renal function is compromised. The normal counterregulatory response to hypoglycemia may be impaired, leading to an even more dangerous situation with increased morbidity and mortality. As Drs Alsahli and Gerich discuss, episodes of hypoglycemia can be reduced in severity and occurrence with intensive education of patients.

Drs Maletkovic and Drexler describe the effect of poorly controlled diabetes, namely diabetic ketoacidotic (DKA) and hyperosmolar states (HHS). Despite the widespread use of insulin in type 1 patients as well as a panoply of oral agents for type 2 patients, these acute conditions are still prevalent today. Both conditions present with hyperglycemia and dehydration; however, the complete absence of insulin in type 1 patients leads to excess lipolysis and ketoacidosis. Often the cause is an intermittent stressful condition. DKA is often more rapid in onset, whereas HHS is more insidious. There are established protocols for fluid, insulin, and electrolyte replacement, and while most patients recover, this is unfortunately not always the outcome.

Drs Vlassara and Striker discuss the role of advanced glycosylation end products (AGEs) in the chronic complications of diabetes, both type 1 and type 2. The source of AGEs, pro-oxidant molecules, is primarily from the diet, particularly from so-called "fast-food" meals and heat-processed foods. AGEs function via their receptors on the cell called RAGE, whose activation causes an increase in oxidative stress and increased cellular inflammation. The authors consider this process to be the major pathogenic mechanism for diabetic vascular complications, both microvascular and macrovascular.

Another important microvascular complication is retinopathy, a leading cause of new blindness in the United States. Dr Rosberger reminds us of the various trials demonstrating that tight glycemic control in both type 1 (DCCT) and in type 2 diabetic

Endocrinol Metab Clin N Am 42 (2013) xiii–xv
http://dx.doi.org/10.1016/j.ecl.2013.07.008
0889-8529/13/$ – see front matter © 2013 Published by Elsevier Inc.

endo.theclinics.com

patients (eg, UKPDS) controls retinopathy progression. Two serious conditions, the macular edema and proliferative retinopathy, are treated using laser photocoagulation that can save the patient's eyesight.

Diabetic neuropathy, especially peripheral neuropathy, is a very common and extremely troublesome complication of diabetes. There is both a vascular and a metabolic component in the pathogenesis. Painful neuropathy can be treated with agents like pregabalin and/or duloxetine, but the relief of pain is incomplete in many patients. Drs Vinik, Nevoret, Casellini, and Parson detail the pathophysiology, symptomatology, and clinical signs in detail and also stress that autonomic neuropathy often coexists and should be screened for in all these cases. Furthermore, they detail the various agents that have been tested for the condition and proven to be essentially ineffective. The mainstay of prevention and even reversal of early peripheral neuropathy remains tight glycemic control.

The connection of the cardiovascular system and the kidney in the development of diabetic complications such as impaired renal function and end-stage renal disease is now well described as the cardio-renal syndrome. It posits that elements of the cardiovascular system, such as hypertension and the lack of nocturnal blood pressure "dipping," are risk factors for the development and progression of renal disease. In their article, Drs Jindal, Garcia-Touza, Jindal, Whaley-Connell, and Sowers discuss the importance of controlling both blood pressure and blood glucose levels to retard the early renal complications seen in diabetes.

Gastrointestinal complications are quite common in diabetic patients with the most troublesome being due to autonomic neuropathy as well as those caused by medications. Some of the conditions include esophageal motility dysfunction, reflux, esophageal candidiasis, and gastroparesis. As Drs Boland, Edelman, and Wolosin discuss, in addition to the symptomatology there is also the problem of glycemic control that is affected by the GI complications, in both type 1 and type 2 diabetes. Furthermore, autoimmune disorders such as celiac disease are increased in type 1 patients. In obese and type 2 patients non-alcoholic fatty liver disease (NAFLD) has been recognized as a major complication and, if left untreated, may progress to steatohepatitis and cirrhosis; the incidence or detection of NALFD has increased recently and has become a major health concern.

Diabetic foot complications can be devastating, as they can result in amputation that can further complicate the patient's metabolic control as well as the effect on lifestyle. Drs Kim and Steinberg describe how peripheral vascular changes and peripheral neuropathy together can lead to lower limb ulceration and, if left untreated, can eventuate in gangrene and amputation. They also describe how the pressure of the lower limb adds to the sensitivity of the tissues to ulceration. Standard therapeutic regimens, including debridement, antibiotics, and foot care, with an emphasis on a team approach, can prevent devastating complications.

A less well-known complication of diabetes is periodontitis. Dr Preshaw discusses how the relationship between periodontal disease and diabetes is bidirectional. Diabetic individuals are three times more at risk for periodontal disease, due in part to poor glycemic control and a tendency to inflammatory processes. Periodontal disease itself makes glycemic control worse probably through the effects of inflammatory cytokines. Indeed, when periodontal disease is treated efficiently, HbA1c levels fall by almost 0.5%. This relationship should be brought to the attention of health care providers and dentists as well as patients.

Drs Murphy-Chutorian and Cohen describe the numerous skin manifestations that are seen in diabetic patients. These include specific conditions, such as necrobiosis lipoidica diabeticorum, generalized granuloma annulare, bullosa diabeticorum, scleredema diabeticorum, acanthosis nigricans, and others. Commonly, the skin conditions are named according to certain observed characteristics and, while in some cases the etiology involves a vascular abnormality, often the underlying cause is unknown. Similarly, therapy can be either specific depending on the known etiologic factors or empiric. Diabetic patients are also prone to infections, both bacterial and fungal, and here the therapy is more directed. In addition, lipodystrophy and lipohypertrophy may present at the sites of insulin injections, the latter probably due to the direct effect of insulin on adipocytes, whereas the former from unknown reasons.

Drs Gaunay, Nagler, and Stember describe the effect of diabetes on male sexual function. The two major complications involve sexual dysfunction and hypogonadism, the former due to vascular changes and neuropathy, while the latter more commonly secondary to hypothalamic-pituitary effects. Erectile dysfunction is the most worrisome problem and the authors describe the multiple methods of treatment, not all being totally successful. Ejaculatory dysfunction may also require medical or surgical interventions. In regard to hypogonadism, testosterone replacement is recommended, again with varying success rates.

Insulin plays an important role in the female reproductive system. Acting via its own cognate receptor insulin stimulates ovarian steroidogenesis, at least partially, by synergizing with gonadotrophins. Other effects of insulin are mediated by its inhibition of sex hormone binding globulin synthesis, thereby increasing the proportion of free sex hormone in the circulation. Similarly it decreases insulin-like growth factor bondingprotein 1 (IGFBP-1) production, freeing IGF-1 to also enhance ovarian steroidogenesis. Drs Nandi and Poretsky explain in their article how these peripheral and central effects of insulin often lead to infertility and especially to polycystic ovarian syndrome; not surprising then, that metformin and thiazolidinediones are effective in this condition.

Drs Corathers, Peavie, and Salehi discuss the various antidiabetic agents used to manage diabetes and to prevent the long-term complications. Their article covers both the known mechanisms of each class of agents and the potential side effects. Thus, metformin has gastrointestinal side effects and may possibly cause lactic acidosis, particularly in patients with renal impairment. Thiazolidinediones cause weight gain, edema, and bone fractures and may precipitate heart failure in susceptible patients. Insulin secretagogues cause weight gain and hypoglycemia. Incretins (GLP-1 mimetics and DPP-IV inhibitors) have recently been described as possibly associated with pancreatitis and pancreatic cancer; however, the evidence supporting this is still debatable. Other agents also discussed are sodium-glucose cotransporter 2 (SGLT-2) inhibitors, amylin, and α-glucosidase inhibitors.

The reader is encouraged to partake of this menu of outstanding and up-to-date articles on important clinical problems and await the next issue that promises to be equally important.

We thank the issue editors, Drs Liao and Poretsky, for their hard work in designing and editing this issue as well as for recruiting the best authors.

Derek LeRoith, MD, PhD
Director of Research
Division of Endocrinology, Metabolism, and Bone Diseases
Department of Medicine
Mount Sinai School of Medicine
One Gustave L. Levy Place
Box 1055, Altran 4-36
New York, NY 10029, USA

E-mail address:
derek.leroith@mssm.edu

Preface

Why Focus on Complications?

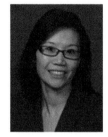 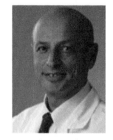

Emilia Pauline Liao, MD   Leonid Poretsky, MD
Editors

KEYWORDS

• Complications • Pathogenesis • Diabetes

Hyperglycemia is asymptomatic until the glucose concentration surpasses the renal threshold for reabsorbing glucose, resulting in glucosuria, osmotic diuresis, and dehydration. Diabetes is largely asymptomatic until complications develop. Because of this, nearly one-third of people with diabetes are not aware that they have the disease. This poses a question: if a patient is asymptomatic, then why treat? Diabetes is dangerous because of its complications, which are often present at the time of diagnosis.[1] The rate of some complications can be reduced with appropriate glycemic control, even in an asymptomatic patient.

At either extreme of glycemia, acute complications such as hypoglycemia, diabetic ketoacidosis, and hyperosmolar state can be life threatening. Chronic complications such as retinopathy, nephropathy, neuropathy, and atherosclerosis cause significant morbidity and reduced quality of life. Diabetes is the leading cause of blindness in persons aged 20 to 74 years and is the leading cause of kidney failure, accounting for 44% of new cases.[2] In addition, 60% to 70% of people with diabetes have mild to severe forms of neuropathy.

In both type 1 and type 2 diabetes, microvascular complications increase with duration of diabetes and higher hemoglobin A1c (HbA1c). The United Kingdom Prospective Diabetes Study (UKPDS) 35 showed a 37% reduction in microvascular complications with 1% reduction in HbA1c.[3] The Diabetes Control and Complications Trial (DCCT) similarly showed reductions in retinopathy (by 70%), microalbuminuria (by 39%),

Endocrinol Metab Clin N Am 42 (2013) xvii–xxii
http://dx.doi.org/10.1016/j.ecl.2013.06.006
0889-8529/13/$ – see front matter © 2013 Elsevier Inc. All rights reserved.

endo.theclinics.com

and neuropathy (by 60%) comparing groups with HbA1c of 7.2% versus 9.1% over 6.5 years.[4]

The cells affected in diabetic microvascular complications, namely retinal endothelial cells, glomerular mesangial cells, and peripheral neurons and Schwann cells, are particularly susceptible to hyperglycemia because these cells are unable to downregulate glucose transport into the cell.[5,6] The resulting intracellular hyperglycemia leads to mitochondrial production of superoxide and reactive oxygen species (ROS). ROS triggers a cascade of events, described by Brownlee[7] as the "unifying mechanism of hyperglycemia-induced cellular damage." Free radicals induce DNA strand breaks, which activate poly-ADP ribose polymerase (PARP), a DNA repair enzyme. PARP modifies glyceraldehyde-3-phosphate dehydrogenase (GADPH), decreasing its activity, which activates further pathways that are damaging to vasculature (**Fig. 1**). Increased polyol pathway activity leads to greater aldose reductase activity, which consumes nicotinamide adenine dinucleotide phosphate hydrogen (NADPH), leaving less NADPH available to reduce glutathione, an intracellular antioxidant. Thus, cells become more susceptible to oxidative stress. Protein kinase C is also activated, which leads to reduction of endothelial nitric oxide synthase activity, increasing endothelin-1, transforming growth factor beta (TGF-β), plasminogen activator inhibitor-1 (PAI-1), vascular endothelial growth factor (VEGF), and nuclear factor kappa B. ROS also activates the hexosamine pathway, which increases TGF-β andPAI-1.[7] In addition, intracellular hyperglycemia leads to increased production of advanced glycation end products (AGE), which have intracellular and extracellular effects.[8] Glycation of proteins alters structure and function (extracellular effects), and AGE bind to receptors (receptor for AGE) to promote inflammation, thrombogenesis, and apoptosis (intracellular effects).

Even intermittent and mild increases in circulating glucose concentrations that are less than the diabetes diagnosis threshold can cause diabetes complications. The

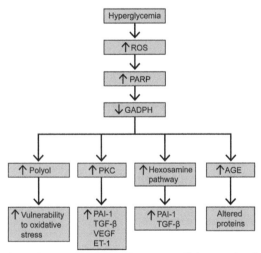

Fig. 1. How hyperglycemia causes cellular damage: unifying mechanism. AGE, advanced glycation end products; ET, endothelin; PAI, plasminogen activator inhibitor; PKC, protein kinase C; TGF, transforming growth factor; VEGF, vascular endothelial growth factor. (*Adapted from* Brownlee M. The pathobiology of diabetic complications: a unifying mechanism. Diabetes 2005;54:1615–25.)

prevalence of diabetic neuropathy increases significantly among groups of normal glucose tolerance (7.4%), impaired fasting glucose (11.3%), impaired glucose tolerance (13%), and type 2 diabetes (28%).[9] Higher rates of microalbuminuria were similarly reported in individuals with impaired fasting glucose, and each millimole per liter increase in average fasting glucose was associated with a 27% increase in albuminuria.[10] Microalbuminuria was also more common in individuals with metabolic syndrome, with higher rates of microalbuminuria in those with more components of the metabolic syndrome.[11]

Cardiovascular disease is the leading cause of death in patients with diabetes. Hyperglycemia increases the risk of macrovascular disease. UKPDS and DCCT follow-up studies showed risk reduction for myocardial infarction in the intensively treated arms that were maintained for years, despite similar HbA1c levels at study end.[12] In contrast, recent large clinical trials such as Action to Control Cardiovascular Risk in Diabetes (ACCORD), Action in Diabetes and Vascular Disease: Preterax and Diamicron MR Controlled Evaluation (ADVANCE), and Veterans Affairs Diabetes Trial (VADT), have not shown reduced cardiovascular mortality with intense glucose control.[13] Thus, for macrovascular disease, there may be additional factors beyond hyperglycemia accelerating atherosclerosis. In the 10-year follow-up for the Pittsburgh Epidemiology of Diabetes Complications (EDC) study, glycemia did not predict future coronary artery disease events,[14] and estimated glucose disposal rate, a marker of insulin resistance, showed inverse association. In UKPDS, patients on metformin showed 39% risk reduction, despite nonsignificant differences in HbA1c levels, suggesting that metformin confers benefit beyond glucose reduction.

Metformin is an insulin sensitizer and inhibitor of AGE formation. Both insulin resistance and AGE are contributors to diabetes and its complications. As mentioned earlier, AGE inflict cellular damage through multiple mechanisms. Insulin resistance is a main contributor to diabetes and is associated with systemic inflammation. Increased levels of inflammatory markers, such as C-reactive protein (CRP), PAI-1, and monocyte chemoattractant protein-1 (MCP-1) are also reported to predict diabetes.[15] Inflammatory markers are associated with high rates of nephropathy and retinopathy.

Insulin resistance is accompanied by hypertriglyceridemia and excess free fatty acids. Visceral fat releases free fatty acids directly into the portal vein, then to the liver and pancreas, contributing further to insulin resistance.[16] Insulin resistance at the liver level results in increased very-low-density lipoprotein (VLDL) synthesis, which is especially prominent in the postprandial state. Individuals with high waist circumference and hyperlipidemia have higher fasting glucose and different responses to oral glucose tolerance testing compared with age-matched and weight-matched subjects with normal waist circumference.[17] Adipose tissue and endothelial cells stressed by hyperglycemia, excess free fatty acids, and AGE release cytokines that promote inflammation and coagulation pathways.

Low-density lipoprotein (LDL) cholesterol has also been shown to be toxic to beta cells. Pancreatic islet cells have LDL receptors, and LDL particles may increase beta cell apoptosis,[18,19] leading to beta cell dysfunction. The interplay between insulin resistance, dyslipidemia, and type 2 diabetes is summarized in **Fig. 2**.

In summary, the final common pathways in the pathogenesis of diabetes complications involve inflammation and thrombogenesis, which are triggered and fueled by hyperglycemia, oxidative stress, dyslipidemia, and AGE. Acute and chronic complications of diabetes are reviewed in detail elsewhere in this issue. The role of AGE in contributing to diabetes and its complications are discussed. In addition, gastrointestinal, reproductive, dermatologic, and dental complications are presented, as well as

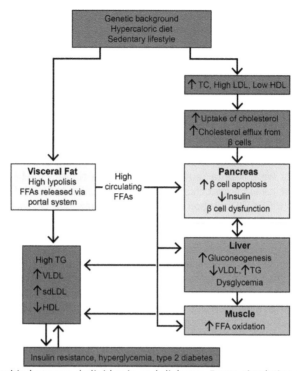

Fig. 2. Relationship between dyslipidemia and diabetes. Excess circulating free fatty acids (FFAs) from diet and visceral fat lead to beta cell dysfunction, increased gluconeogenesis, and high triglycerides (TGs), causing insulin resistance and hyperglycemia. HDL, high-density lipoprotein; sdLDL, small dense LDL; TC, total cholesterol. (*Adapted from* Bardini G, Rotella CM, Giannini S. Dyslipidemia and diabetes: reciprocal impact of impaired lipid metabolism and beta cell dysfunction on micro and macrovascular complications. Rev Diabet Stud 2012;9:87.)

potential complications of diabetes treatment. In the next issue, conditions associated (and often coexisting with) diabetes, such as metabolic syndrome, heart disease, sleep apnea, cancer, and dementia, will be examined, including common pathogenic mechanisms and treatment.

In the past decade, more individuals with diabetes reached the recommended goals for HbA1c reduction (<7.0%), LDL (<100 mg/dl), and blood pressure (130/80 mm Hg), but 30% to 50% of patients with diabetes still do not reach recommended treatment goals.[20] At dedicated centers using diabetes team care, studies have shown declining rates of complications. In patients with type 1 diabetes for 20 years, the incidence of nephropathy decreased from 28% for those diagnosed between 1961 and 1965, to 5.8% in those diagnosed between 1976 and 1980.[21] The improvement was attributed to aggressive glycemic control by the diabetes team. In addition, the survival from onset of diabetic kidney disease increased from 6 to 7 years in the 1970s to 21 years in 2005.[22] With the prevalence of diabetes continuing to increase, and people living longer with the disease, an increase in complications of diabetes is a concern. It is hoped that this and the following issues will help improve understanding of the pathogenesis and treatment of diabetes and its complications, thus helping more patients reach their goals and reduce the rate of serious complications of this common disease.

Emilia Pauline Liao, MD
Department of Medicine
Albert Einstein College of Medicine
1300 Morris Park Avenue
Bronx, NY 10461, USA

Endocrinology
Beth Israel Medical Center
16th Street, First Avenue
New York, NY 10003, USA

Leonid Poretsky, MD
Department of Medicine
Albert Einstein College of Medicine
1300 Morris Park Avenue
Bronx, NY 10461, USA

Endocrinology
Beth Israel Medical Center
16th Street, First Avenue
New York, NY 10003, USA

E-mail addresses:
eliao@chpnet.org (E.P. Liao)
LPoretsk@chpnet.org (L. Poretsky)

REFERENCES

1. Spijkerman AM, Dekker JM, Adriaanse MC, et al. Microvascular complications at time of diagnosis of type 2 diabetes are similar among diabetic patients detected by targeted screening and patients newly diagnosed in general practice. Diabetes Care 2003;26:2604–8.
2. Centers for Disease Control and Prevention. National diabetes fact sheet: national estimates and general information on diabetes and prediabetes in the United States, 2011. Atlanta (GA): US Department of Health and Human Services, Centers for Disease Control and Prevention; 2011.
3. Stratton IM, Adler AI, Neil HA, et al. Association of glycaemia with macrovascular and microvascular complications of type 2 diabetes (UKPDS 35): prospective observational study. BMJ 2000;321:405–12.
4. Diabetes Control and Complications Trial Research Group. The effect of intensive treatment of diabetes on the development and progression of long-term complications in insulin-dependent diabetes mellitus. N Engl J Med 1993;329:977–86.
5. Kaiser N, Sasson S, Feener EP, et al. Differential regulation of glucose transport and transporters by glucose in vascular endothelial and smooth muscle cells. Diabetes 1993;42:80–9.
6. Heilig CW, Concepcion LA, Riser BL, et al. Overexpression of glucose transporters in rat mesangial cells cultures in a normal glucose milieu mimics the diabetic phenotype. J Clin Invest 1995;96:1802–14.
7. Brownlee M. The pathobiology of diabetic complications: a unifying mechanism. Diabetes 2005;54:1615–25.

8. Poretsky LP. Looking beyond overnutrition for causes of epidemic metabolic disease. Proc Natl Acad Sci U S A 2012;109(39):15537–8.
9. Ziegler D, Rathmann W, Dickhaus T, KORA Study Group. Prevalence of polyneuropathy in pre-diabetes and diabetes is associated with abdominal obesity and macroangiopathy. The MONICA/KORA Augsburg Surveys S2 and S3. Diabetes Care 2008;31:464–9.
10. Zacharias JM, Young TK, Riediger ND, et al. Prevalence, risk factors and awareness of albuminuria on a Canadian First Nation: a community based screening study. BMC Public Health 2012;12:290.
11. Sheng C, Hu B, Fan W, et al. Microalbuminuria in relation to the metabolic syndrome and its components in a Chinese populations. Diabetol Metab Syndr 2011;3:6.
12. Khardori R, Nguyen DD. Glucose control and cardiovascular outcomes: reorienting approach. Front Endocrinol (Lausanne) 2012;3:110.
13. Skyler J, Bergenstal R, Bonow RO, et al. Intensive glycemic control and the prevention of cardiovascular events: implications of the ACCORD, ADVANCE and VA diabetes trials. Diabetes Care 2009;32:187–92.
14. Orchard TJ, Olson JC, Erbey JR, et al. Insulin resistance-related factors, but not glycemia, predict coronary artery disease in type 1 diabetes. Diabetes Care 2003;26:1374–9.
15. Goldberg RB. Cytokine and cytokine-like inflammation markers, endothelial dysfunction, and imbalanced coagulation in development of diabetes and its complications. J Clin Endocrinol Metab 2009;94:3171–82.
16. Bardini G, Rotella CM, Giannini S. Dyslipidemia and diabetes: reciprocal impact of impaired lipid metabolism and beta cell dysfunction on micro and macrovascular complications. Rev Diabet Stud 2012;9:82–93.
17. Giannini S, Bardini G, Dicembrini I, et al. Lipid levels in obese and nonobese subjects as predictors of fasting and postload glucose metabolism. J Clin Lipidol 2012;6:132–8.
18. Brunham LR, Kruit JK, Verchere CB, et al. Cholesterol in islet dysfunction and type 2 diabetes. J Clin Invest 2008;118:403–8.
19. Kruit JK, Kremer PH, Dai L, et al. Cholesterol efflux via ATP-binding cassette transporter A1 (ABCA1) and cholesterol uptake via the LDL receptor influences cholesterol-induced impairment of beta cell function in mice. Diabetologia 2010;53:1110–9.
20. Ali MK, Bullard KM, Saaddine JB, et al. Achievement of goals in U.S. diabetes care, 1999-2010. N Engl J Med 2013;368:1613–24.
21. Bojestig M, Arnqvist HF, Hermansson G, et al. Declining incidence of nephropathy in insulin-dependent diabetes mellitus. N Engl J Med 1994;330:15–8.
22. Astrup AS, Tarnow L, Rossing P, et al. Improved prognosis in type 1 diabetic patients with nephropathy: a prospective follow up study. Kidney Int 2005;68:1250–7.

Hypoglycemia

Mazen Alsahli, MD[a,b], John E. Gerich, MD[c,*]

KEYWORDS

- Type 1 diabetes • Type 2 diabetes • Hypoglycemia
- Hypoglycemia counterregulation

KEY POINTS

- Hypoglycemia is a frequent occurrence for many patients with type 1 or type 2 diabetes treated with insulin or insulin secretagogues and those with renal insufficiency.
- Episodes of hypoglycemia have significant morbidity and mortality and are the main limiting factor for achieving near optimal glycemic control.
- Impaired glucose counterregulation and hypoglycemia unawareness are the major risk factors for severe hypoglycemia.
- Risk factors, including impaired glucose counterregulation and hypoglycemia unaware-ness, are largely preventable and/or reversible.
- Management and prevention of hypoglycemia should focus on reducing risk factors through patient education, individualization of glycemic targets, and judicious use of anti-diabetic regimens.

GENERAL CONSIDERATIONS

Normally, plasma glucose concentrations are maintained within a relatively narrow range throughout the day (usually between 55 and 165 mg/dL, ~3.0 and 9.0 mM/L) despite wide fluctuations in the delivery (eg, meals) and removal (eg, exercise) of glucose from the circulation. This is accomplished by a tightly linked balance between glucose production and glucose utilization regulated by complex mechanisms.

Disclosures: Dr Alsahli has nothing to disclose.
Funding Sources: Dr Gerich: University of Rochester Senior Faculty Associates Program.
Conflict of Interest: Dr Gerich: Consultant: AstraZeneca, Boehringer Ingelheim, Bristol-Myers Squibb, Eli Lilly, Merck, Sanofi-Aventis, and Janssen Pharmaceuticals.
Speakers' Bureau: AstraZeneca, Boehringer Ingelheim, Bristol-Myers Squibb, Eli Lilly, Merck, Sanofi-Aventis, and Janssen Pharmaceuticals.
[a] Division of Endocrinology, Department of Medicine, Southlake Regional Health Center, 309-531 Davis Drive, Newmarket, Ontario L3Y 6P5, Canada; [b] Faculty of Medicine, Department of Medicine, University of Toronto, 1 King's College Cir, Toronto, Ontario M5S 1A8, Canada; [c] Division of Endocrinology, Department of Medicine, University of Rochester School of Medicine, 601 Elmwood Avenue, Rochester, NY 14642, USA
* Corresponding author. 403 Woodcrest Road, Wayne, PA 19087.
E-mail address: johngerich@compuserve.com

Hypoglycemia is to be avoided to protect the brain and prevent cognitive dysfunction. Because of limited availability of ketone bodies and amino acids and the limited transport of free fatty acids across the blood brain barrier, glucose can be considered to be the sole source of energy for the brain except under conditions of prolonged fasting. In the latter situation, ketone bodies increase several fold so that these may be used as an alternative fuel.[1]

The brain cannot store or produce glucose and therefore requires a continuous supply of glucose from the circulation. At physiologic plasma glucose levels, phosphorylation of glucose is rate limiting for its use; however, because of the kinetics of glucose transfer across the blood brain barrier, uptake becomes rate limiting as plasma glucose concentrations decrease below the normal range. Consequently, maintenance of the plasma glucose concentration above some critical level is essential to the survival of the brain and thus the organism. It is therefore not surprising that a complex physiologic mechanism has evolved to prevent or correct hypoglycemia (vide infra). Nevertheless, for many patients with type 1 or type 2 diabetes, hypoglycemia is a frequent occurrence. Because of its possible detrimental effects on the central nervous system and the fear thereof by patients and caregivers, hypoglycemia is considered to be the main limiting factor for achieving near optimal glycemic control.[2]

EPIDEMIOLOGY OF HYPOGLYCEMIA

The reported incidence of hypoglycemia varies considerably among studies. For the purpose of reporting hypoglycemia in clinical trials, the American Diabetes Association and the Endocrine Society have developed 5 categories, as outlined in **Table 1**.[3] The incidence of one category, severe hypoglycemia, has been determined more precisely, as it is defined as that associated with unconsciousness or requiring external assistance. The complete detection of chemical hypoglycemia (commonly

Table 1
Hypoglycemia categories as defined by the American Diabetes Association and the Endocrine Society

Category	Definition
Documented symptomatic	An event during which typical symptoms of hypoglycemia are associated by a measured plasma glucose concentration ≤70 mg/dL[a]
Severe	An event requiring assistance of another person to administer carbohydrate, glucagon, or other resuscitative actions[b]
Asymptomatic	An event not accompanied by typical symptoms of hypoglycemia but with a measured plasma glucose concentration ≤70 mg/dL[a]
Probable symptomatic	An event during which symptoms of hypoglycemia are not accompanied by a plasma glucose measurement but that was presumably caused by a plasma glucose concentration ≤70 mg/dL[a]
Pseudo-hypoglycemia	An event during which the person with diabetes reports any of the typical symptoms of hypoglycemia with a measured plasma glucose concentration >70 mg/dL but approaching that level

[a] 70 mg/dL equals 3.9 mmol/L.
[b] If plasma glucose measurements are not available during such an event; the neurologic recovery attributable to the restoration of plasma glucose to normal is considered sufficient evidence that the event was induced by hypoglycemia.
Data from Seaquist ER, Anderson J, Childs B, et al. Hypoglycemia and diabetes: a report of a Workgroup of the American Diabetes Association and the Endocrine Society. Diabetes Care 2013;36:1384–95.

defined as a capillary blood glucose concentration <50 mg/dL, ~3.0 mM/L[4]) would require continuous blood glucose measurements over prolonged periods. The few studies using this approach have generally found that the frequency and duration of hypoglycemia, especially the nocturnal hypoglycemia, is greater than what was previously thought.[5,6]

In general, the frequency is greater in patients with type1 diabetes than in those with type 2 diabetes.[7–10] For example, in a review comparing intensively treated patients in clinical trials with comparable treatment goals, the incidence of severe hypoglycemia, defined as any event requiring the assistance of another individual, in patients treated with insulin averaged approximately 3 to 4 per 100 patient-years in type 2 diabetic patients versus 62 per 100 patient-years in type 1 diabetic patients in the Diabetes Control and Complication Trial (DCCT).[11]

Hypoglycemia occurs more often during intensified insulin therapy than during conventional insulin therapy. For example during the 6.5-year follow-up in the DCCT trial,[12] 35% of patients in the conventional treatment group and 65% of patients in the intensive treatment group had at least 1 episode of severe hypoglycemia.

Among patients with type 2 diabetes, the frequency of hypoglycemia will vary by treatment modality. In patients treated with sulfonylureas, the incidence of severe hypoglycemia has been reported to be approximately 1.5 episodes per 100 patient-years[13] and is more common with long-acting sulfonylureas, such as glyburide and chlorpropamide.[14] Prandial insulins (short-acting insulins taken before meals to limit postprandial hyperglycemia) are associated with a greater frequency of hypoglycemia than are the long-acting so-called basal insulins.[15] Metformin, thiazolidinediones, dipeptidyl-peptidase-4 inhibitors, glucagonlike 1 mimetics, and sodium glucose cotransporter 2 inhibitors do not increase the risk of hypoglycemia when used without insulin or insulin secretagogues (sulfonylureas and meglitinides).[16]

RISK FACTORS FOR HYPOGLYCEMIA

Risk factors for hypoglycemia are summarized in **Box 1**. Conventional risk factors relate to absolute or relative insulin excess. These include insulin doses that are excessive or ill-timed, missed meals or snacks, lack of compensation for increased exercise, alcohol ingestion, or mistaken insulin administration. However, a thorough analysis of a large number of episodes of severe hypoglycemia in the DCCT has indicated that such conventional risk factors explained only a minority of the episodes[17,18]; indeed, mathematical models incorporating many of these factors were found to have little predictive power.[17] Instead, it is now well established that impaired glucose counterregulation and hypoglycemia unawareness (vide infra) are the major risk factors for severe hypoglycemia in type 1 and type 2 diabetes.[2,19] These defects are particularly common in patients with a long diabetes duration,[20,21] tight glycemic control,[20,22,23] antecedent hypoglycemia,[24,25] and autonomic neuropathy.[26–28] Hypoglycemia awareness may also be compromised by the use of β-blockers.[29] The risk of severe hypoglycemia is increased 25-fold in patients with impaired hypoglycemia counterregulation[30] and increased 6-fold in those with hypoglycemia unawareness.[31] Other risk factors for severe hypoglycemia due to diabetes complications include renal insufficiency, gastroparesis, which causes unpredictable and delayed food absorption, poor vision, and (rarely) insulin antibodies. In the latter condition, hypoglycemia occurs via dissociation of insulin from antibodies, causing prolonged hyperinsulinemia.[21]

In addition to impaired glucose counterregulation and hypoglycemia unawareness, multiple other factors may be simultaneously involved. These include liver disease, malnutrition, sepsis, burns, total parenteral nutrition, malignancy, and administration

---

Box 1
Hypoglycemia causes and risk factors

Absolute or relative insulin or insulin secretagogues excess

- Excessive doses
- Decreased clearance (eg, renal impairment, liver failure, and hypothyroidism)
- Decreased glucose production (eg, liver or kidney disease and alcohol ingestion)
- Increased glucose use (eg, exercise)
- Increased insulin sensitivity (eg, exercise, weight loss, and use of insulin sensitizers)
- Intentional hypoglycemia (overdose)

Mismatch between insulin or insulin secretagogues and food absorption

- Ill-timed insulin doses
- Missed meals
- Gastroparesis
- Post gastric bypass surgery
- Gastrointestinal disease with malabsorption (eg, celiac disease)

Glucose counterregulation factors

- Defective hypoglycemia counterregulation
- Hypoglycemia unawareness
- Autonomic neuropathy
- Deficiency of hormones needed for hypoglycemia counterregulation (eg, adrenal insufficiency and growth hormone deficiency)

*Drugs (listed in **Table 2**)*

- Drugs capable of causing hypoglycemia by themselves (eg, alcohol, insulin, sulfonylureas)
- Drugs that could cause hypoglycemia only in combination with insulin or insulin secretagogues (eg, metformin, angiotensin-converting enzyme inhibitors)
- Drugs that can compromise hypoglycemia awareness (eg, β-blockers)
- Sudden decrease in drugs that cause hyperglycemia (eg, discontinuing glucocorticosteroids or glucose infusion during hospitalization in insulin-treated patients)

Errors and medication administration issues

- Lack of diabetes education (eg, injecting insulin into lipohypertrophy or intramuscularly)
- Poor adherence to regimen or distraction (eg, miscalculated carbohydrate content or taking wrong type of insulin)
- Functional neurologic deficit (eg, cognitive or visual impairment leading to incorrect dosing)

Tumor-associated hypoglycemia

- Increased insulin (insulinomas)
- Decreased gluconeogenesis (eg, advanced metastatic tumor in the liver)
- Insulinlike growth factor II–mediated hypoglycemia (eg, secreting fibrosarcoma)

Autoimmune hypoglycemia

- Insulin-binding antibodies
- Activating insulin receptor antibodies

Other

- Extremes of age (children and elderly)
- Pregnancy (usually first trimester)
- Hospitalization (eg, new NPO [nothing by mouth] status, sedation, medication dispensing errors, and interruption of tube feeding or parenteral nutrition)
- Malnutrition
- Total parenteral nutrition
- Severe infections and sepsis
- Burns
- Macroalbuminuria

of certain medications known to reduce plasma glucose concentrations (**Table 2**).[32] Another recently prospectively identified risk factor is the presence of baseline macro-albuminuria[33] in diabetic patients with apparently normal or minimally decreased renal function (eg, estimated glomerular filtration rate >60 mL/min/1.73 m²). Over a 10-year follow-up period, approximately 13% of patients developed severe hypoglycemia (1.55 per 100 patient-years), 5% of whom died.

Table 2
Drug-induced hypoglycemia

Drugs Capable of Causing Hypoglycemia by Themselves		Drugs Probably Causing Hypoglycemia Only in Combination with Insulin/Sulfonylurea/Meglitinides	
Antidiabetic Drugs	**Other**	**Antidiabetic Drugs**	**Other**
Insulin	Alcohol	Metformin	ACE-inhibitors
Sulfonylureas	Salicylates	Thiazolidinediones	Angiotensin II receptor
Meglitinides	Propranolol	Alpha-glucosidase	antagonists
	Pentamidine	inhibitors	Phenylbutazone
	Sulfamethoxazole	Glucagonlike peptide-1	Lidocaine
	Vacor	agonists	Coumadin
	Quinine	Dipeptidyl peptidase-4	Ranitidine
	Propoxyphene	inhibitors	Cimetidine
	Para-aminobenzoic	Pramlintide	Doxepin
	acid		Danazol
	Perhexiline		Azopropazone
			Oxytetracycline
			Clofibrate
			Benzofibrate
			Colchicine
			Ketoconazole
			Chloramphenicol
			Haloperidol
			Monoamine oxidase
			inhibitors
			Thalidomide
			Orphenadrine
			Selegiline

Abbreviation: ACE, angiotensin-converting enzyme.

Gastric bypass surgery is becoming more common as a treatment for morbid obesity. Many of these patients have type 2 diabetes. Hypoglycemia has been reported to occur in some patients, usually in the second or third hour postprandially.[34–37] The exact mechanism is currently being investigated but could be multifactorial and related to the changes that follow surgery, such as decreased caloric intake, weight loss, and a change in the nutrient composition, flora, and transit time in the gastrointestinal tract.[38–40] Studies have also shown decreased ghrelin secretion, exaggerated release of glucagonlike peptide-1 (GLP-1), and possibly other gastrointestinal hormone changes.[41–45] These hormonal changes should enhance the release of insulin and inhibit the release of glucagon. Additionally, several severe cases of hyperinsulinemic hypoglycemia presenting as postprandial hypoglycemia after Roux-en-Y gastric bypass surgery have been published.[46–48] The mechanism by which this occurs is not entirely clear. Examination of pancreatic specimens obtained following partial pancreatectomy performed to treat these cases implicated nesidioblastosis or islet cell hyperplasia as a possible cause.[46,47] A subsequent report, however, found no evidence of increased islet cell mass or neogenesis when some of these specimens were reexamined and compared with those of well-matched subjects.[49] The report suggests that hypoglycemia in these patients is related to a combination of gastric dumping and inappropriately increased insulin secretion due to either failure of beta cells to adapt to changes after gastric bypass or as an acquired phenomenon. It is also not clear whether patients with diabetes are more or less likely to suffer from post–gastric-bypass hypoglycemia when compared with other patients.

HYPOGLYCEMIA COUNTERREGULATION
Normal Hypoglycemia Counterregulation and Hypoglycemia Awareness

Glucose counterregulation refers to the sum of the body's defense mechanisms that prevent hypoglycemia from occurring and that restore euglycemia. Hypoglycemia awareness refers to the symptomatic responses of hypoglycemia that alert the patient of declining blood glucose levels.

In healthy postabsorptive humans (ie, after an overnight fast), the sum of glucose release by liver and kidney nearly equals systemic glucose utilization so that plasma glucose concentrations remain relatively stable. Because insulin suppresses both hepatic and renal glucose release[50,51] and stimulates glucose uptake, exogenous insulin administration causes systemic glucose utilization to exceed systemic glucose release so that plasma glucose concentrations decrease.

As the plasma glucose levels decrease, there is a characteristic hierarchy of responses (**Fig. 1**).[52] Reduction of insulin secretion, the first in the cascade of hypoglycemia counterregulation,[2] derepresses glucose production and reduces glucose utilization. When plasma glucose levels decline to approximately 70 mg/dL (3.8 mM/L), there is an increase in the secretion of counterregulatory hormones (glucagon, epinephrine, growth hormone, cortisol).[26,52–54] Glucagon and epinephrine have immediate effects on glucose kinetics, whereas the effects of growth hormone and cortisol are delayed by several hours.[55,56]

Under normal physiologic conditions, these responses prevent a further decrease in plasma glucose concentrations and restore normoglycemia. Decreases to approximately 60 mg/dL (3.4 mM/L) usually evoke the so-called autonomic warning symptoms[57,58] (hunger, anxiety, palpitations, sweating, nausea), which, if interpreted correctly, lead a person to eat and prevent more serious hypoglycemia. However, clues of hypoglycemia may vary considerably from person to person.[59] If, for some reason, plasma glucose levels decrease to about 55 mg/dL (~3.0 mM/L),

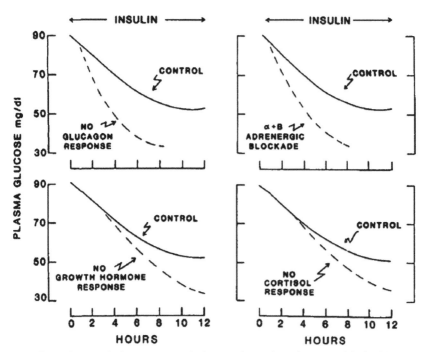

Fig. 1. Effect of lack of glucagon, catecholamine (α- and β-adrenergic blockade), growth hormone, and cortisol responses on insulin-induced hypoglycemia in nondiabetic volunteers studied with pituitary-adrenal-pancreatic clamp. (*From* Gerich J. Glucose counterregulation and its impact on diabetes mellitus. Diabetes 1988;37:1611. Copyright © 1988 The American Diabetes Association; with permission.)

neuroglycopenic signs/symptoms of brain dysfunction (blurred vision, slurred speech, glassy-eyed appearance, confusion, difficulty in concentrating) would occur.[57,58] Further decreases can produce coma and values less than 30 mg/dL (~1.6 mM/L), if prolonged, can cause seizures, permanent neurologic deficits, and death. However, it should be pointed out that in otherwise healthy/young (<45 years) individuals, glucose levels averaging 35 mg/dL (~2.0 mM/L) have been maintained for as long as 8 hours without any long-term adverse effects[60] and chronic levels as low as 24 mg/dL (1.3 mM/L) in patients with insulinoma have been observed in association with apparently normal cerebral function.[61]

Hypoglycemia Counterregulation and Hypoglycemia Awareness in Type 1 Diabetes

In type 1 diabetes, the physiology of the defense against hypoglycemia is seriously deranged. First, as endogenous insulin secretion becomes totally deficient over the first few years of type 1 diabetes, the appearance of insulin in the circulation becomes unregulated, as it relies on absorption from subcutaneous injection sites. Consequently, as plasma glucose levels are falling, insulin levels do not decrease. Second, glucagon responses to hypoglycemia are lost early in the course of type 1 diabetes.[21,62] This defect coincides with the loss of insulin secretion and is therefore the rule in people with type 1 diabetes.[63] Nonetheless, glucose counterregulation appears to be adequate in such patients, probably because of compensatory counterregulation by epinephrine.[64] After a few more years, epinephrine responses to hypoglycemia are also commonly reduced.[21,65,66] When compared with patients with a defective glucagon response but normal epinephrine responses, patients with a combined defect in glucagon and epinephrine responses have at least a 25-fold increased risk for severe iatrogenic hypoglycemia.[30,67] The combined defect in glucagon and epinephrine responses is therefore considered as the syndrome of impaired hypoglycemia counterregulation.[2] This is now known to be associated with impaired glucose production in both liver and kidney.[68] Pathophysiologic mechanisms might be different when only glucagon responses are impaired and epinephrine responses are intact. Because glucagon affects exclusively the liver whereas epinephrine has a temporary effect on the liver but a sustained effect on the kidney, only hepatic glucose production might be decreased under these conditions.

In addition to impaired glucose counterregulation, people with type 1 diabetes often suffer from hypoglycemia unawareness. These patients no longer have autonomic warning symptoms of developing hypoglycemia that previously prompted them to take appropriate action (ie, food intake before severe hypoglycemia with neuroglyco-penia occurs). Hypoglycemia unawareness has been reported to occur in about 50% of patients with long-standing diabetes and is estimated to affect 25% overall.[19,31,69,70] Hypoglycemia unawareness is associated with sixfold increased risk for severe hypoglycemia.[31]

The mechanisms of impaired hypoglycemia counterregulation and hypoglycemia unawareness are not entirely clear but several factors have been proposed. These include altered intra-islet structure and altered cell-cell interaction (reduced glucagon responses),[71,72] autonomic neuropathy (reduced catecholamine responses),[26–28] upregulation of glucose transporters in the central nervous system by antecedent hypoglycemia, which prevents central hypoglycemia during subsequent hypoglycemia (reduced hormone and symptom responses),[73] and impaired β-adrenergic sensitivity to catecholamines, which reduces autonomic warning symptoms of hypoglycemia.[74]

Studies in animals have shown that the ventromedial hypothalamus (VMH) plays a major role in controlling the counterregulatory responses to hypoglycemia and that AMP-activated protein kinase plays a key role in the glucose-sensing mechanism used by VMH neurons.[75] These studies also suggest that increased urocortin I, an endogenous type 2 corticotropin-releasing factor receptor (CRFR2) agonist, in the VMH during antecedent hypoglycemia, could explain a decreased sympathoadrenal response to subsequent hypoglycemia.[76]

Hypoglycemia Counterregulation and Hypoglycemia Awareness in Type 2 Diabetes

In type 2 diabetes, the hormonal glucose counterregulation is usually less impaired than in type 1 diabetes.[77–79] Nevertheless, defects can be seen when patients become markedly insulin deficient.[80] One important factor for the nearly intact hormonal glucose counterregulation in type 2 diabetes may be some residual, albeit abnormal, insulin secretion. Normally, insulin directly suppresses glucagon secretion. There is now experimental evidence to suggest that the glucagon response to hypoglycemia may depend on the decrease in insulin secretion because the latter would derepress glucagon secretion.[72] Because antecedent hypoglycemia is one of the main factors for impaired epinephrine responses to hypoglycemia and because hypoglycemia rarely occurs in people with type 2 diabetes because of their intact glucagon response, epinephrine responses usually also remain intact.

Once patients with type 2 diabetes become markedly insulin deficient, glucagon responses are commonly impaired. However, in contrast to patients with type 1 diabetes, the epinephrine responses usually remain intact and in fact may partially compensate for the reduced glucagon responses to hypoglycemia.[79,81] This may explain the reduced risk for severe hypoglycemia in patients with type 2 diabetes compared with patients with type 1 diabetes.

MANIFESTATIONS OF HYPOGLYCEMIA

Manifestations of hypoglycemia are nonspecific and can sometimes be noted by observers rather than patients themselves. They can be categorized as neurogenic (mostly due to sympathetic neural activation) and neuroglycopenic (due to brain glucose deprivation) (**Box 2**). Neurogenic manifestations, also called autonomic or sympathoadrenal, precede neuroglycopenic symptoms and allow patients to recognize and self-treat hypoglycemia. Patients with hypoglycemia unawareness are likely to have hypoglycemia manifesting at an advanced stage with neuroglycopenic symptoms that may prevent self-treatment. Nocturnal hypoglycemia can manifest with disturbed sleep, nightmares, and "waking in sweat." Acute severe hypoglycemia can present with a range of neurologic and cardiovascular complications as detailed in the following section.

COMPLICATIONS OF HYPOGLYCEMIA

An episode of severe hypoglycemia can be detrimental or even fatal mostly due to its effects on the central nervous system. At plasma glucose concentration of approximately 55 mg/dL ($\sim$3 mM/L), cognitive impairment and electroencephalogram changes are demonstrable. Decreases below 40 mg/dL ($\sim$2.5 mM/L) result in sleepiness and gross behavioral (eg, combativeness) abnormalities. Further decreases can produce coma, and values less than 30 mg/dL ($\sim$1.6 mM/L), if prolonged, can cause seizures, permanent neurologic deficits, and death.[82–85]

Box 2
Manifestations of hypoglycemia

Neurogenic (autonomic or sympathoadrenal)

- Anxiety and irritability
- Fine tremor
- Tachycardia
- Hunger
- Cold sweats
- Paresthesias
- Headache

Neuroglycopenic

- Cognitive impairment
- Mood and behavioral changes
- Fatigue and weakness
- Lightheadedness and dizziness
- Visual changes (blurred vision, diplopia)
- Slurred speech
- Seizures
- Coma

Hypoglycemia also affects the cardiovascular system, creating cardiac repolarization abnormalities with lengthening of the QT interval and also ST wave changes. It is also thought to promote a prothrombotic state. In individuals with underlying cardiovascular disease, life-threatening arrhythmias, myocardial infarction, and strokes may be precipitated.[86–88]

Moreover, in patients with underlying eye disease, hypoglycemia has been shown to trigger retinal hemorrhages.[89] It has been suggested that repeated episodes of severe hypoglycemia may lead to subtle permanent cognitive dysfunction.[90] In addition to its physical morbidity and mortality, recurrent hypoglycemia may be also associated with psychosocial morbidity. In fact, many patients with diabetes are as much afraid of severe hypoglycemia as they are of blindness or renal failure.[69]

Severe hypoglycemia has been reported to be at least a contributing factor to the cause of death in 3% to 13% of patients with type 1 diabetes, which include, for example, motor vehicle accidents and injuries at work.[91,92] Severe hypoglycemia due to sulfonylureas has been shown to have a mortality between 4% and 7%.[93,94]

Hypoglycemia is also associated with more short-term disability and higher health care costs.[95,96]

MANAGEMENT OF HYPOGLYCEMIA
Treatment

Treatment is aimed at restoring euglycemia, preventing recurrences, and, if possible, alleviating the underlying cause.

In an insulin-taking diabetic patient with mild hypoglycemia due to a skipped meal, 15 to 20 g of oral carbohydrate every 15 to 20 minutes until the blood glucose is above 80 mg/dL (4.5 mM/L) constitutes adequate treatment (**Box 3**).[97,98] Examples for oral carbohydrate source are presented in **Box 4**. In a patient with more severe hypoglycemia resulting in obtundation, in whom oral administration of carbohydrate might result in aspiration, 1 mg of glucagon administered subcutaneously or intramuscularly might be sufficient to raise the blood glucose and revive the patient so that oral carbohydrate may be given. Comatose patients should receive intravenous glucose (25-g bolus, followed by an infusion at an initial rate of 2 mg/kg/min, roughly 10 g/h) for as long as necessary for the insulin or sulfonylurea to wear off (**Box 5**). Sulfonylurea

---

Box 3
Treatment of hypoglycemia in nonhospitalized patients

1. Patient conscious and able to swallow

   a. Consume 15–20 g of rapidly absorbed carbohydrates (see **Box 4** for examples)

   b. Check blood glucose 15–20 minutes later and retreat if hypoglycemia not reversed

   c. Follow successful treatment (blood glucose above 70–80 mg/dL [3.8–4.5 mM/L]) with a meal or snack within 30–60 minutes

2. Patient cannot swallow/at risk for aspiration, combative, or with decreased level of consciousness

   a. Administer glucagon 0.5–1 mg subcutaneously or intramuscularly. Glucagon may cause nausea and vomiting. Turn patient on his or her side during treatment to avoid aspiration

   b. Check blood glucose 15–20 minutes later and retreat if hypoglycemia not reversed (patient may be able to take oral carbohydrates then)

   c. Follow successful treatment with a meal or snack within 30–60 minutes

---

Box 4
Examples of 15–20 g oral carbohydrates for treatment of hypoglycemia

- Pure glucose or dextrose (eg, glucose tablet, glucose gel, or glucose liquid) is the preferred choice especially for patients on alpha-glucosidase inhibitors that will slow digestion and absorption of other forms of carbohydrates

- Beverages containing rapidly absorbed carbohydrates (eg, 1/3–1/2 cup of fruit juice or regular soft drink, 1 cup of skim milk or sports drink)

- Food containing carbohydrates with minimal fat, protein, or fiber content (eg, 1 tablespoon table sugar or honey, 2 tablespoons raisins, 2–3 pieces of hard candy, 3 squares graham crackers, 7 lifesavers, 7 gummy bears, or 7 jelly beans)

---

overdose can result in prolonged hypoglycemia requiring sustained intravenous glucose infusion aimed at keeping the blood glucose at approximately 80 mg/dL (~4.5 mM/L) to avoid hyperglycemia, which would cause further stimulation of insulin secretion, thus setting in motion a vicious cycle. Blood glucose levels should be monitored initially every 15 to 20 minutes and subsequently at 1-hour to 2-hour intervals. Rarely, diazoxide or a somatostatin analog may be needed to inhibit insulin secretion.[99] Where other drugs may be involved, they should be discontinued, if possible (ie, sulfonamides in a patient with renal insufficiency). In other conditions, the underlying disorder should be treated (eg, sepsis, heart failure, endocrine deficiency) and the blood glucose supported.

Prevention of Recurrences

Conventional measures
For prevention of recurrences, it is important to determine whether hypoglycemia was an isolated event or whether it has occurred before. If so, how frequently? Is

---

Box 5
Treatment of hypoglycemia in hospitalized patients

1. Assess level of consciousness, swallowing, NPO status, and availability of venous access

   - Patient alert and able to swallow → 15–20 g oral carbohydrates or 25 g of 50% dextrose IV bolus

   - Patient alert and NPO → 25 g of 50% dextrose IV bolus

   - Patient with decreased level of consciousness or unable to swallow → 25 g of 50% dextrose IV bolus

   - Patient with decreased level of consciousness or unable to swallow or is NPO and has no venous access → glucagon 1 mg SC or IM plus establish venous access for further treatment. Glucagon may cause nausea and vomiting. Turn patient on his or her side during treatment to avoid aspiration

2. Recheck blood glucose every 15–20 minutes and retreat until euglycemia is restored (blood glucose >70–80 mg/dL [3.8–4.5 mM/L])

3. Follow successful treatment with a meal or snack within 30–60 minutes unless the patient is NPO

4. Glucose infusion at initial rate of 2 mg/kg/min aimed at keeping the blood glucose at ~80 mg/dL (~4.5 mM/L) should be considered soon following initial treatment if patient is NPO or recurrent or prolonged hypoglycemia is expected

Abbreviations: IM, intramuscular; IV, intravenous; NPO, nothing by mouth; SC, subcutaneous.

---

there any pattern to occurrences, that is, always at night? For how long have the hypoglycemic episodes been occurring? Are they associated with hypoglycemic warning symptoms? If so, usually at what level of glycemia is hypoglycemia recognized? Are there any precipitating factors, for example, exercise, skipped meal, erroneous insulin injection, alcohol ingestion, recent weight loss, or other precipitating factors (see earlier in this article)? Did the patient spontaneously recover? What did the patient do to prevent recurrences or relieve symptoms? What is the patient's occupation?

Obviously, if these questions reveal precipitating factors for hypoglycemia, these should be eliminated (**Box 6**). However, if careful testing does not reveal any apparent precipitating factors but reveals hypoglycemia unawareness instead, chances are relatively high that there is also impaired hypoglycemia counterregulation, especially in a patient with frequent hypoglycemic episodes. Consequently, the question arises how to treat the affected patients.

The principles of intensive therapy (patient education, self-monitoring of blood glucose [SMBG], and an insulin regimen that provides basal insulin levels with prandial increments) still apply to most patients who require insulin to control their diabetes. However, glycemic goals must be individualized according to the frequency of hypoglycemia. Because the prevention or correction of hypoglycemia normally involves dissipation of insulin and activation of counterregulatory hormones, as discussed previously, it follows that patients with impaired glucose counterregulation are extremely sensitive to very little insulin in excess of its requirement resulting in hypoglycemia. It is, therefore, generally accepted that normoglycemia is not a reasonable goal for such patients.[100,101] The American Diabetes Association's most recent practice guidelines still recommend A1C goal for most adults to be less than 7%, but also recognize that less stringent goals (such as <8%) may be appropriate for patients with a history of severe hypoglycemia, limited life expectancy, advanced complications, and comorbid conditions.[102] Approximately 25 to 35 mg/dL (1.5–2.0 mM/L) upward adjustment of SMBG goals is needed to increase the A1C by 1%.

Box 6
Measures to reduce hypoglycemia

- Identification and management of risk factors
- Education programs for patients and as needed for their family members, friends, or coworkers
- Individualization of glycemic goals for both A1C and self-monitoring of blood glucose
- At-risk patients should carry or wear emergency medical identification
- Continuous glucose monitoring for appropriate patients
- Judicious management of insulin therapy
  - Adjusting regimen according to glycemic pattern and lifestyle
  - Avoiding sliding scales and insulin stacking
  - Switching from regular to rapid insulin with meals and from neutral protamine Hagedorn (NPH) to long-acting analogues as basal insulin
  - Considering basal-bolus with correction scale instead of fixed-ratio regimens
  - Carbohydrate counting for appropriate patients
  - Insulin pump therapy for appropriate patients

Diabetes education in general and programs that focus on hypoglycemia have proven to be helpful and should be implemented to involve patients and their family or friends.[103–105] Patients need to learn basic skills, such as the need to check blood glucose regularly, to carry supplies for treating hypoglycemia with them all the time, to have a glucagon emergency kit available, to carry or wear medical alert identification, and to plan better for exercise. Advanced skills, such as insulin dose adjustments and the use of continuous glucose monitors and/or insulin pumps, can also be taught for many motivated and capable patients.

Substitution of preprandial short-acting (regular) insulin for rapid insulin (lispro, aspart, glulisine) may reduce the frequency of hypoglycemic episodes by reducing prolonged postprandial hyperinsulinemia.[106] Furthermore, substitution of intermediate-acting insulin (neutral protamine Hagedorn [NPH]) for long-acting insulin analogue (glargine or detemir) has been shown to reduce the frequency of hypoglycemia in patients with type 1 or type 2 diabetes.[107–109] In appropriate candidates, hypoglycemia can be reduced by insulin pump therapy despite that glycemic control could actually improve with such therapy.[110,111] Additionally, implementation of continuous glucose monitoring systems has shown promising results in preventing hypoglycemia[112–114] and should be considered for appropriate patients.

If these measures result in strict avoidance of hypoglycemia, hypoglycemia awareness may be restored.[115] This might be due to an improvement in β-adrenergic sensitivity.[116] Although strict avoidance of hypoglycemia does not improve glucagon responses to hypoglycemia in type 1 diabetes,[115,117–120] it does increase epinephrine responses.[117,120] This, however, seems to be limited to patients with a diabetes duration of fewer than approximately 15 years. In patients with type 1 diabetes of more than 15 years' duration, epinephrine responses may remain markedly impaired.[115,118] Thus, there is unfortunately no conventional therapy available to reverse impaired hypoglycemia counterregulation in such patients. Although the effects of avoidance of hypoglycemia have not been studied in patients with type 2 diabetes, it seems likely that these are similar to those in type 1 diabetes.

Pancreas/islet transplantation

Because of the irreversibly impaired hypoglycemia counterregulation in long-standing type 1 diabetes, pancreas or islet transplantation has been proposed as a possible treatment in patients who suffer from recurrent severe hypoglycemia despite all conventional measures.[121–123] Pancreatic transplantation is usually reserved for patients undergoing simultaneous kidney transplantation. It has been found to improve glucagon responses to hypoglycemia in most studies[124–130] and to improve or normalize epinephrine responses.[126–128,130–132] Furthermore, it has been reported to improve hypoglycemia awareness in type 1 diabetes.[130]

Experience in the effects of islet transplantation on hypoglycemia counterregulation and awareness is limited and inconsistent. It seems that glucagon responses remain impaired after islet transplantation,[121,128,133] possibly because of the transplantation site.[134] However, in one study, epinephrine responses and hypoglycemia awareness were reported to improve in long-standing type 1 diabetes,[122] whereas a later larger study found no evidence of improvement in epinephrine or hypoglycemia awareness despite prolonged insulin independence and near normal glycemic control in 7 patients with islet transplantation.[133]

Although pancreas transplantation and islet transplantation may be promising alternatives for some patients with recurrent severe hypoglycemia, risk benefit ratios should be very carefully analyzed because of the invasive nature of these forms of therapy and the necessity for potent long-term immunosuppression.

REFERENCES

1. Owen O, Morgan A, Kemp H, et al. Brain metabolism during fasting. J Clin Invest 1967;46:1589–95.
2. Cryer P. Banting lecture: hypoglycemia, the limiting factor in the management of IDDM. Diabetes 1994;43:1378–89.
3. Seaquist ER, Anderson J, Childs B, et al. Hypoglycemia and diabetes: a report of a Workgroup of the American Diabetes Association and The Endocrine Society. Diabetes Care 2013;36(5):1384–95.
4. Foster D, Rubenstein A. Hypoglycemia. In: Wilson J, Braunwald E, Isselbacher K, editors. Harrison's principles of internal medicine. New York: McGraw-Hill; 1991. p. 1759.
5. Guillod L, Comte-Perret S, Monbaron D, et al. Nocturnal hypoglycaemias in type 1 diabetic patients: what can we learn with continuous glucose monitoring? Diabetes Metab 2007;33:360–5.
6. Wentholt IM, Maran A, Masurel N, et al. Nocturnal hypoglycaemia in Type 1 diabetic patients, assessed with continuous glucose monitoring: frequency, duration and associations. Diabet Med 2007;24:527–32.
7. Leese GP, Wang J, Broomhall J, et al. Frequency of severe hypoglycemia requiring emergency treatment in type 1 and type 2 diabetes: a population-based study of health service resource use. Diabetes Care 2003;26:1176–80.
8. UK Hypoglycemia Study Group. Risk of hypoglycemia in types 1 and 2 diabetes: effects of treatment modalities and their duration. Diabetologia 2007; 50:1140–7.
9. Akram K, Pedersen-Bjergaael U, Borch-Johnson K, et al. Frequency and risk factors of severe hypoglycemia in insulin-treated type 2 diabetes: a literature survey. J Diabet Complications 2006;20:402–8.
10. Amiel SA, Dixon T, Mann R, et al. Hypoglycemia in type 2 diabetes. Diabet Med 2008;25:245–54.
11. Gerich J. Hypoglycemia and counterregulation in type 2 diabetes. Lancet 2000; 356(9246):19467.
12. DCCT Research Group. The effect of intensive treatment of diabetes on the development and progression of long-term complications in insulin dependent diabetes mellitus. N Engl J Med 1993;329:977–86.
13. van Staa T, Abenhaim L, Monette J. Rates of hypoglycemia in users of sulfonylureas. J Clin Epidemiol 1997;50:735–41.
14. Gangji AS, Cukierman T, Gerstein HC, et al. A systematic review and meta-analysis of hypoglycemia and cardiovascular events: a comparison of glyburide with other secretagogues and with insulin. Diabetes Care 2007;30:389–94.
15. Holman RR, Farmer AJ, Davies MJ, et al, 4-T Study Group. Three-year efficacy of complex insulin regimens in type 2 diabetes. N Engl J Med 2009;361:1736–47.
16. Zammitt NN, Frier BM. Hypoglycemia in type 2 diabetes. Diabetes Care 2005; 28:2948–61.
17. DCCT Research Group. Epidemiology of severe hypoglycemia in the diabetes control and complications trial. Am J Med 1991;90:450–9.
18. Nilsson A, Tideholm B, Kalen J, et al. Incidence of severe hypoglycemia and its causes in insulin- treated diabetics. Acta Med Scand 1988;224:257–62.
19. Amiel S. R.D. Lawrence Lecture 1994. Limits of normality: the mechanisms of hypoglycemia unawareness. Diabet Med 1994;11:918–24.
20. Mokan M, Mitrakou M, Veneman T, et al. Hypoglycemia unawareness in IDDM. Diabetes Care 1994;17:1397–403.

21. Bolli G, DeFeo P, Compagnucci P, et al. Abnormal glucose counterregulation in insulin-dependent diabetes mellitus: interaction of anti-insulin antibodies and impaired glucagon and epinephrine secretion. Diabetes 1983;32:134–41.
22. Amiel S, Tamborlane W, Simonson D, et al. Defective glucose counterregulation after strict control of insulin-dependent diabetes mellitus. N Engl J Med 1987; 316:1376–83.
23. Simonson D, Tamborlane W, DeFronzo R, et al. Intensive insulin therapy reduces counterregulatory responses to hypoglycemia in type I diabetes. Ann Intern Med 1985;103:184–8.
24. Davis M, Mellman M, Shamoon H. Further defects in counterregulatory responses induced by recurrent hypoglycemia in IDDM. Diabetes 1992;41:1335–40.
25. Lingenfelser T, Renn W, Sommerwerck U, et al. Compromised hormonal counter-regulation, symptom awareness, and neurophysiologic function after recurrent short-term episodes of insulin-induced hypoglycemia in IDDM patients. Diabetes 1993;42:610–8.
26. Meyer C, Grosmann R, Mitrakou A, et al. Effects of autonomic neuropathy on counterregulation and awareness of hypoglycemia in type 1 diabetic patients. Diabetes Care 1998;21:1960–6.
27. Horie H, Hanafusa T, Matsuyama T, et al. Decreased response of epinephrine and norepinephrine to insulin-induced hypoglycemia in diabetic autonomic neuropathy. Horm Metab Res 1984;16:398–401.
28. Hoeldtke R, Boden G, Shuman C, et al. Reduced epinephrine secretion and hypoglycemic unawareness in diabetic autonomic neuropathy. Ann Intern Med 1982;96:459–62.
29. Hirsch I, Boyle P, Craft S, et al. Higher glycemic thresholds for symptoms during beta-adrenergic blockade in IDDM. Diabetes 1991;40:1177–86.
30. White N, Skor D, Cryer P, et al. Identification of type I diabetic patients at increased risk for hypoglycemia during intensive therapy. N Engl J Med 1983; 308:485–91.
31. Gold A, MacLeod K, Frier B. Frequency of severe hypoglycemia in patients with type 1 diabetes with impaired awareness of hypoglycemia. Diabetes Care 1994; 17:697–703.
32. Gerich J. Hypoglycemia. In: DeGroot L, editor. Endocrinology. Philadelphia: W. B. Saunders; 2001. p. 921–40.
33. Yun JS, Ko SH, Ko SH, et al. Presence of macroalbuminuria predicts severe hypoglycemia in patients with type 2 diabetes mellitus. Diabetes Care 2013;36(5): 1283–9.
34. Miholic J, Orskov C, Holst J, et al. Emptying of the gastric substitute, glucagon-like peptide-1 (GLP-1), and reactive hypoglycemia after total gastrectomy. Dig Dis Sci 1991;36:1361–70.
35. Wapnick S, Jones JJ. Changes in glucose tolerance and serum insulin following partial gastrectomy and intestinal resection. Gut 1972;13:871–3.
36. Leichter S, Permutt M. Effect of adrenergic agents on postgastrectomy hypoglycemia. Diabetes 1975;24:1005–10.
37. Shultz KT, Neelon FA, Nilsen LB, et al. Mechanism of postgastrectomy hypoglycemia. Arch Intern Med 1971;128:240–6.
38. Guidone C, Manco M, Valera-Mora E, et al. Mechanisms of recovery from type 2 diabetes after malabsorptive bariatric surgery. Diabetes 2006;55:2025–31.
39. Gumbs AA, Modlin IM, Ballantyne GH. Changes in insulin resistance following bariatric surgery: role of caloric restriction and weight loss. Obes Surg 2005; 15:462–73.

40. Maggard MA, Shugarman LR, Suttorp M, et al. Meta-analysis: surgical treatment of obesity. Ann Intern Med 2005;142:547–59.

41. Gebhard B, Holst JJ, Biegelmayer C, et al. Postprandial GLP-1, norepinephrine, and reactive hypoglycemia in dumping syndrome. Dig Dis Sci 2001;46:1915–23.

42. Lawaetz O, Blackburn AM, Bloom SR, et al. Gut hormone profile and gastric emptying in the dumping syndrome. A hypothesis concerning the pathogenesis. Scand J Gastroenterol 1983;18:73–80.

43. Dube PE, Brubaker PL. Nutrient, neural and endocrine control of glucagon-like peptide secretion. Horm Metab Res 2004;36:755–60.

44. Kellum JM, Kuemmerle JF, O'Dorisio TM, et al. Gastrointestinal hormone responses to meals before and after gastric bypass and vertical banded gastroplasty. Ann Surg 1990;211:763–70.

45. Cummings DE, Weigle DS, Frayo RS, et al. Plasma ghrelin levels after diet-induced weight loss or gastric bypass surgery. N Engl J Med 2002;346:1623–30.

46. Patti ME, McMahon G, Mun EC, et al. Severe hypoglycaemia post-gastric bypass requiring partial pancreatectomy: evidence for inappropriate insulin secretion and pancreatic islet hyperplasia. Diabetologia 2005;48:2236–40.

47. Service GJ, Thompson GB, Service FJ, et al. Hyperinsulinemic hypoglycemia with nesidioblastosis after gastric-bypass surgery. N Engl J Med 2005;353:249–54.

48. Won JG, Tseng HS, Yang AH, et al. Clinical features and morphological characterization of 10 patients with noninsulinoma pancreatogenous hypoglycaemia syndrome (NIPHS). Clin Endocrinol (Oxf) 2006;65:566–78.

49. Meier JJ, Butler AE, Galasso R, et al. Hyperinsulinemic hypoglycemia after gastric bypass surgery is not accompanied by islet hyperplasia or increased beta-cell turnover. Diabetes Care 2006;29:1554–9.

50. Cersosimo E, Garlick P, Ferretti J. Renal glucose production during insulin-induced hypoglycemia in humans. Diabetes 1999;48:261–6.

51. Meyer C, Dostou J, Gerich J. Role of the human kidney in glucose counterregulation. Diabetes 1999;48:943–8.

52. Schwartz N, Clutter W, Shah S, et al. The glycemic thresholds for activation of glucose counterregulatory systems are higher than the threshold for symptoms. J Clin Invest 1987;79:777–81.

53. Mitrakou A, Ryan C, Veneman T, et al. Hierarchy of glycemic thresholds for counterregulatory hormone secretion, symptoms, and cerebral dysfunction. Am J Physiol 1991;260:E67–74.

54. Fanelli C, Pampanelli S, Epifano L, et al. Relative roles of insulin and hypoglycemia on induction of neuroendocrine responses to, symptoms of, and deterioration of cognitive function in hypoglycemia in male and female humans. Diabetologia 1994;37:797–807.

55. DeFeo P, Perriello G, Torlone E, et al. Demonstration of a role of growth hormone in glucose counterregulation. Am J Physiol 1989;256:E835–43.

56. DeFeo P, Perriello G, Torlone E, et al. Contribution of cortisol to glucose counterregulation in humans. Am J Physiol 1989;257:E35–42.

57. Hepburn D, Deary I, Frier B, et al. Symptoms of acute insulin-induced hypoglycemia in humans with and without IDDM. Factor-analysis approach. Diabetes Care 1991;14:949–57.

58. Towler D, Havlin C, Craft S, et al. Mechanism of awareness of hypoglycemia: perception of neurogenic (predominantly cholinergic) rather than neuroglycopenic symptoms. Diabetes 1993;42:1791–8.

59. Cox D, Gonder-Frederick L, Antoun B, et al. Perceived symptoms in the recognition of hypoglycemia. Diabetes Care 1993;16:519–27.

60. Bolli G, DeFeo P, Perriello G, et al. Role of hepatic autoregulation in defense against hypoglycemia in humans. J Clin Invest 1985;75:1623–31.
61. Mitrakou A, Fanelli C, Veneman T, et al. Reversibility of unawareness of hypoglycemia in patients with insulinomas. N Engl J Med 1993;329:834–9.
62. Gerich J, Langlois M, Noacco C, et al. Lack of glucagon response to hypoglycemia in diabetes: evidence for an intrinsic pancreatic alpha-cell defect. Science 1973;182:171–3.
63. Fukuda M, Tanaka A, Tahara Y, et al. Correlation between minimal secretory capacity of pancreatic β-cells and stability of diabetic control. Diabetes 1988;37:81–8.
64. Rizza R, Cryer P, Gerich J. Role of glucagon, epinephrine and growth hormone in glucose counterregulation. J Clin Invest 1979;64:62–71.
65. Hirsch B, Shamoon H. Defective epinephrine and growth hormone responses in type I diabetes are stimulus specific. Diabetes 1987;36:20–6.
66. Dagogo-Jack S, Craft S, Cryer P. Hypoglycemia-associated autonomic failure in insulin dependent diabetes mellitus. J Clin Invest 1993;91:819–28.
67. Bolli G, DeFeo P, DeCosmo S, et al. A reliable and reproducible test for adequate glucose counterregulation in Type I diabetes mellitus. Diabetes 1984;33:732–7.
68. Cersosimo E, Ferretti J, Sasvary D, et al. Adrenergic stimulation of renal glucose release is impaired in type 1 diabetes. Diabetes 2001;50(Suppl 2):A54.
69. Pramming S, Thorsteinsson B, Bendtson I, et al. Symptomatic hypoglycemia in 411 type I diabetic patients. Diabet Med 1991;8:217–22.
70. Hepburn D, Patrick A, Eadington D, et al. Unawareness of hypoglycemia in insulin-treated diabetic patients: prevalence and relationship to autonomic neuropathy. Diabet Med 1990;7:711–7.
71. Raju B, Cryer PE. Loss of the decrement in intraislet insulin plausibly explains loss of the glucagon response to hypoglycemia in insulin-deficient diabetes: documentation of the intraislet insulin hypothesis in humans. Diabetes 2005;54:757–64.
72. Unger R. Insulin-glucagon relationships in the defense against hypoglycemia. Diabetes 1983;32:575–83.
73. Boyle P, Kempers S, O'Connor A, et al. Brain glucose uptake and unawareness of hypoglycemia in patients with insulin-dependent diabetes mellitus. N Engl J Med 1995;333:1726–31.
74. Fritsche A, Stumvoll M, Grüb M, et al. Effect of hypoglycemia on beta-adrenergic sensitivity in normal and type 1 diabetic subjects. Diabetes Care 1998;21:1505–10.
75. McCrimmon RJ, Shaw M, Fan X, et al. Key role for AMP-activated protein kinase in the ventromedial hypothalamus in regulating counterregulatory hormone responses to acute hypoglycemia. Diabetes 2008;57:444–50.
76. McCrimmon RJ, Song Z, Cheng H, et al. Corticotrophin-releasing factor receptors within the ventromedial hypothalamus regulate hypoglycemia-induced hormonal counterregulation. J Clin Invest 2006;116:1723–30.
77. Heller S, MacDonald I, Tattersall R. Counterregulation in type 2 (noninsulin-dependent) diabetes mellitus: normal endocrine and glycemic responses, up to 10 years after diagnosis. Diabetologia 1987;30:924–9.
78. Levy C, Kinsley B, Bajaj M, et al. Effect of glycemic control on glucose counterregulation during hypoglycemia in NIDDM. Diabetes Care 1998;21:1330–8.
79. Shamoon H, Friedman S, Canton C, et al. Increased epinephrine and skeletal muscle responses to hypoglycemia in non-insulin-dependent diabetes mellitus. J Clin Invest 1994;93:2562–71.

80. Segel S, Paramore D, Cryer P. Hypoglycemia-associated autonomic failure in advanced type 2 diabetes. Diabetes 2002;51:724–33.
81. Bolli G, Tsalikian E, Haymond M, et al. Defective glucose counterregulation after subcutaneous insulin in noninsulin-dependent diabetes mellitus. J Clin Invest 1984;73:1532–41.
82. Silas J, Grant D, Maddocks J. Transient hemiparetic attacks due to unrecognised nocturnal hypoglycaemia. BMJ 1981;282:132–3.
83. Wredling R, Levander S, Adamson U, et al. Permanent neuropsychological impairment after recurrent episodes of severe hypoglycaemia in man. Diabetologia 1990;33:152–7.
84. Patrick A, Campbell I. Fatal hypoglycaemia in insulin-treated diabetes mellitus: clinical features and neuropathological changes. Diabet Med 1990;7:349–54.
85. Perros P, Frier B. The long-term sequelae of severe hypoglycemia on the brain in insulin-dependent diabetes mellitus. Horm Metab Res 1997;29:197–202.
86. Fisher B, Quin J, Rumley A, et al. Effects of acute insulin-induced hypoglycaemia on haemostasis, fibrinolysis and haemorheology in insulin-dependent diabetic patients and control subjects. Clin Sci 1991;80:525–31.
87. Frier BM, Schernthaner G, Heller SR. Hypoglycemia and cardiovascular risks. Diabetes Care 2011;34(Suppl 2):S132–7.
88. Duh E, Feinglos M. Hypoglycemia-induced angina pectoris in a patient with diabetes mellitus. Ann Intern Med 1994;121:945–6.
89. Kohner E, McLeod D, Marshall J. Complications of diabetes. London: Edward Arnold; 1982.
90. Deary I, Crawford J, Hepburn D, et al. Severe hypoglycemia and intelligence in adult patients with insulin-treated diabetes. Diabetes 1993;42:341–4.
91. Paz-Guevara A, Hsu T-H, White P. Juvenile diabetes mellitus after forty years. Diabetes 1975;24:559–65.
92. Nabarro J, Mustaffa B, Morris D, et al. Insulin deficient diabetes. Contrasts with other endocrine deficiencies. Diabetologia 1979;16:5–12.
93. Seltzer H. Severe drug-induced hypoglycemia: a review. Compr Ther 1979;5:21–9.
94. Berger W, Caduff F, Pasquel M, et al. Die relative haufigkeit der schweren Sulfonylharnstoff- hypoglykamie in den letzten 25 Jahren in der Schweiz. Schweiz Med Wochenschr 1986;116:145–51 [in German].
95. Rhoads GG, Orsini LS, Crown W, et al. Contribution of hypoglycemia to medical care expenditures and short-term disability in employees with diabetes. J Occup Environ Med 2005;47:447–52.
96. Curkendall SM, Natoli JL, Alexander CM, et al. Economic and clinical impact of inpatient diabetic hypoglycemia. Endocr Pract 2009;15:302–12.
97. Gaston S. Outcomes of hypoglycemia treated by standardized protocol in a community hospital. Diabetes Educ 1992;18:491–4.
98. Slama G, Traynard P, Desplanque N, et al. The search for an optimized treatment of hypoglycemia. Carbohydrates in tablets, solution, or gel for the correction of insulin reactions. Arch Intern Med 1990;150:589–93.
99. Palatnick W, Meatherall R, Tenenbein M. Clinical spectrum of sulfonylurea overdose and experience with diazoxide therapy. Arch Intern Med 1991;151:1859–62.
100. Cryer P, Gerich J. Glucose counterregulation, hypoglycemia, and intensive insulin therapy in diabetes mellitus. N Engl J Med 1985;313:232–41.
101. Bolli G. How to ameliorate the problem of hypoglycemia in intensive as well as non-intensive treatment of type 1 diabetes. Diabetes Care 1999;22(Suppl 2):B43–52.

102. American Diabetes Association. Standards of medical care in diabetes-2013. Diabetes Care 2013;36(Suppl 1):S4–10.
103. Cox D, Ritterband L, Magee J, et al. Blood glucose awareness training delivered over the Internet. Diabetes Care 2008;31(8):1527–8.
104. Samann A, Muhlhauser I, Bender R, et al. Glycaemic control and severe hypoglycaemia following training in flexible, intensive insulin therapy to enable dietary freedom in people with type 1 diabetes: a prospective implementation study. Diabetologia 2005;48:1965–70.
105. The DAFNE Study Group. Training in flexible intensive insulin management to enable dietary freedom in people with type 1 diabetes: dose adjustment for normal eating (DAFNE) randomized controlled trial. BMJ 2002;325:746–52.
106. Brunelle R, Llewelyn J, Anderson J, et al. Meta-analysis of the effect of insulin lispro on severe hypoglycemia in patients with type 1 diabetes. Diabetes Care 1998;21:1726–31.
107. Home P, Bartley P, Russell-Jones D, et al. Insulin detemir offers improved glycemic control compared with NPH insulin in people with type 1 diabetes: a randomized clinical trial. Diabetes Care 2004;27:1081–7.
108. Rosenstock J, Dailey G, Massi-Benedetti M, et al. Reduced hypoglycemia risk with insulin glargine: a meta-analysis comparing insulin glargine with human NPH insulin in type 2 diabetes. Diabetes Care 2005;28:950–5.
109. Hermansen K, Davies M, Derezinski T, et al. A 26-week, randomized, parallel, treat-to-target trial comparing insulin detemir with NPH insulin as add-on therapy to oral glucose-lowering drugs in insulin-naive people with type 2 diabetes. Diabetes Care 2006;29:1269–74.
110. Boland E, Grey M, Oesterle A, et al. Continuous subcutaneous insulin infusion. A new way to lower risk of severe hypoglycemia, improve metabolic control, and enhance coping in adolescents with type 1 diabetes. Diabetes Care 1999;22: 1779–84.
111. Pickup JC, Sutton AJ. Severe hypoglycaemia and glycaemic control in type 1 diabetes: meta-analysis of multiple daily insulin injections compared with continuous subcutaneous insulin infusion. Diabet Med 2008;25:765–74.
112. Juvenile Diabetes Research Foundation Continuous Glucose Monitoring Study Group. Effectiveness of continuous glucose monitoring in a clinical care environment: evidence from the Juvenile Diabetes Research Foundation Continuous Glucose Monitoring (JDRF-CGM) trial. N Engl J Med 2010;363:311–20.
113. Bergenstal RM, Tamborlane WV, Ahmann A, et al, STAR 3 Study Group. Effectiveness of sensor augmented insulin-pump therapy in type 1 diabetes. N Engl J Med 2010;363:311–20.
114. Battelino T, Phillip M, Bratina N, et al. Effect of continuous glucose monitoring on hypoglycemia in type 1 diabetes. Diabetes Care 2011;34(4):795–800.
115. Dagogo-Jack S, Rattarason C, Cryer P. Reversal of hypoglycemia unawareness, but not defective glucose counterregulation in IDDM. Diabetes 1994;43:1426–34.
116. Fritsche A, Stumvoll M, Haring H, et al. Reversal of hypoglycemia unawareness in a long-term type 1 diabetic patient by improvement of beta-adrenergic sensitivity after prevention of hypoglycemia. J Clin Endocrinol Metab 2000;85:523–5.
117. Fanelli C, Epifano L, Rambotti A, et al. Meticulous prevention of hypoglycemia normalizes the glycemic thresholds and magnitude of most of neuroendocrine responses to, symptoms of, and cognitive function during hypoglycemia in intensively treated patients with short-term IDDM. Diabetes 1993;42:1683–9.
118. Fanelli C, Pampanelli S, Epifano L, et al. Long-term recovery from unawareness, deficient counterregulation and lack of cognitive dysfunction during

hypoglycemia, following institution of rational, intensive insulin therapy in IDDM. Diabetologia 1994;37:1265–76.

119. Cranston I, Lomas J, Maran A, et al. Restoration of hypoglycemia unawareness in patients with long- duration insulin-dependent diabetes. Lancet 1994;344: 283–7.

120. Davis M, Mellman M, Friedman S, et al. Recovery of epinephrine response but not hypoglycemic symptom threshold after intensive therapy in type 1 diabetes. Am J Med 1994;97:535–42.

121. Kendall D, Teuscher A, Robertson R. Defective glucagon secretion during sustained hypoglycemia following successful islet allo- and autotransplantation in humans. Diabetes 1997;46:23–7.

122. Meyer C, Hering B, Grosmann R, et al. Improved glucose counterregulation and autonomic symptoms after intraportal islet transplants alone in patients with long-standing type I diabetes mellitus. Transplantation 1998;66:233–40.

123. Federlin K, Pozza G. Indications for clinical islet transplantation today and in the foreseeable future—the diabetologist's point of view. J Mol Med 1999;77: 148–52.

124. Bosi E, Piatti P, Secchi A, et al. Response of glucagon and insulin secretion to insulin-induced hypoglycemia in diabetic patients after pancreatic transplantation. Diabetes Nutr Metab 1988;1:21–7.

125. Diem P, Redman J, Abid M, et al. Glucagon, catecholamine, and pancreatic polypeptide secretion in type I diabetic recipients of pancreas allografts. J Clin Invest 1990;86:2008–13.

126. Bolinder J, Wahrenberg H, Persson A, et al. Effect of pancreas transplantation on glucose counterregulation in insulin-dependent diabetic patients prone to severe hypoglycaemia. J Intern Med 1991;230:527–33.

127. Bolinder J, Wahrenberg H, Linde B, et al. Improved glucose counterregulation after pancreas transplantation in diabetic patients with unawareness of hypoglycemia. Transplant Proc 1991;23:1667–9.

128. Landgraf R, Nusser J, Riepl R, et al. Metabolic and hormonal studies of Type 1 (insulin-dependent) diabetic patients after successful pancreas and kidney transplantation. Diabetologia 1991;34(Suppl 1):S61–7.

129. Barrou Z, Seaquist E, Robertson R. Pancreas transplantation in diabetic humans normalizes hepatic glucose production during hypoglycemia. Diabetes 1994; 43:661–6.

130. Kendall D, Rooney D, Smets Y, et al. Pancreas transplantation restores epinephrine response and symptom recognition during hypoglycemia in patients with long-standing type 1 diabetes and autonomic neuropathy. Diabetes 1997;46: 249–57.

131. Luzi L, Battezzati A, Perseghin G, et al. Lack of feedback inhibition of insulin secretion in denervated human pancreas. Diabetes 1992;41:1632–9.

132. Battezzati A, Luzi L, Perseghin G, et al. Persistence of counter-regulatory abnormalities in insulin-dependent diabetes mellitus after pancreas transplantation. Eur J Clin Invest 1994;24:751–8.

133. Paty BW, Ryan EA, Shapiro AM, et al. Intrahepatic islet transplantation in type 1 diabetic patients does not restore hypoglycemic hormonal counterregulation or symptom recognition after insulin independence. Diabetes 2002;51:3428–34.

134. Gupta V, Wahoff D, Rooney D, et al. The defective glucagon response from transplanted intrahepatic pancreatic islets during hypoglycemia is transplantation site-determined. Diabetes 1997;46:28–33.

Diabetic Ketoacidosis and Hyperglycemic Hyperosmolar State

Jelena Maletkovic, MD*, Andrew Drexler, MD

KEYWORDS

- Diabetes mellitus • Ketoacidosis • Hyperosmolar state • Hyperglycemic crisis

KEY POINTS

- Diabetic ketoacidosis and the hyperglycemic hyperosmolar state are potentially fatal hyperglycemic crises that occur as acute complications of uncontrolled diabetes mellitus.
- The discovery of insulin in 1921 changed the life expectancy of patients with diabetes.

BACKGROUND AND EPIDEMIOLOGY

Diabetic ketoacidosis (DKA) and the hyperglycemic hyperosmolar state (HHS) are potentially fatal hyperglycemic crises that occur as acute complications of uncontrolled diabetes mellitus.

Because of the improved awareness, prevention, and treatment guidelines, the age-adjusted death rate for hyperglycemic crises in 2009 was less than half the rate in 1980 (7.5 vs 15.3 per 1,000,000 population); however, hyperglycemic crises still caused 2417 deaths in 2009 in the United States.[1] The mortality rate from HHS is much higher than that of DKA and approaches 20%.[2] On the other hand, the incidence of HHS is less than 1 case per 1000 person-years. The annual incidence of DKA varies in different reports and is related to the geographic location.[3-7] It has been reported to be as low as 12.9 per 100,000 in the general population in Denmark[3]; in Malaysia the rate of DKA is high, with 26.3 per 100 patient-years.[4]

The incidence of DKA is increasing in the United States (**Fig. 1**). The National Diabetes Surveillance Program of the Centers for Disease Control and Prevention estimated that from 1988 to 2009, the age-adjusted hospital discharge rate for DKA per 10,000 population consistently increased by 43.8%, so the number of hospital discharges with DKA as the first-listed diagnosis increased from about 80,000 in 1988 to about 140,000 in 2009.[1]

Disclosures: The authors have no conflict of interest regarding this article.
Department of Endocrinology, UCLA School of Medicine, Gonda Diabetes Center, 200 UCLA Medical Plaza, Suite 530, Los Angeles, CA 90095, USA
* Corresponding author.
E-mail address: jmaletkovic@mednet.ucla.edu

Endocrinol Metab Clin N Am 42 (2013) 677–695
http://dx.doi.org/10.1016/j.ecl.2013.07.001
0889-8529/13/$ – see front matter © 2013 Elsevier Inc. All rights reserved.

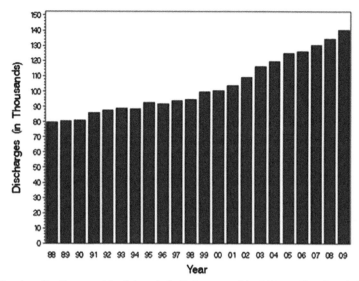

Fig. 1. Number (in thousands) of hospital discharges with DKA as first-listed diagnosis, United States, 1988 to 2009. The number of hospital discharges with DKA as the first-listed diagnosis increased from about 80,000 discharges in 1988 to about 140,000 in 2009. (*From* Centers for Disease Control and Prevention. National hospital discharge survey. Available at: http://www.cdc.gov/nchs/nhds.htm. Accessed April 25, 2013.)

DEFINITION AND DIAGNOSIS

Both DKA and HHS are severe complications of diabetes mellitus and are found to occur simultaneously in about one-third of cases.[8] Although both represent acute hyperglycemic states, DKA is more characterized by ketonemia and anion-gap acidosis and HHS by hyperosmolarity and dehydration.

HHS used to be named *hyperglycemic hyperosmolar nonketotic coma*, but it was found that it frequently presents without coma. It was also named *hyperglycemic hyperosmolar nonketotic state*, but findings of moderate ketonemia in several patients lead to the acceptance of its current term *HHS*. Laboratory findings differ, but some features overlap and are given in **Table 1**:

1. Anion-gap acidosis: Although this is the most important feature of DKA, with serum pH less than 7.3, serum bicarbonate less than 15 mEq/L, and anion gap greater than 10, it is not the finding typical for HHS.

Table 1 Laboratory findings in DKA and HHS		
	DKA	HHS
Anion-gap acidosis	pH <7.3 Bicarbonate <18 Anion gap >10	pH >7.3 Bicarbonate >18 Anion-gap variable
Osmolality	<320	>320
Hyperglycemia	>250	>600
Ketonemia/ketonuria	Present	Rare

2. Ketonemia and ketonuria are more pronounced in DKA but can be present in HHS.
3. Hyperglycemia is elevated in both conditions but more pronounced in HHS, with glucose concentrations frequently greater than 600 mg/dL. Cases of euglycemic DKA have been reported and occur more frequently in pregnancy.[9,10]
4. Osmolality is usually normal in DKA, but may be elevated, and is invariably elevated in hyperosmolar state to above 320 mOsm/kg.

DKA most commonly occurs in patients with type 1 diabetes mellitus although it can occur with type 2 diabetes after serious medical or surgical illness.[11] On the other hand, HHS is more frequently associated with type 2 diabetes, however it has also been reported in type 1 diabetes as a simultaneous occurrence with DKA.[12–14] Many investigators report ketosis-prone type 2 diabetes,[15–17] which is also called Flatbush diabetes after the area in the city of Brooklyn, New York where this type of diabetes was first described and is most frequently diagnosed. These patients are commonly African American and obese with acute defects in insulin secretion and no islet cell autoantibodies.[18–20] Following treatment, some insulin secretory capacity is recovered, and many of them do not require insulin therapy in the future.[21,22]

PRECIPITATING FACTORS

Newly diagnosed individuals with type 1 diabetes mellitus account for 15% of cases of DKA. The frequency of DKA at the diagnosis of type 1 diabetes also varies across different countries,[23] with some extremes, such as United Arab Emirates where it has been reported to be 80%[4] or Sweden where it is 12.8%.[7] Data from Europe reported an inverse correlation between the background incidence of type1 diabetes and the frequency of DKA.[24,25] Most DKA events occur in patients with known diabetes at times of extreme stress, especially infection, such as pneumonia or urinary tract infection, but also myocardial ischemia or any other medical or surgical illness. These cases account for about 40% of all DKA events. The second most important contributor to development of DKA is inadequate insulin treatment, commonly seen as a result of noncompliance, especially in the young population.[26,27] DKA has also been reported with the mismanagement of insulin pumps and undetected leakage of the infusion system or[28] at the time of religious fasting.[29,30] In some cases, medications, such as corticosteroids, pentamidine, and terbutaline, have been identified as triggers for DKA.[31–33] Recent reports from the United States and Canada point to a significant role of atypical antipsychotic medications in the development of fatal cases of DKA.[34–37] Cocaine use is associated with frequent omissions of insulin administration, but it also has significant effects on counter-regulatory hormones. It was found to be an important contributor in the development of DKA and HHS together with alcohol and other abused substances.[27,38–41] In a small number of cases, the workup does not identify any precipitating factor. A rough estimate of most common precipitating factors in development of DKA is given in **Fig. 2**.

In HHS, the most common precipitating events are also inadequate insulin therapy and underlying illness, such as infection, ischemia, or surgery. Because HHS develops more slowly and in a more subtle way, the important contributor to this complication is decreased water intake, especially in elderly patients, that leads to gradual but severe dehydration.[8,42] These patients have either a reduced thirst mechanism or they are unable to access water because of physical or neurologic limitations.

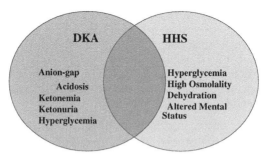

Fig. 2. Major characteristics of DKA and HHS and their estimated overlap.

PATHOGENESIS

The pathogenesis of HHS results from disturbances in glucose metabolism and fluid balance. In DKA, a third component, ketogenesis also contributes to the condition. Both conditions present with hyperglycemia and dehydration.

HORMONES

Both DKA and HHS result from diminished or absent insulin levels and elevated counter-regulatory hormone levels. Insulin deficiency causes glycogenolysis, gluconeogenesis, lipolysis, and protein catabolism. The counter-regulatory hormones present in both of these conditions are glucagon, norepinephrine, epinephrine, cortisol, and growth hormone. Glucagon is the most important of these, whereas growth hormone is probably the least important. DKA is much less likely to occur in the absence of glucagon, but cases of DKA have been reported in patients with complete pancreatectomy. Norepinephrine increases ketogenesis not only by stimulating lipolysis but also by increasing intrahepatic ketogenesis. Catecholamines stimulate lipolysis and fatty acid release even in the presence of insulin. Growth hormone has little effect in the presence of insulin but can enhance ketogenesis in insulin deficiency. The difference between DKA and HHS is that in the latter, the insulin levels do not decrease to a level whereby unrestrained ketogenesis occurs.

Hyperglycemia results from increases in glucose levels obtained from 4 sources:

- Intestinal absorption
- Gluconeogenesis (from carbohydrate, protein, fat)
- Glycogenolysis
- Decreased utilization of glucose by cells, primarily muscle and fat cells

The fate of glucose in the cell can be different depending of the current metabolic needs of the body. It can be stored or it can enter glycolysis and form pyruvate. Pyruvate can be reduced to lactate, transaminated to alanine, or converted to acetyl coenzyme A (CoA). Acetyl CoA can be oxidized to carbon dioxide and water, converted to fatty acids, or used for ketone body or cholesterol synthesis.

Insulin deficiency, absolute or relative, is present in both conditions and results in increased gluconeogenesis and glycogenolysis. Insulin deficiency prevents glucose from entering cells and being metabolized. One of the consequences of insulin deficiency is protein, primarily muscle, breakdown with the provision of precursors for gluconeogenesis. Gluconeogenesis is the crucial action in the development of severe hyperglycemia that is found in DKA and HHS.

Gluconeogenic enzymes are stimulated by the actions of glucagon, catecholamines, and cortisol.[43] The lack of inhibitory action of insulin further drives gluconeogenesis and glycogenolysis and causes increased glucagon activity.[43–45] The end result of insulin deficiency is impairment in carbohydrate utilization, and energy must be obtained from an alternative source, namely, fatty acid metabolism.

Lipid

Lipid mobilization and metabolism are affected by insulin deficiency. In normal subjects, insulin affects fat metabolism by different mechanisms.[46–48] Insulin increases the clearance of triglyceride-rich chylomicrons from the circulation, stimulates creation of triglycerides from free fatty acids (FFA), and inhibits lipolysis of triglycerides.[49–51] In insulin deficiency, fat mobilization is accelerated, resulting in an abundant supply of FFA to the liver. An increase in FFA availability increases ketone production not only by a mass effect but also by a diversion of hepatic fatty acid metabolism toward ketogenesis.[52] FFA levels may be as high in HHS as in DKA.

Ketogenesis

Ketogenesis depends on the amount of FFA supplied to the liver and on the hepatic metabolic fate of fatty acids in the direction of either oxidation and ketogenesis or reesterification.[52] Ketogenesis occurs inside hepatic mitochondria. The glucagon/insulin ratio activates carnitine palmitoyltransferase I, the enzyme that allows FFA in the form of CoA to cross mitochondrial membranes after their esterification with carnitine. In HHS, this ratio does not reach a level whereby unrestrained ketoacidosis occurs. This increase in carnitine palmitoyltransferase I occurs associated with a decrease in malonyl CoA. Fatty acids that are in the mitochondria are converted to acetyl CoA. Most of the acetyl CoA is used in the synthesis of beta-hydroxybutyric acid and acetoacetic acid.[53] Acetoacetate is converted to acetone through nonenzymatic decarboxylation in linear relation to its concentration. Ketones are filtered by the kidney and partially excreted in urine. Progressive volume depletion leads to a reduced glomerular filtration and the shift of acetoacetate to beta-hydroxybutyrate.[54]

Hyperosmolar

Hyperosmolar state develops as a result of osmotic diuresis caused by hyperglycemia, which then creates severe fluid loss. The total body deficit of water is usually about 7 to 12 L in HHS, which represents a loss of about 10% to 15% of body weight. Although mild ketosis can be seen with HHS, it is generally absent in this state. It is considered that patients with HHS who are usually older patients with type 2 diabetes still do have enough insulin to be protected from exaggerated lipolysis and the consequent abundance of FFA.[55] They do not, however, have enough insulin to prevent hyperglycemia.[56]

CLINICAL PRESENTATION

DKA and HHS can have similar clinical presentations. There are usually signs and symptoms of hyperglycemia and a general unwell feeling with malaise, fatigue, and anorexia. Patients can present with symptoms of the preceding illness, such as infection (pneumonia, urinary tract infection, and so forth) or myocardial ischemia. DKA will usually develop faster than HHS, sometimes in less than 24 hours. HHS takes days to weeks to develop in most patients.

Some of the differences in the clinical presentations result from the state of metabolic acidosis in DKA. Patients with DKA will frequently have hyperventilation (Kussmaul ventilation) as a compensatory mechanism for acidosis that is rarely seen with HHS. DKA will also present with abdominal pain that is associated with the level of acidosis.[57] Sometimes the presentation with significant abdominal pain is associated with an underlying abdominal process, such as acute pancreatitis.[58] Abdominal pain is frequently associated with acidosis only and no underlying pathological condition can be identified; however, it always requires a workup for acute abdominal process.

Most patients with HHS will have some degree of neurologic disturbance, whereas only patients with more advanced DKA will be comatose. If they present early in the course of the disease, patients with DKA will frequently have a normal neurologic examination. This difference is caused by greater hyperosmolality in HHS caused by osmotic diuresis and free water loss.[59–62] Hyperosmolar state causes cellular dehydration produced by osmotic shifts of water from the intracellular fluid space to the extracellular space.[63,64] If osmolality is normal and patients show severe neurologic deficit, further workup is indicated to rule out underlying neurologic pathologic condition. Elderly patients are particularly susceptible to these disturbances. Some possible neurologic presentations include irritability, restlessness, stupor, muscular twitching, hyperreflexia, spasticity, seizures, and coma.[65–68] The clinical signs and symptoms reflect both the severity of the hyperosmolality and the rate at which it develops.[69]

Free water deficit is more pronounced in HHS, as compared with DKA; patients with HHS will have more evidence of severe dehydration. An additional source of dehydration is impaired water intake, particularly in elderly patients with ongoing lethargy and confusion.[70] Evaluation of volume status is one of the initial assessments of patients with DKA or HHS. **Table 2** shows some of the important clinical features of DKA and HHS.

INITIAL EVALUATION

Both DKA and HHS are medical emergencies with improved, but high, mortality rates that require careful evaluation. As a first step in evaluating patients who present with a hyperglycemic emergency, the physician should secure the airway and ensure adequate ventilation and oxygenation. Patients should also have secure intravenous (IV) access, with at least 2 ports, and continuous cardiac monitoring. A Foley catheter should be placed for strict monitoring of intake and output.

The initial laboratory investigation should include the following: serum glucose, metabolic panel, serum phosphate and magnesium, arterial blood gas analysis, complete blood count (CBC) with differential, hepatic enzymes, serum ketones, urinalysis, cardiac enzymes, hemoglobin A1C, and coagulation profile. Additional laboratory values that should be considered are infectious workup with urine and blood cultures,

Table 2 Clinical features of DKA and HHS		
Clinical Presentation	**DKA**	**HHS**
Development of Symptoms	Hours to Days	Days to Weeks
Polydipsia/polyuria	+	+
Nausea/vomiting	+	+
Abdominal pain	+	−
Anorexia	+	+
Fatigue/malaise	+	+
Neurologic abnormalities	±	+ +
Hyperventilation	+	−
Dehydration	+	+ +

lumbar puncture in selected cases, serum lipase, and amylase. Other investigations should include electrocardiogram and chest radiograph, and selected cases will require additional chest/abdomen/brain or other imaging depending on the clinical presentation. Serum glucose and electrolytes should be repeated every 1 to 2 hours until patients are stable and then every 4 to 6 hours. The most important points in the initial evaluation of DKA and HHS are given in **Table 3**. The initial calculations include serum sodium correction, serum osmolality, anion gap, and free water deficit.

Basic considerations in the evaluation of DKA and HHS laboratory values are given in the following text.

Serum Glucose

Serum glucose is usually more elevated in HHS than in DKA. This elevation is partly caused by the acidosis of DKA leading to an earlier diagnosis of the condition before glucoses levels have increased as high. Also contributing is the fact that about a half of the patients with type 1 diabetes mellitus have glomerular hyperfiltration in the first years in the course of their disease. Patients with type 2 diabetes mellitus also initially have an increased glomerular filtration rate of about 2 standard deviations more than their age-matched nondiabetic and obese controls, but the degree of hyperfiltration is less than that of patients with type 1 diabetes. These differences allow for an increased glucose excretion degree in DKA and less hyperglycemia as compared with HHS.[71] In

Table 3	
Initial evaluation of patients with hyperglycemic emergency (DKA/HHS)	
First steps	IV line (at least 2 ports, consider central access)
	Airway and adequate ventilation/oxygenation
	Cardiac monitor
	In and out monitoring (Foley catheter)
Initial laboratory test results	Serum glucose
	Basic metabolic panel with electrolytes
	Arterial blood gas analysis
	BUN/creatinine
	CBC with differential
	Serum phosphate
	Liver enzymes
	Urinalysis
	Cardiac enzymes
	Coagulation profile
	Serum ketones
	Hemoglobin A1C
Additional laboratory test results (case-by-case basis)	Blood and urine culture
	Lumbar puncture
	Amylase and lipase
	Other laboratory tests based on clinical presentation
Initial imaging	CXR
	Optional imaging based on clinical presentation (CT head/chest/abdomen)
Initial calculations	Anion gap
	Corrected serum sodium
	Free water deficit
	Serum osmolality

Abbreviations: BUN, serum urea nitrogen; CT, computed tomography; CXR, chest X-ray.

HHS, the glucose level is more than 600 mg/dL and can frequently be more than 1000 mg/dL.[72] The degree of hyperglycemia reflects the degree of dehydration and hyperosmolality.[73] Cases of normoglycemic DKA have been described in pregnant patients.[74,75] Patients with renal failure usually have severe hyperglycemia because of poor renal clearance of glucose. These patients, however, usually do not develop hyperosmolality because of the lack of osmotic diuresis, and their mental status with HHS tends to be less affected than with patients who have preserved renal function.[76–79]

Serum Sodium

Serum sodium levels are affected in both DKA and HHS. In the setting of hyperglycemia, osmotic forces drive water into the vascular space and cause dilution with resulting hyponatremia. Each 100 mg/dL of the glucose level more than normal lowers the serum sodium level by about 1.6 mEq/L. The treatment of DKA and HHS with insulin causes reversal of this process and drives water back into the extravascular space with a subsequent increase in serum sodium level. Corrected serum sodium is calculated with the following formula:

Corrected sodium = serum sodium (mEq/L) + (1.6 mEq/L for each 100 mg/dL of glucose more than 100 mg/dL)

One study suggested that a more accurate correction factor in extreme hyperglycemic states is 2.4 mEq/L for each 100 mg/dL because of the nonlinear relationship between the glucose and sodium concentration.[80] An additional decrease in serum sodium is present with confounding pseudohyponatremia that occurs with hyperlipidemia or hyperproteinemia with some laboratory assays.[81,82] Thus, most patients will present with hyponatremia. In some cases of HHS, patients may present with hypernatremia secondary to osmotic diuresis and more severe dehydration.[83,84] Hypernatremia indicates a profound degree of water loss. The measured, and not the calculated, serum sodium level should be used to calculate the anion gap.[85]

Serum Potassium

Serum potassium is frequently paradoxically elevated despite the total body deficit in DKA and HHS. This elevation is caused by the extracellular shift of potassium in exchange for the hydrogen ions accumulated in acidosis, reduced renal function, release of potassium from cells caused by glycogenolysis, insulin deficiency, and hyperosmolality.[86,87] It is thought that the water deficit from the cells creates passive potassium flux to the extracellular space leading to relative hyperkalemia without having significant acidosis in HHS.[88] The body deficit of potassium occurs with diuresis but also with gastrointestinal losses.[89] Treatment with insulin shifts potassium into the cell and causes a rapid decrease of the serum potassium levels. Hypokalemia is frequently encountered after starting insulin treatment. Careful monitoring and potassium supplementing are required in patients with DKA and HHS, especially if they initially present with a normal or low potassium level.[90–93]

Serum Phosphate

Serum phosphate is lost by diuresis in DKA and HHS, and its typical deficit is usually up to 7 mmol/kg.[94,95] Similarly, as in the case of potassium deficit, patients may present with normal or even high levels of phosphate because insulin deficiency drives phosphate out of the cells. The level of serum phosphate will start decreasing as soon as insulin treatment is established. Hyperphosphatemia, on the first presentation, also reflects volume depletion. Acidosis is another mechanism that causes falsely normal or high phosphate levels. Patients who present with profound acidosis are at higher risk of developing hypophosphatemia when insulin administration is started. The severity of subsequent hypophosphatemia can be predicted by the degree of metabolic acidosis on presentation.[38] Untreated hypophosphatemia can lead to serious complications, including cardiac arrest.[39–41]

Serum Bicarbonate

Serum bicarbonate is typically more than 18 mEq/L in HHS. Because DKA is characterized by acidosis, the serum bicarbonate is lower than 18 mEq/L and frequently lower than 15 mEq/L. A decrease of bicarbonate to less than 10 mEq/L indicates severe DKA.[96,97]

Serum Ketones

Serum ketones are used as an energy source when glucose is not readily available and are increased in DKA, as a response to low insulin levels and high levels of counter-regulatory hormones.[98] Acetoacetate is a ketoacid, whereas beta-hydroxybutyrate represents a hydroxy acid that is formed by the reduction of acetoacetate. The third ketone body, acetone, is the least abundant of all and is formed by decarboxylation of acetic acid. Although ketones are always present, their levels increase in certain conditions, such as starvation, pregnancy, and exercise. DKA causes the most prominent increase in ketone body levels compared with the other common conditions. Serum ketone testing is performed when a urinary dipstick tests positive for urine ketones. The most commonly used test for serum ketones is nitroprusside. However, it detects only acetoacetate and acetone and not hydroxybutyrate. Because beta-hydroxybutyrate is the most prominent ketone body and is disproportionally so in DKA, it is possible to have a negative testing for serum ketones in the presence of severe ketoacidosis.[99] Cases of children who developed DKA, that could have potentially been prevented, as a consequence of false-negative home ketone test-strip readings with nitroprusside have been described.[100]

The initiation of treatment with insulin causes a conversion of beta-hydroxybutyrate to acetoacetate while the overall levels of ketone bodies are decreasing.[101] This effect can potentially create a false observation that DKA is worsening, although, in fact, it is improving; subsequent unnecessary increases in insulin treatment could lead to other complications.[102] Quantitative enzymatic tests have been developed and can be used as point-of-care tests that identify beta-hydroxybutyrate.[99,103,104] On the other hand, false-positive results for serum ketone bodies have been identified in patients using drugs with sulfhydryl groups.[105–109] The risk of inappropriate therapy with insulin caused by false-positive ketones in serum is low but existing.

Anion Gap

Anion gap represents unmeasured anions in serum (ketones) after subtracting the major measured anions from the major measured cation.

$$AG = (\text{serum sodium}) - (\text{chloride} + \text{bicarbonate})$$

where AG is anion gap

Measured, not corrected, serum sodium levels should be used to estimate the anion gap.[110] The anion gap is usually more than 20 mEq/L in DKA, and it reflects the production and accumulation of acetoacetate and beta-hydroxybutyrate in the serum. It inversely reflects the rate of excretion of acids that will be impaired with renal failure.[112] Patients admitted with diabetic ketoacidosis have a mean bicarbonate deficit that is approximately equal to the excess anion gap.

Arterial Blood

Arterial blood gas measurement is recommended in all cases of hyperglycemic complications of diabetes mellitus. Acidosis is one of the main features of DKA and is included in the diagnostic criteria, with arterial pH of less than 7.3. Arterial pH in HHS is usually more than 7.3. In order to avoid the painful and more difficult procedure of arterial blood drawing, in patients with normal oxygen saturation on room air, venous blood gas is sometimes used to estimate acidosis. It has been found that there is a high degree of correlation and agreement with the arterial value, with acceptably narrow 95% limits of agreement.[111] Arterial blood gas analysis can, on the other hand, indicate an underlying disease associated with DKA or HHS. Hypoxemia may be found with cardiac or pulmonary trigger diseases, and low carbon dioxide may represent hyperventilation as a compensatory mechanism for metabolic acidosis.

Serum Osmolality

The serum osmolality elevation correlates with the degree of neurologic disturbance.[112] The serum osmolality is determined by the concentrations of the different solutes in the plasma. In normal subjects, sodium salts, glucose, and urea are the primary circulating solutes. Increased serum osmolality to more than 320 mosmol/kg is seen in patients with neurologic abnormalities and is typical for HHS. Rarely, serum osmolality can be more than 400 mOsm/kg. Neurologic deficits ranging from confusion to coma can be seen with DKA, with a less significant increase in serum osmolality, which then reflect the degree of acidosis.[113] The formula for the calculation of serum osmolality is given next[114–116]:

$$\text{Serum osmolality} = (2 \times \text{serum [Na]}) + (\text{glucose, in mg/dL})/18 + (\text{BUN in mg/dL})/2.8$$

where *BUN* is serum urea nitrogen
The formula with all units in millimoles per liter is the following:

$$\text{Serum osmolality} = (2 \times \text{serum [Na]}) + (\text{glucose}) + (\text{urea})$$

The serum osmolal gap represents the difference between the measured and calculated serum osmolality. In normal individuals, the osmolal gap was not significant and was found to be 1.9 ± 3.7 mosmol/kg and -1.7 ± 1.7 mosmol/kg in 2 studies.[117] The measured serum osmolality can be significantly higher than the calculated value in the presence of an additional solute, such as ethylene glycol, methanol, ethanol, formaldehyde, isopropyl alcohol, diethyl ether, glycine, sorbitol, or mannitol, or in presence of significant pseudohyponatremia caused by severe hyperproteinemia or hyperlipidemia.[118–120]

Leukocytosis

Leukocytosis is present in hyperglycemic emergencies even in the absence of infection. This presence is explained by elevated stress hormones, such as cortisol and catecholamines, and cytokines and is proportional to the degree of ketonemia.[121–123] True leukocytosis is also frequent, and a source of infection should be investigated in all cases. White blood cell counts of greater than 25,000/μL were independently associated with altered sensorium in one study.[124]

Amylase and Lipase

Amylase and lipase can be elevated with DKA in the absence of pancreatitis. An increase in lipase correlates with plasma osmolality, and an increase in amylase correlates with plasma osmolality and pH.[125] True pancreatitis is also a frequent precipitating factor for hyperglycemic emergencies and can be confirmed with other clinical characteristics and imaging **Fig. 3**.[59]

TREATMENT

The management of DKA and HHS consists of fluid and electrolyte repletion, insulin administration, and the treatment of the precipitating cause if one can be identified. Patients should be admitted to a monitored unit where close observation of mental status, blood pressure, heart rate and rhythm, and urine output can be done.

Fluid Replacement

Fluid replacement should be the initial therapy in DKA and HHS, with the goal of correcting a fluid deficit in the first 24 hours. The initial fluid should be normal saline. The rate in the first hours should be 10 to 15 mL/kg. Once patients are euvolemic, switching to half-normal saline is appropriate for those with normal sodium or hypernatremia. This change allows for more efficient replacement of the free water deficit induced by the glucose osmotic diuresis. Half-normal saline should be administered at a rate of 4 to 14 mL/kg. Five percent dextrose with half-normal saline should be started when the blood glucose level decreases less than 250 mg/dL in DKA and 300 mg/dL in HHS.[56]

Cerebral edema is a serious complication of DKA treatment with a high mortality of 21% to 24% that is primarily seen in children when hyperosmolality was corrected too rapidly.[126] Symptomatic cerebral edema occurs in 0.5% to 1.0% of pediatric DKA episodes, and 15% to 26% of children remain with permanent neurologic sequelae.[127] Children who presented with higher osmolality and higher serum urea nitrogen (BUN) demonstrated a more severe clinical picture, with the most profound acidosis and hypocapnia.[128]

Treating patients with renal or cardiac compromise is challenging because a fine balance needs to be established between the volume deficit and the volume overload. These patients require frequent monitoring of volume status and parameters of fluid

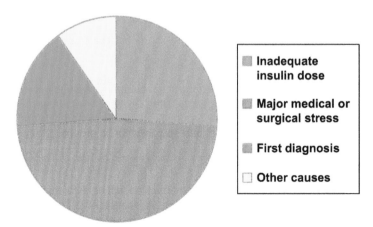

Fig. 3. Estimated prevalence of precipitating factors in development of DKA.

homeostasis, such as osmolality, serum sodium, BUN and creatinine, blood glucose, and urine output, as well as frequent clinical monitoring for signs of respiratory compromise caused by volume overload.

Potassium

Potassium may initially be elevated because of the extracellular shift caused by insulin deficiency, acidosis, and proteolysis.[129] This elevation will rapidly correct with the administration of fluids that create dilution and insulin treatment that will allow for potassium to be shifted back to the cell. Urinary and gastrointestinal loss of potassium also causes an overall deficit in potassium concentration. Glucosuria results in the loss of 70 mEq of sodium and potassium for each liter of fluid lost. The correction of actual deficit of potassium should be started when the potassium level is less than 5.3 mEq/L. The potassium level should be maintained between 4 and 5 mEq/L.

Insulin

Insulin at a low dose should be started approximately 1 hour after the initiation of fluid replacement therapy, with regular insulin as a treatment of choice. This treatment should be further delayed if serum potassium is less than 3.3 mEq/L because of the risk of hypokalemia. The administration of an initial bolus dose of insulin is not associated with a significant benefit to patients with DKA.[130] As an alternative to IV regular insulin, an intramuscular regimen with rapid-acting analogues has been reported to decrease the cost of DKA treatment.[131] When the plasma glucose level is less than 250 mg/dL in DKA or 300 mg/dL in HHS, the insulin rate should be decreased and maintained to keep blood glucose between 150 to 200 mg/dL in DKA and 250 to 300 mg/dL in HHS, until the ketoacidosis and/or hyperosmolar states are resolved.[129,132] It is critical that insulin therapy be based on the correction of the anion gap and not the serum glucose level. In some cases, it may be necessary to give IV 50% dextrose solution to allow adequate insulin therapy.

Bicarbonate therapy is controversial given the potential problems, such as hypokalemia, acidosis, hypoxia, hypernatremia, and the lack of a therapeutic effect.[133,134] There is insufficient data to confirm a benefit of treatment. It should be reserved only for severe cases of ketoacidosis with a very low bicarbonate of less than 10 and severe acidosis. In similar fashion, phosphate repletion is not recommended in all patients. Studies do not show a clear benefit of this treatment, and it may only be of some use in patients who are symptomatic for hypophosphatemia with heart or skeletal muscle involvement.[135–137] The main risk of phosphate therapy is hypocalcemia, especially as the pH normalizes.

SUMMARY

The discovery of insulin in 1921 changed the life expectancy of patients with diabetes mellitus dramatically. Today, almost a century later, DKA and HHS remain a significant economic burden and, most importantly, a significant cause of morbidity and mortality across different countries, ages, races, and socioeconomic groups.

REFERENCES

1. Centers for Disease Control and Prevention. National hospital discharge survey. Available at: www.cdc.gov/nchs/nhds.htm. Accessed April 25, 2013.
2. Wachtel TJ, Tctu-Mouradjian LM, Goldman DL, et al. Hyperosmolarity and acidosis in diabetes mobility. J Gen Intern Med 1991;6:495–502.

3. Henriksen OM, Roder ME, Prahl JB, et al. Diabetic ketoacidosis in Denmark incidence and mortality estimated from public health registries. Diabetes Res Clin Pract 2007;76(1):51–6.
4. Craig ME, Jones TW, Silink M, et al. Diabetes care, glycemic control, and complications in children with type 1 diabetes from Asia and the Western Pacific region. J Diabetes Complications 2007;21(5):280–7.
5. Campbell-Stokes PL, Taylor BJ. Prospective incidence study of diabetes mellitus in New Zealand children aged 0 to 14 years. Diabetologia 2005;48(4): 643–8.
6. Pronina EA, Petraikina EE, Antsiferov MB, et al. A 10-year (1996–2005) prospective study of the incidence of type 1 diabetes. Diabet Med 2008;25(8):956–9.
7. Samuelsson U, Stenhammar L. Clinical characteristics at onset of type 1 diabetes in children diagnosed between 1977 and 2001 in the south-east region of Sweden. Diabetes Res Clin Pract 2005;68:49–55.
8. Wachtel TJ. The diabetic hyperosmolar state. Clin Geriatr Med 1990;6(4):797.
9. John R, Yadav H, John M. Euglycemic ketoacidosis as a cause of a metabolic acidosis in the intensive care unit. Acute Med 2012;11(4):219–21.
10. Guo RX, Yang LZ, Li LX, et al. Diabetic ketoacidosis in pregnancy tends to occur at lower blood glucose levels: case-control study and a case report of euglycemic diabetic ketoacidosis in pregnancy. J Obstet Gynaecol Res 2008;34(3): 324–30.
11. Bowden SA, Duck MM, Hoffman RP. Young children (<5 yr) and adolescents (>12 yr) with type 1 diabetes mellitus have low rate of partial remission: diabetic ketoacidosis is an important risk factor. Pediatr Diabetes 2008;9(3 Pt 1): 197–201.
12. DeFronzo R, Matsuda M, Barrett E. Diabetic ketoacidosis: a combined metabolic nephrologic approach to therapy. Diabetes Rev 1994;2:209–38.
13. Rosenbloom A. Hyperglycemic hyperosmolar state: an emerging pediatric problem. J Pediatr 2010;156:180–4.
14. Lotz M, Geraghty M. Hyperglycemic, hyperosmolar, nonketotic coma in a ketosis-prone juvenile diabetic. Ann Intern Med 1968;69(6):1245–6 No abstract available.
15. Umpierrez GE, Casals MM, Gebhart SP, et al. Diabetic ketoacidosis in obese African-Americans. Diabetes 1995;44:790–5.
16. Kitabchi AE. Ketosis-prone diabetes-A new subgroup of patients with atypical type 1 and type 2 diabetes? J Clin Endocrinol Metab 2003;88:5087–9.
17. Mauvais-Jarvis F, Sobngwi E, Porcher R, et al. Ketosis-prone type 2 diabetes in patients of sub-Saharan African origin: clinical pathophysiology and natural history of beta-cell dysfunction and insulin resistance. Diabetes 2004;53:645–53.
18. Banerji MA. Diabetes in African Americans: unique pathophysiologic features. Curr Diab Rep 2004;4(3):219–23.
19. Banerji MA. Impaired beta-cell and alpha-cell function in African-American children with type 2 diabetes mellitus–"Flatbush diabetes". J Pediatr Endocrinol Metab 2002;15(Suppl 1):493–501.
20. Banerji MA, Chaiken RL, Huey H, et al. GAD antibody negative NIDDM in adult black subjects with diabetic ketoacidosis and increased frequency of human leukocyte antigen DR3 and DR4. Flatbush diabetes. Diabetes 1994;43(6): 741–5.
21. Rodacki M, Zajdenverg L, Lima GA, et al. Case report: diabetes Flatbush - from ketoacidosis to non pharmacological treatment. Arq Bras Endocrinol Metabol 2007;51(1):131–5 [in Portuguese].

22. Maldonado M, Hampe CS, Gaur LK, et al. Ketosis-prone diabetes: dissection of a heterogeneous syndrome using an immunogenetic and beta-cell functional classification, prospective analysis, and clinical outcomes. J Clin Endocrinol Metab 2003;88:5090–8.

23. Kitabchi AE, Umpierrez GE, Murphy MB, et al. Management of hyperglycemic crises in patients with diabetes. Diabetes Care 2001;24(1):131–53.

24. Lévy-Marchal C, Patterson CC, Green A. Geographical variation of presentation at diagnosis of type I diabetes in children: the EURODIAB study. European and Diabetes. Diabetologia 2001;44(Suppl 3):B75–80.

25. Ellis D, Naar-King S, Templin T, et al. Multisystemic therapy for adolescents with poorly controlled type 1 diabetes: reduced diabetic ketoacidosis admissions and related costs over 24 months. Diabetes Care 2008;31(9):1746–7.

26. Umpierrez GE, Kelly JP, Navarrete JE, et al. Hyperglycemic crises in urban blacks. Arch Intern Med 1997;157(6):669–75.

27. Walter H, Günther A, Timmler R, et al. Ketoacidosis in long-term therapy with insulin pumps. Incidence, causes, circumstances. Med Klin 1989;84(12):565–8.

28. Hanas R, Lindgren F, Lindblad B. A 2-yr national population study of pediatric ketoacidosis in Sweden: predisposing conditions and insulin pump use. Pediatr Diabetes 2009;10(1):33–7.

29. Friedrich I, Levy Y. Diabetic ketoacidosis during the Ramadan fast. Harefuah 2000;138(1):19–21, 86.

30. Ahmedani MY, Haque MS, Basit A, et al. Ramadan Prospective Diabetes Study: the role of drug dosage and timing alteration, active glucose monitoring and patient education. Diabet Med 2012;29(6):709–15.

31. Herchline TE, Plouffe JF, Para MF. Diabetes mellitus presenting with ketoacidosis following pentamidine therapy in patients with acquired immunodeficiency syndrome. J Infect 1991;22(1):41–4.

32. Ramaswamy K, Kozma CM, Nasrallah H. Risk of diabetic ketoacidosis after exposure to risperidone or olanzapine. Drug Saf 2007;30(7):589–99.

33. Tibaldi JM, Lorber DL, Nerenberg A. Diabetic ketoacidosis and insulin resistance with subcutaneous terbutaline infusion: a case report. Am J Obstet Gynecol 1990;163(2):509–10.

34. Ely SF, Neitzel AR, Gill JR. Fatal diabetic ketoacidosis and antipsychotic medication. J Forensic Sci 2012 [Epub ahead of print]. Available at: http://www ncbi. nlm.nih.gov/pubmed/23278567.

35. Guenette MD, Giacca A, Hahn M, et al. Atypical antipsychotics and effects of adrenergic and serotonergic receptor binding on insulin secretion in-vivo: an animal model. Schizophr Res 2013;146(1–3):162–9.

36. Bobo WV, Cooper WO, Epstein RA Jr, et al. Positive predictive value of automated database records for diabetic ketoacidosis (DKA) in children and youth exposed to antipsychotic drugs or control medications: a Tennessee Medicaid study. BMC Med Res Methodol 2011;11:157.

37. Makhzoumi ZH, McLean LP, Lee JH, et al. Diabetic ketoacidosis associated with aripiprazole. Pharmacotherapy 2008;28(9):1198–202.

38. Warner EA, Greene GS, Buchsbaum MS, et al. Diabetic ketoacidosis associated with cocaine use. Arch Intern Med 1998;158(16):1799–802.

39. Ng RS, Darko DA, Hillson RM. Street drug use among young patients with type 1 diabetes in the UK. Diabet Med 2004;21(3):295–6.

40. Nyenwe EA, Loganathan RS, Blum S, et al. Active use of cocaine: an independent risk factor for recurrent diabetic ketoacidosis in a city hospital. Endocr Pract 2007;13(1):22–9.

41. Isidro ML, Jorge S. Recreational drug abuse in patients hospitalized for diabetic ketosis or diabetic ketoacidosis. Acta Diabetol 2013;50(2):183–7.
42. Wachtel TJ, Silliman RA, Lamberton P. Predisposing factors for the diabetic hyperosmolar state. Arch Intern Med 1987;147(3):499–501.
43. Taborsky GJ Jr. The physiology of glucagon. J Diabetes Sci Technol 2010;4(6):1338–44.
44. Miles JM, Gerich JE. Glucose and ketone body kinetics in diabetic ketoacidosis. Clin Endocrinol Metab 1983;12(2):303–19.
45. Fanelli CG, Porcellati F, Rossetti P, et al. Glucagon: the effects of its excess and deficiency on insulin action. Nutr Metab Cardiovasc Dis 2006;16(Suppl 1):S28–34.
46. Farese RV Jr, Yost TJ, Eckel RH. Tissue-specific regulation of lipoprotein lipase activity by insulin/glucose in normal-weight humans. Metabolism 1991;40(2):214.
47. Fielding BA, Frayn KN. Lipoprotein lipase and the disposition of dietary fatty acids. Br J Nutr 1998;80(6):495.
48. Zimmermann R, Lass A, Haemmerle G. Fate of fat: the role of adipose triglyceride lipase in lipolysis. Biochim Biophys Acta 2009;1791(6):494.
49. Lass A, Zimmermann R, Oberer M, et al. Lipolysis - a highly regulated multi-enzyme complex mediates the catabolism of cellular fat stores. Prog Lipid Res 2011;50(1):14.
50. Enoksson S, Degerman E, Hagström-Toft E, et al. Various phosphodiesterase subtypes mediate the in vivo antilipolytic effect of insulin on adipose tissue and skeletal muscle in man. Diabetologia 1998;41(5):560.
51. Strålfors P, Honnor RC. Insulin-induced dephosphorylation of hormone-sensitive lipase. Correlation with lipolysis and cAMP-dependent protein kinase activity. Eur J Biochem 1989;182(2):379.
52. Beylot M. Regulation of in vivo ketogenesis: role of free fatty acids and control by epinephrine, thyroid hormones, insulin and glucagon. Diabetes Metab 1996;22(5):299–304.
53. Chiasson JL, Aris-Jilwan N, Bélanger R, et al. Diagnosis and treatment of diabetic ketoacidosis and the hyperglycemic hyperosmolar state. CMAJ 2003;168(7):859–66.
54. Adrogue HJ, Eknoyan G, Suki WK. Diabetic ketoacidosis: role of the kidney in the acid-base homeostasis re-evaluated. Kidney Int 1984;25:591–8.
55. Kitabchi AE, Umpierrez GE, Miles JM, et al. Hyperglycemic crises in adult patients with diabetes. Diabetes Care 2009;32(7):1335–43.
56. Smiley D, Chandra P, Umpierrez G. Update on diagnosis, pathogenesis and management of ketosis-prone type 2 diabetes mellitus. Diabetes Manag (Lond) 2011;1(6):589–600.
57. Umpierrez G, Freire AX. Abdominal pain in patients with hyperglycemic crises. J Crit Care 2002;17(1):63.
58. Pant N, Kadaria D, Murillo LC, et al. Abdominal pathology in patients with diabetes ketoacidosis. Am J Med Sci 2012;344(5):341–4.
59. Park BE, Meacham WF, Netsky MG. Nonketotic hyperglycemic hyperosmolar coma. Report of neurosurgical cases with a review of mechanisms and treatment. J Neurosurg 1976;44(4):409–17.
60. Braaten JT. Hyperosmolar nonketotic diabetic coma: diagnosis and management. Geriatrics 1987;42(11):83–8, 92.
61. Lorber D. Nonketotic hypertonicity in diabetes mellitus. Med Clin North Am 1995;79(1):39.

62. Gaglia JL, Wyckoff J, Abrahamson MJ. Acute hyperglycemic crisis in the elderly. Med Clin North Am 2004;88(4):1063–84, xii.

63. Verbalis JG. Control of brain volume during hypoosmolality and hyperosmolality. Adv Exp Med Biol 2006;576:113–29.

64. Derr RF, Zieve L. Weakness, neuropathy, and coma following total parenteral nutrition in underfed or starved rats: relationship to blood hyperosmolarity and brain water loss. J Lab Clin Med 1978;92(4):521–8.

65. Arieff AI. Central nervous system manifestations of disordered sodium metabolism. Clin Endocrinol Metab 1984;13:269–94.

66. Star RA. Hyperosmolar states. Am J Med Sci 1990;300(6):402–12.

67. Butts DE. Fluid and electrolyte disorders associated with diabetic ketoacidosis and hyperglycemic hyperosmolar nonketotic coma. Nurs Clin North Am 1987; 22(4):827–36.

68. Ellis EN. Concepts of fluid therapy in diabetic ketoacidosis and hyperosmolar hyperglycemic nonketotic coma. Pediatr Clin North Am 1990;37(2):313–21.

69. Palevsky PM. Hypernatremia. Semin Nephrol 1998;18(1):20–30.

70. Levine SN, Sanson TH. Treatment of hyperglycaemic hyperosmolar non-ketotic syndrome. Drugs 1989;38(3):462–72.

71. Jerums G, Premaratne E, Panagiotopoulos S, et al. The clinical significance of hyperfiltration in diabetes. Diabetologia 2010;53(10):2093–104.

72. Delaney MF, Zisman A, Kettyle WM. Diabetic ketoacidosis and hyperglycemic hyperosmolar nonketotic syndrome. Endocrinol Metab Clin North Am 2000;29: 683–705.

73. Nugent BW. Hyperosmolar hyperglycemic state. Emerg Med Clin North Am 2005;23(3):629–48, vii.

74. Chico M, Levine SN, Lewis DF. Normoglycemic diabetic ketoacidosis in pregnancy. J Perinatol 2008;28(4):310–2.

75. Cullen MT, Reece EA, Homko CJ, et al. The changing presentations of diabetic ketoacidosis during pregnancy. Am J Perinatol 1996;13(7):449–51.

76. Al-Kudsi RR, Daugirdas JT, Ing TS, et al. Extreme hyperglycemia in dialysis patients. Clin Nephrol 1982;17(5):228.

77. Popli S, Sun Y, Tang HL, et al. Acidosis and coma in adult diabetic maintenance dialysis patients with extreme hyperglycemia. Int Urol Nephrol 2013. [Epub ahead of print].

78. Tzamaloukas AH, Ing TS, Elisaf MS, et al. Abnormalities of serum potassium concentration in dialysis-associated hyperglycemia and their correction with insulin: review of published reports. Int Urol Nephrol 2011;43(2):451–9.

79. Tzamaloukas AH, Ing TS, Siamopoulos KC, et al. Body fluid abnormalities in severe hyperglycemia in patients on chronic dialysis: review of published reports. J Diabetes Complications 2008;22(1):29–37.

80. Hiler TA, Abbott D, Barrett EJ. Hyponatremia: evaluating the correction factor for hyperglycemia. Am J Med 1999;106:399–403.

81. Weisberg LS. Pseudohyponatremia: a reappraisal. Am J Med 1989;86(3): 315–8.

82. Dhatt G, Talor Z, Kazory A. Direct ion-selective electrode method is useful in diagnosis of pseudohyponatremia. J Emerg Med 2012;43(2):348–9.

83. Liamis G, Gianoutsos C, Elisaf MS. Hyperosmolar nonketotic syndrome with hypernatremia: how can we monitor treatment? Diabetes Metab 2000;26(5):403–5.

84. Milionis HJ, Liamis G, Elisaf MS. Appropriate treatment of hypernatraemia in diabetic hyperglycaemic hyperosmolar syndrome. J Intern Med 2001;249(3): 273–6.

85. Beck LH. Should the actual or the corrected serum sodium be used to calculate the anion gap in diabetic ketoacidosis? Cleve Clin J Med 2001;68(8):673–4.
86. Uribarri J, Oh MS, Carroll HJ. Hyperkalemia in diabetes mellitus. J Diabet Complications 1990;4(1):3–7.
87. Adrogué HJ, Lederer ED, Suki WM, et al. Determinants of plasma potassium levels in diabetic ketoacidosis. Medicine (Baltimore) 1986;65(3):163.
88. Arieff AI, Carroll HJ. Nonketotic hyperosmolar coma with hyperglycemia: clinical features, pathophysiology, renal function, acid-base balance, plasma-cerebrospinal fluid equilibria and the effects of therapy in 37 cases. Medicine (Baltimore) 1972;51(2):73.
89. Schultze RG. Recent advances in the physiology and pathophysiology of potassium excretion. Arch Intern Med 1973;131(6):885–97.
90. Abramson E, Arky R. Diabetic acidosis with initial hypokalemia. Therapeutic implications. JAMA 1966;196(5):401.
91. Greenberg A. Hyperkalemia: treatment options. Semin Nephrol 1998;18(1):46–57.
92. Kim HJ, Han SW. Therapeutic approach to hyperkalemia. Nephron 2002;92(Suppl 1):33–40.
93. Unwin RJ, Luft FC, Shirley DG. Pathophysiology and management of hypokalemia: a clinical perspective. Nat Rev Nephrol 2011;7(2):75–84.
94. Ennis ED, Stahl EJ, Kreisberg RA. The hyperosmolar hyperglycemic syndrome. Diabetes Rev 1994;2:115–26.
95. Ennis ED, Kreisberg RA. Diabetic ketoacidosis and hyperosmolar syndrome. In: Leroith D, Taylor SI, Olefsky JM, editors. Diabetes mellitus. A fundamental and clinical text. 3rd edition. Philadelphia: Lippincott Williams & Wilkins; 2004. p. 627–42.
96. Kitabchi AE, Fisher JN, Murphy MB, et al. Diabetic ketoacidosis and the hyperglycemic hyperosmolar nonketotic state. In: Kahn CR, Weir GC, editors. Joslin's diabetes mellitus. 13th edition. Philadelphia: Lea & Febiger; 1994. p. 738–70.
97. Kitabchi AE, Murphy MB. Hyperglycemic crises in adult patients with diabetes mellitus. In: Wass JA, Shalet SM, Amiel SA, editors. Oxford textbook of endocrinology. New York: Oxford University Press; 2002. p. 1734–47.
98. Laffel L. Ketone bodies: a review of physiology, pathophysiology and application of monitoring to diabetes. Diabetes Metab Res Rev 1999;15(6):412–26.
99. Meas T, Taboulet P, Sobngwi E, et al. Is capillary ketone determination useful in clinical practice? In which circumstances? Diabetes Metab 2005;31(3 Pt 1):299–303.
100. Rosenbloom AL, Malone JI. Recognition of impending ketoacidosis delayed by ketone reagent strip failure. JAMA 1978;240(22):2462–4.
101. Davidson M. Diabetic ketoacidosis and hyperosmolar nonketotic syndrome. In: Davidson M, editor. Diabetes mellitus: diagnosis and treatment. 4th edition. Philadelphia: W.B Saunders Co; 1998. p. 159–94.
102. Kitabchi AE, Young R, Sacks H, et al. Diabetic ketoacidosis: reappraisal of therapeutic approach. Annu Rev Med 1979;30:339–57.
103. Arora S, Henderson SO, Long T, et al. Diagnostic accuracy of point-of-care testing for diabetic ketoacidosis at emergency-department triage: {beta}-hydroxybutyrate versus the urine dipstick. Diabetes Care 2011;34(4):852–4.
104. Naunheim R, Jang TJ, Banet G, et al. Point-of-care test identifies diabetic ketoacidosis at triage. Acad Emerg Med 2006;13(6):683–5.
105. Csako G. False-positive results for ketone with the drug mesna and other free-sulfhydryl compounds. Clin Chem 1987;33:289–92.

106. Csako G. Causes, consequences, and recognition of false-positive reactions for ketones. Clin Chem 1990;36:1388–9.
107. Viar M, Wright R. Spurious ketonemia after mesna therapy. Clin Chem 1987;33: 913.
108. Csako G, Elin RJ. Spurious ketonuria due to captopril and other free sulfhydryl drugs. Diabetes Care 1996;19:673–4.
109. Csako G, Benson CC, Elin RJ. False-positive ketone reactions in CAP surveys. Clin Chem 1993;39:915–7.
110. Adrogué HJ, Wilson H, Boyd AE 3rd. Plasma acid-base patterns in diabetic ketoacidosis. N Engl J Med 1982;307(26):1603–10.
111. Kelly AM, McAlpine R, Kyle E. Venous pH can safely replace arterial pH in the initial evaluation of patients in the emergency department. Emerg Med J 2001; 18(5):340–2.
112. Kitabchi AE, Wall BM. Diabetic ketoacidosis. Med Clin North Am 1995;79(1): 9–37.
113. Nyenwe EA, Razavi LN, Kitabchi AE, et al. Acidosis: the prime determinant of depressed sensorium in diabetic ketoacidosis. Diabetes Care 2010;33(8):1837.
114. Rasouli M, Kalantari KR. Comparison of methods for calculating serum osmolality: multivariate linear regression analysis. Clin Chem Lab Med 2005;43(6): 635.
115. Worthley LI, Guerin M, Pain RW. For calculating osmolality, the simplest formula is the best. Anaesth Intensive Care 1987;15(2):199.
116. Lynd LD, Richardson KJ, Purssell RA, et al. An evaluation of the osmole gap as a screening test for toxic alcohol poisoning. BMC Emerg Med 2008;8:5.
117. Schelling JR, Howard RL, Winter SD, et al. Increased osmolal gap in alcoholic ketoacidosis and lactic acidosis. Ann Intern Med 1990;113(8):580.
118. Glasser L, Sternglanz PD, Combie J, et al. Serum osmolality and its applicability to drug overdose. Am J Clin Pathol 1973;60(5):695.
119. Gennari FJ. Current concepts. Serum osmolality. Uses and limitations. N Engl J Med 1984;310(2):102.
120. Robinson AG, Loeb JN. Ethanol ingestion–commonest cause of elevated plasma osmolality? N Engl J Med 1971;284(22):1253.
121. Razavi L, Taheri E, Larijani B, et al. Catecholamine-induced leukocytosis in acute hypoglycemic stress. J Investig Med 2007;55:S262.
122. Karavanaki K, Kakleas K, Georga S, et al. Plasma high sensitivity C-reactive protein and its relationship with cytokine levels in children with newly diagnosed type 1 diabetes and ketoacidosis. Clin Biochem 2012;45(16–17):1383–8.
123. Stentz FB, Umpierrez GE, Cuervo R. Proinflammatory cytokines, markers of cardiovascular risks, oxidative stress, and lipid peroxidation in patients with hyperglycemic crises. Diabetes 2004;53(8):2079.
124. Ekpebegh C, Longo-Mbenza B. Determinants of altered sensorium at presentation with diabetic ketoacidosis. Minerva Endocrinol 2011;36(4):267–72.
125. Yadav D, Nair S, Norkus EP, et al. Nonspecific hyperamylasemia and hyperlipasemia in diabetic ketoacidosis: incidence and correlation with biochemical abnormalities. Am J Gastroenterol 2000;95(11):3123.
126. Orlowski JP, Cramer CL, Fiallos MR. Diabetic ketoacidosis in the pediatric ICU. Pediatr Clin North Am 2008;55(3):577–87.
127. Wolfsdorf J, Glaser N, Sperling MA. Diabetic ketoacidosis in infants, children, and adolescents. A consensus statement from the American Diabetes Association. Diabetes Care 2006;29:1150–9.

128. Glaser NS, Wootton-Gorges SL, Marcin JP, et al. Mechanism of cerebral edema in children with diabetic ketoacidosis. J Pediatr 2004;145:164–71.
129. Kitabchi AE, Nyenwe EA. Hyperglycemic crises in diabetes mellitus: diabetic ketoacidosis and hyperglycemic hyperosmolar state. Endocrinol Metab Clin North Am 2006;35(4):725–51, viii.
130. Goyal N, Miller JB, Sankey SS, et al. Utility of initial bolus insulin in the treatment of diabetic ketoacidosis. J Emerg Med 2010;38(4):422–7.
131. Kaiserman K, Rodriguez H, Stephenson A. Continuous subcutaneous infusion of insulin lispro in children and adolescents with type 1 diabetes mellitus. Endocr Pract 2012;18(3):418–24.
132. Tridgell DM, Tridgell AH, Hirsch IB. Inpatient management of adults and children with type 1 diabetes. Endocrinol Metab Clin North Am 2010;39(3):595–608.
133. White NH. Diabetic ketoacidosis in children. Endocrinol Metab Clin North Am 2000;29(4):657–82.
134. Bureau MA, Begin R, Berthiaume Y, et al. Cerebral hypoxia from bicarbonate infusion in diabetic acidosis. J Pediatr 1980;96:968–73.
135. Fisher JN, Kitabchi AE. A randomized study of phosphate therapy in the treatment of diabetic ketoacidosis. J Clin Endocrinol Metab 1983;57:177–80.
136. Amanzadeh J, Reilly RF Jr. Hypophosphatemia: an evidence-based approach to its clinical consequences and management. Nat Clin Pract Nephrol 2006; 2(3):136–48.
137. Shiber JR, Mattu A. Serum phosphate abnormalities in the emergency department. J Emerg Med 2002;23(4):395–400.

Advanced Glycation Endproducts in Diabetes and Diabetic Complications

Helen Vlassara, MD[a],*, Gary E. Striker, MD[b]

KEYWORDS

- Advanced glycation endproduct • Diabetes • Metabolism • Insulin resistance

KEY POINTS

- Advanced glycation endproducts (AGEs) are prooxidants that increase intracellular oxidative stress.
- Prolonged exposure to high AGE levels is a major factor underlying chronically increased oxidative stress in people with and without diabetes mellitus.
- AGEs bind to multiple receptors, which are either part of the antioxidant defenses or the prooxidant/inflammatory processes. AGER1 is an important member of the antioxidant defense system, because it removes AGEs from the extracellular spaces and detoxifies them in lysosomes. There are many prooxidant AGE receptors, RAGE being the best studied. These receptors mediate intracellular oxidative stress and inflammation.
- Chronic exposure to high levels of AGEs, either from food or intracellular sources, results in downregulation of antioxidant defenses. This is true of those at the cell surface (AGER1) and those within the cell (Nrf2, SIRT1, glyoxalase 1, glutathione, and many others).
- Because the kidneys are an important site for removal of AGEs from the circulation, reduced renal function is a major contributor to increased oxidative stress in the body. As a result, reduced renal function is the most important cause of mortality across the age spectrum.
- Reduced levels of critical antioxidant defenses can be reversed by restricting the amount of AGEs in the diet. There are also drugs that either prevent AGE entry into the body, AGE formation, or break AGE-induced cross-links.

[a] Departments of Geriatrics and Medicine, Division of Experimental Diabetes and Aging, Icahn School of Medicine at Mount Sinai, 1 Gustave Levy Place, Annenberg Building, Box 1640, New York, NY 10029, USA; [b] Departments of Geriatrics and Medicine, Division of Nephrology, Experimental Diabetes and Aging, Icahn School of Medicine at Mount Sinai, 1 Gustave Levy Place, Annenberg Building, Box 1640, New York, NY 10029, USA
* Corresponding author.
E-mail address: helen.vlassara@mssm.edu

Endocrinol Metab Clin N Am 42 (2013) 697–719
http://dx.doi.org/10.1016/j.ecl.2013.07.005
0889-8529/13/$ – see front matter © 2013 Elsevier Inc. All rights reserved.
endo.theclinics.com

INTRODUCTION
Relationship Between AGEs and Diabetes

It was initially believed that advanced glycation end products (AGEs) arose primarily from endogenous sources, and that excess amounts were only present in patients with diabetes mellitus or in aging.[1,2] It is now clear that the diet is a principal source of AGEs in normal individuals,[3] as well as those with diabetes mellitus.[4–6] AGEs are present in the body as a part of normal metabolism, but their levels are tightly controlled. It is only when their levels become high and remains chronically increased, as in diabetes and aging, that they are associated with organ damage.

It has long been recognized that patients with diabetes (both type 1 [T1D] and type 2 [T2D]) have high circulating and tissue levels of AGEs.[7,8] Furthermore, the levels of AGEs have been shown to be associated with the development of complications and mortality in experimental models[9] and possibly in humans. A large study of patients in Canada and the United Kingdom showed that the number of individuals with diabetes increased by approximately 50% from 1996 to 2003.[10] When the investigators compared mortality in a population with and without diabetes, they found an excess risk of mortality primarily in those with diabetes. However, the excess risk decreased over a period of 13 years. This was interpreted to be partly due to earlier detection of diabetes, which contributed to a higher prevalence of prediabetes, and to improvements in the management of diabetes. An increased prevalence of diabetes has also been found in the United States and other parts of the world,[11] and it parallels the increase in obesity (**Fig. 1**). With respect to AGEs, the increase in obesity is associated with the change in food habits in the developed world. Namely, there has been increased consumption of foods that are high in AGES, such as red meat, fast food, and heat-processed foods.[12] AGEs may be a significant factor underlying the risk of developing both T1D and T2D and their complications.[12] One particularly disturbing fact is that T2D is becoming more frequent in the young, in whom it has been found to be much more aggressive, and is characterized by an early and more rapid loss of β cell function.[11] AGEs have been shown to directly injure β cells,[13] which potentially gives them a role in the induction of both T1D and T2D. Because AGEs can be controlled by dietary modifications or drugs, AGE control has now become a high priority across the age spectrum.

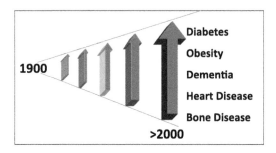

...CURRENT EPIDEMICS ARE FOOD RELATED

Fig. 1. Epidemiologic evidence clearly documents a marked increase in the prevalence of chronic diseases, which can no longer be explained by genetic causes, aging, or nutritional overload. Socioeconomic shifts in the last century have generated new environmental risk factors, a major one being food-derived AGEs or glycotoxins.

The appearance of insulin-dependent T1D (and latent T1D) in aging, although not as frequent as T2D, is now a recognized entity,[14] and may be related to loss of β cell function. Although the mechanisms are complex, the fact that AGEs are directly toxic to β cells and there is a documented increase of AGEs with aging suggest that AGEs may be an underlying contributing factor.

For instance, insulin resistance in patients with T2D can be reduced by the restriction of AGE intake.[15] Excess AGEs in ingested food may play a role in changes in the gut microbiome, which may influence the development of β cell injury. Namely, AGE restriction reduces the incidence of T1D in NOD mice.[16–18] Although the gut microbiome was not investigated in these studies, the importance of both the microbiome and gender were recently explored.[17]

This review presents insights from studies of AGEs in humans and mice. Although the emphasis is on the effects of exogenous AGEs and the suppression of specific host defense mechanisms, AGEs are also formed intracellularly, where they are critical for several normal intracellular functions. It is only when the overall levels of AGEs in the extracellular and the intracellular spaces exceeds the ability of the native antioxidant (and AGE) defenses that they pose a problem. This is most evident in chronic disease conditions in which there are sustained high levels of oxidative stress.

Insights from studies of humans and mice are discussed with emphasis on the effects of chronic high levels of exogenous AGEs and that the chronicity of exposure is the major factor underlying the suppression of specific host defense mechanisms and factors. Loss in defenses is likely a driving force behind the increased oxidative stress and the pathogenesis of both T1D and T2D and their complications.[3] New links have been found between cellular AGE receptors (AGER1) and the NAD^+-dependent deacetylase sirtuin 1 (SIRT1), 2 components of a complex and powerful homeostasis system that has cell-protective effects. Thus, a potential cause of the epidemic nature of diabetes and obesity may be the imbalance between depleted host defenses and overt exposure to oxidants (AGEs) from the environment, mainly the diet (**Fig. 2**).[12] The results include β cell injury that predisposes to the clinical syndrome of diabetes mellitus. Therefore, restricting or blocking the effects of sustained exposure to AGEs in the diet could be a novel and cost-efficient strategy in the prevention and treatment of diabetes.

Over the past decade, it has become apparent that the interactions between AGEs, advanced lipoxidation end products (ALEs), and oxidized lipids are far more prevalent in vivo than previously estimated. Substantial amounts of oxidized lipids are generated by AGE precursors.[19] Oxidized lipids were studied in patients with T2D, in whom consumption of a test meal with either a low or high oxidized fatty acid content showed that the levels of conjugated dienes in serum chylomicrons were increased in those with poor glycemic control and remained increased for longer periods of time, compared with those with better glycemic control (HbA1c<10). The levels in patients with T2D with good control did not differ from nondiabetic controls. Although unsaturated fatty acids from exogenous sources can act as major donors of reactive carbonyls and are more efficient catalysts of AGE or ALE production than glucose, this fact seems to have escaped serious attention. However, Staprans and colleagues[20] showed that oxidized cholesterol in the diet can accelerate atherosclerosis by increasing oxidized cholesterol content in circulating low-density lipoprotein (LDL) and chylomicron remnants. Oxidized fatty acids were not found to play a role in the formation of oxidized cholesterol fractions in this study. However, because ALEs can also interact with AGE receptors, these compounds could underlie processes currently attributed to free fatty acids, such as β cell injury, insulin resistance, and atherosclerosis.[21] Also although fatty acids,

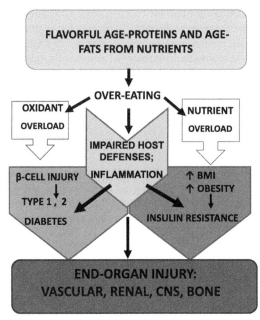

Fig. 2. A paradigm shift: the modern (Western-style) diet promotes overeating and a high content of AGEs, many of which are flavor-enhancing compounds. Chronic consumption of AGE-enriched foods can cause oxidant overload, β-cell injury, suppression of host defense systems, and increased inflammation. AGE-enriched heat-processed food products are highly palatable and can cause overnutrition, high body mass index (BMI), obesity, insulin resistance, and T2D. These effects simultaneously incite insulin resistance, diabetes and its complications. CNS, central nervous system.

like AGEs, are believed to play a major part in atherosclerosis,[22,23] the fact that fatty acids have a low affinity for certain receptors (including toll-like receptor 4 [TLR4]) suggests that free fatty acids at circulating levels may play a lesser role, whereas TLR4 could directly interact with AGEs.[21,24] Intracellular AGE formation is usually tightly controlled, partly by the balance between nascent oxidants and antioxidants, and by the glyoxalase system and other enzymes that reduce oxidative stress and inhibit AGE formation.[25] Extracellular AGE-modified proteins, including those liberated from tissues, are sequestered by AGE receptors,[26] internalized, and degraded by proteolytic digestion. The resulting products are normally excreted by the kidneys.[27,28] Therefore, AGE levels are increased in tissues and cells when renal function is decreased. Another reason for delayed AGE detoxification is that proteins and lipids modified by AGEs are resistant to degradation, which delays their turnover and interferes with tissue repair.

This review focuses on methylglyoxal (MG), a reactive AGE, and two new aspects of the cellular anti–oxidative stress host (innate) defense system, AGER1 and the NAD^+-dependent SIRT1. These two components are part of a complex and powerful cellular antioxidant defense system that controls cellular oxidative stress at physiologic levels. The major prooxidant AGE receptor (RAGE) mediates increased cellular inflammation and oxidative stress, and a secreted form circulates and is able to bind circulating AGEs.[29] As host defenses are breached by a chronic excess of oxidants from the environment and AGEs are allowed to accumulate in tissues and cells, the result is a sustained increase of oxidative stress, leading to cell injury. This sustained change in homeostasis could underlie the increased susceptibility to diabetes mellitus and its complications.

Thus, AGEs may play a central role in the induction of diabetes and its complications, and their control may need to be reassessed in the management of both T1D and T2D.

BRIEF DEFINITION OF BIOREACTIVE AGEs
General Comments

AGEs are prooxidant metabolic derivatives of nonenzymatic reactions between reducing sugars and free amines of proteins, largely α-NH2 or ε-NH2 groups, as well as of aminolipids and nucleic acids.[30–32] Extracellular and intracellular reactive carbonyl precursors (i.e. glyoxal, 3-deoxyglucosone or MG) generate AGEs or glycoxidants (including Nε-carboxymethyl-lysine [CML], MG-imidazolone-H1 (MG-H1 or crosslink-forming end products such as pentosidine.[33,34] The chemical process of glycation, initially identified by Maillard in 1912, is sensitive to pH, high temperature, hydration, type of sugar, and acid or base buffering conditions.[35] Although this reaction is slow and strictly regulated in vivo, under supraphysiologic conditions, AGE formation may occur at greatly accelerated rates. The amount of AGEs formed depends on the substrate source (animal or plant), temperature applied, and the time of exposure to the increased temperature.[36]

AGEs are formed by the nonenzymatic interaction of hydroxyl groups (typically from sugars) and amino groups, preferably lysine or arginine. Many intermediates are unstable and spontaneously degrade or undergo redox cyclization reactions, releasing reactive oxygen species (ROS) that can modify proteins, lipids, or nucleic acids either in the intracellular or extracellular spaces, as well as in mixtures of nutrients, at high temperature. This review focuses on one of the active AGE precursors (MG), which readily modifies proteins containing arginine residues to form the derivative MG-imidazolone-H1 (MG-H1). The modification of proteins by MG is particularly important because it is directed to arginine residues, which have a high probability of location at functional sites.[37] Unlike some of the early AGE precursors, MG derivatives are relatively stable. For these reasons, MG-H1 may be quantitatively one of the more important derivatives in the pathogenesis of diseases, especially diabetes and diabetes-associated complications.

AGE Targets

Rather than consider each individual organ/cell type targeted by AGEs, some representative examples are provided and the reader is directed to the literature. The examples serve mainly to familiarize the reader with the broad clinical significance of AGEs and the importance of keeping their levels as low as possible.

METABOLISM OF INTRACELLULAR MG
General Comments

There are 2 glyoxalase enzymes, glyoxalase-1 (Glo-1) and glyoxalase 2. Because MG is the major substrate for Glo-1, if Glo-1 levels are reduced, the intracellular levels of MG increase to cytotoxic levels. Thus, Glo-1 is an important part of the intracellular antioxidant system, especially glutathione, and the control of MG-derived AGEs.[4] Glo-1 has an antioxidant response element in its promoter region, which binds Nrf2.[38] Therefore, when Nrf2 is acutely upregulated by increased oxidative stress caused by MG, it could bind to the Glo-1 promoter and induce the translation of Glo-1. The result would be reduced intracellular levels of MG. Although this feedback mechanism may control acute changes in MG levels, we have found that Nrf2 levels are decreased in chronic high oxidative stress conditions, such as diabetes with diabetic kidney disease (Gary E. Striker, MD, personal communication, 2013). The net result of this downregulation of an important regulator of intracellular levels of MG could be to promote cell injury and eventually cell death.

CELL SURFACE AGE RECEPTORS
General Comments

There are 2 general types of AGE receptors. One class serves to bind, internalize, and degrade AGEs (**Fig. 3**). AGER1 is the best example in this class.[26] This receptor also serves to control excessive oxidative stress. Therefore, it is a major part of the cellular antioxidant defense system. On the other hand, a second group of receptors also binds AGEs, but instead of detoxifying AGEs, they increase oxidative stress and inflammation.[29] Thus, as a group they are classified as prooxidant receptors. RAGE is the best example of this class. A complete description of these receptors is beyond the scope of this review; elucidation of AGE interactions with AGE receptors has

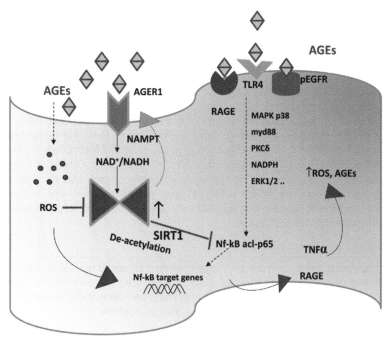

Fig. 3. Host defense cells such as monocytes and macrophages normally endocytose and remove AGEs via AGER1. By blocking the accumulation of AGEs, AGER1 controls many of their proinflammatory effects. This may constitute the basis of the protective synergism between AGER1 and SIRT1, a key deacetylase that controls inflammation and positively regulates metabolic functions in insulin-sensitive tissues. However, a chronic excess of environmental AGEs can suppress AGER1 and NAD$^+$-dependent SIRT1. Chronic suppression of AGER1 can raise intracellular AGEs and reactive oxygen species (ROS) and, thus, suppress SIRT1 levels, leading to abnormal NFkB-enhanced transcription of inflammatory genes, including tumor necrosis factor α (TNFα). However, human and animals studies show that AGER1 and SIRT1 function can be restored to normal levels by AGE restriction. NAMPT, nicotinamide phosphoribosyltransferase; pEGFR, phosphorylated epidermal growth factor receptor.

proved to be complicated. This is because the receptors, other than AGER1, have a relatively low binding affinity for AGEs, bind molecules other than AGEs, and their primary structure is varied. The fact that AGEs, like other oxidant species, can signal through non-AGE receptors, such as scavenger receptors, G-protein–coupled receptors, pattern recognition receptors, and toll-like receptors, as well as via receptor-independent pathways, is underappreciated and has led to considerable confusion in the field. For these reasons, we focus on AGER1 and RAGE.

Receptors that bind AGEs are differentially regulated by ambient levels of both AGEs and oxidative stress. For instance, AGER1 is upregulated by acute increases in AGEs, but is depleted, suppressed, or unresponsive in the presence of chronically high levels of oxidative stress (as in diabetes or diabetic kidney disease). Intracellular antioxidant systems and some of the extracellular host defenses, such as lysozyme and defensins, are also depleted under high oxidative stress. On the other hand, RAGE is induced and remains upregulated in these high oxidative stress states.

AGER1: Defense Against AGE Toxicity

AGE-specific receptors were first recognized on peripheral monocytes.[39-41] AGER1, which is encoded by the gene DDOST, is an evolutionarily conserved type 1 transmembrane protein present on the cell surface, the inner membrane of the endoplasmic membranes, and in mitochondria.[12] AGER1 expression increases after acute exposure to increased levels of AGEs, like many other receptors. However, it becomes downregulated when exposed to persistently increased levels of AGEs, largely arising from ingestion of food containing large amounts of AGEs and/or the presence of diabetes. Thus, under normal conditions, AGER1 levels inversely correlate with intracellular AGEs, and directly with serum AGEs. Because the kidneys are the major site of AGE disposal and AGEs remove AGEs from the blood, AGER1 levels correlate directly with the amount of AGEs present in the urine. This removal of AGEs promotes cell stability and protects against overt oxidative stress. For instance, AGER1 inhibits the activation of NADPH oxidases p47phox (also known as neutrophil cytosol factor 1) and gp91 by suppressing Tyr311 and Tyr332 phosphorylation of protein kinase C δ.[42] These actions prevent NFκB p65 activation and nuclear translocation, processes that are promoted by AGE binding to RAGE. AGER1 also prevents AGE-initiated transactivation of epidermal growth factor receptor (EGFR) caused by high oxidative stress.[43] Thus, AGER1 may also restrict hyperactivity of other G-protein–coupled receptor kinases. Because increased levels of p66Shc are linked to diabetes mellitus, atherosclerosis, and kidney disease, it should be noted that AGER1 inhibits AGE-induced Ser36 phosphorylation of the p66Shc isoform of SHC-transforming protein 1, a major oxidative stress and apoptosis-promoting adaptor protein. AGER1 also inhibits AGE-mediated suppression of the antioxidant effect of FOXO3 on superoxide dismutase 2 (SOD2) expression, perhaps because of its role in the negative regulation of p66Shc activity. These in vitro data were confirmed in mice transgenic for AGER1.[44] These mice had decreased formation of occlusive atheromas following a wire injury, and either a high-fat diet or T2DM. If these findings in mice apply to humans, the significance of reduced levels of AGER1 in diabetes mellitus may explain the increased incidence of atherosclerosis in these patients.

A potentially important protective synergism between AGER1 and SIRT1 has been identified.[15,45] SIRT1 is believed to play a major part in insulin signaling and secretion, insulin resistance, inflammation, lifespan, as well as tissue fibrosis, affecting the cardiovascular system and kidneys in diabetes. Unfortunately, both SIRT1 and AGER1 are suppressed in patients with diabetes mellitus, especially those with complications, that is, conditions characterized by high levels of AGEs and oxidative stress.[12,15] We recently found that AGER1 overexpression blocks AGE-induced suppression of SIRT1, thereby inhibiting NFκB p65 hyperacetylation and inflammatory events. AGER1 also prevents AGE-induced impaired signaling via the insulin receptor and insulin receptor substrate 1 (IRS1) in adipocytes, and results in prevention of an AGE-induced decrease in glucose uptake. These data indicate that AGER1 provides SIRT1 with a shield against a high external oxidant load. This may mitigate inflammation while preserving the metabolic actions of insulin. This conclusion is reinforced by the observation that AGER1 protein levels in peripheral blood mononuclear cells of healthy humans correlate with circulating AGE levels.[3,12]

Thus, because the level of AGER1 expression normally correlates directly with those of intracellular antioxidant systems (SIRT1, nicotinamide phosphoribosyltransferase [NAMPT], SOD2, and glutathione); and negatively with prooxidant pathways (RAGE, NADPH oxidase, and p66shc), AGER1 may be important in the maintenance of normal homeostasis. An obvious corollary is that reduced AGER1 expression levels may presage compromised host defenses.

RAGE: Propagation of AGE Toxicity

In contrast to AGER1, RAGE activation promotes both ROS and inflammation in acute and chronic diseases. Whereas AGER1 is relatively specific for AGEs, RAGE binds multiple ligands, including high-mobility group protein B1, amyloid β protein, and members of the calcium-binding S100 protein group. RAGE is a prominent member of a family of low-affinity pattern recognition receptors that function at the interface of innate and adaptive immunity.[29] Although the binding characteristics for AGEs by AGER1 are well understood, those for multiligand RAGE are not as clear, and have even been debated. Activation of full-length cell-associated RAGE induces an array of signaling events, including MAPK p38-JNK and JAK-STAT, CDC42-RAC and others, many of which may act as both the result and the cause of ROS. Whereas full-length RAGE does not contribute to the endocytosis or removal of AGEs, the extracellular domains of RAGE may be shed as soluble variants possibly contributing to AGE clearance.[46] Even though an association between RAGE and diabetic complications has been reported, it has been difficult to assign a primary role to this receptor other than that as an ROS transducer of ROS. RAGE may be principally modulated by ambient oxidative stress. The best evidence for this supposition is that low oxidative stress, by restricting the availability of external AGEs, markedly suppresses RAGE mRNA and protein levels in diabetic mice.[9,47,48] Similarly, AGE restriction in either healthy humans or those with diabetes mellitus to levels markedly less than their baseline (>60%) reduces RAGE levels in peripheral blood mononuclear cells, indicating that RAGE is regulated by AGEs entering from the external environment. RAGE mRNA and protein levels in peripheral blood mononuclear cells from healthy individuals directly correlate with serum levels of AGEs and oxidative stress, as well as with ingested AGE levels.[3] RAGE levels are only modestly increased in patients with diabetes mellitus without complications. One can conclude that both AGER1 and RAGE respond to the presence of AGEs in the environment, but in discordant directions. These findings in both animals and humans offer new perspectives on the role of RAGE in diabetes mellitus. As with other signal transduction molecules that regulate proinflammatory events, upregulation of RAGE may be a result, rather than a cause of, increased oxidative stress. When host defenses are compromised and basal oxidative stress increases, RAGE may be upregulated and amplify oxidative stress. Other prooxidant scavenger receptors that bind AGEs, such as galectin-3, also seem to function in this manner.[49]

EXAMPLES OF CONDITIONS IN WHICH AGES MAY PLAY A PATHOGENIC ROLE
AGEs and the Induction of T1D in Children

An increasing incidence of T1D in children has been noted throughout the world prompting calls for new prognostic indicators.[50] In a large study, islet cell antibody (ICA)–positive children were evaluated for predictors of T1D.[51] An assay for an AGE (CML) was included, based on evidence implicating the environment in the development of T1D in twins. The investigators studied 7287 unselected school children, of whom 115 were ICA positive, and 32 monozygotic and 32 dizygotic twins discordant for diabetes, and followed them for 7 years. The findings showed that CML was increased in ICA+ and prediabetic children as well as in diabetic and nondiabetic twins and that an increased level of CML was a persistent and independent predictor of diabetes progression, in addition to ICA and HLA risk. The familial environment explained 75% of the CML variance, confirming previous data. The investigators concluded that CML is a potential therapeutic target in ICA-positive children.

AGEs and the Induction of T1D in Adults

Recently, it has been recognized that autoimmune diabetes also occurs in adults.[14] A study of 6156 adults attending adult diabetes clinics in Europe revealed that 541 had autoantibodies, of which most recognized glutamic acid decarboxylase antibodies (GADA; ~90%). Of the total population, ~10% did not require insulin (latent autoimmune diabetes). Most of those with high GADA levels (403/541) were female, lean, and treated with insulin. Overall, latent autoimmune diabetes is much more frequent than adult-onset autoimmune type diabetes. Although AGEs were not examined in these patients, the data from autoimmune diabetes in children[51] would suggest that an increased level of AGEs is a reasonable possibility, and should be examined, because this is a modifiable risk factor.

AGEs and Pancreatic β Cells

The role of β-cell responses to AGEs was examined in mice treated with bovine serum albumin modified by AGEs.[13] The investigators found that treated mice had higher glucose levels and lower insulin levels in response to a glucose challenge than controls, despite normal insulin sensitivity and normal islet morphology. Isolated islets from these mice also had lower glucose-stimulated insulin secretion. In addition, ATP production in isolated islet cells was reduced by AGEs, whereas glucose-stimulated insulin secretion was restored by a sulfonylurea derivative. AGEs also inhibited nitric oxide activity by inducing inducible nitric oxide syntheses (iNOS) activity. Aminoguanidine reversed the inhibitory effects on ATP production and insulin secretion, leading the investigators to conclude that AGEs inhibit cytochrome c oxidase and ATP production, which leads to impaired glucose-stimulated insulin secretion, mediated by iNOS-dependent nitric oxide production.

AGEs as Initiators of Insulin Resistance and T2D

Studies in different models of T2DM (db/db or C57B6 mice fed a high-fat diet as well as C57B6 mice with age-related T2DM), using AGE restriction, are of interest. There was a decrease in oxidative stress and an improvement in insulin resistance, despite hyperglycemia or obesity, high-fat intake, or advanced age. The direct role of food AGEs in insulin resistance was further supported by supplementing a low-AGE diet with or without MG-modified albumin (MG^+ or MG^-). Mice fed an MG^+ diet, as well as mice fed regular mouse chow, but not pair-fed age-matched MG^- mice, had an early onset of age-associated insulin resistance,[52] increased adiposity, and inflammatory changes that could not be attributed to advanced age or overnutrition. Furthermore, MG$^+$ mice, in addition to impaired insulin receptor signaling and low insulin-stimulated glucose uptake, had suppressed tissue expression of key defense factors such as SIRT1, AGER1, and plasma adiponectin.[52] The marked acceleration of T2DM onset in MG$^+$ mice over 5 generations could not be attributed to genetic effects, nor can the doubling of obesity rates in humans in the last generation.

The loss of function in anti-AGE and oxidative stress regulatory genes across generations could reflect epigenetic changes, because of the gradual increase in oxidant levels over several generations. Although further investigation is required, impaired host defenses could gradually result in hyper-responsiveness to inflammatory stimuli and, thus, increased susceptibility to disease.

That AGEs can influence insulin sensitivity was also explored in humans with T2DM and insulin resistance, exposed to AGE restriction for 4 months.[15] Compared with those in the control group, there were substantial reductions in plasma insulin, leptin, and proinflammatory tumor necrosis factor (TNF) and RAGE in patients exposed to AGE restriction, whereas AGER1, SIRT1, and adiponectin were increased. These responses were accentuated by monocytic NFκB p65 hyperacetylation likely caused by suppression of SIRT1. Gene transfer and silencing studies further showed SIRT1 actions to be under the control of AGER1 in monocyte/macrophages, where SIRT1 exerts antiinflammatory functions, or in adipocytes, where it regulates glucose utilization.[53,54]

Further studies exploring this new link between AGEs and diabetes may help to explain how the modern environment depletes host defenses and contributes to the metabolic syndrome and T2D.

Brain

Diabetes is associated with increased risk of clinically verified Alzheimer disease, especially if diagnosed in midlife.[55] This has led to the search for modifiable factors in diabetics and prediabetic individuals. Insulin resistance in an asymptomatic, late middle-aged cohort was found to be associated with progressive atrophy in brain regions associated with Alzheimer disease.[56,57] Because insulin resistance is responsive to reduction of AGEs, this could be an interesting area for further research.[15] After initially proposing that AGEs could be involved in the pathogenesis of Alzheimer disease, it was proposed that MG could be a major contributor to this disease.[55] This postulate was supported by the observation that higher levels of MG in 267 older adults with normal cognitive function at baseline were associated with a faster rate of cognitive decline at serial follow-up.[57] Because MG levels can be modulated by diet and/or drugs, this result could have far-reaching implications. A study of the toxicity of MG for neural cell types revealed that neurons are 6-fold more susceptible to MG injury and Glo-1 had a 9-fold higher expression level in astrocytes compared with neurons.[58] In addition, MG led to glycation of occludin in cerebral microvessels, making them more permeable, thus contributing to the dysfunction of the blood-brain barrier.[59]

Recent unpublished transgenerational studies from our group on mice fed an MG-supplemented diet (MG$^+$) showed that age-related brain dysfunction and SIRT1 deficiency are associated with increased levels of MG in the brain. Cognitive decline was promoted by increased levels of AGEs, in parallel with insulin resistance, via SIRT1 deficiency. AGEs and Aβ, which are known to be toxic to the brain, were increased to levels similar to those found in old mice. However, these changes could not be attributed to aging, because they were absent in pair-fed, genetically identical and age-matched MG$^-$ mice. These findings were consistent with and supported new clinical findings that showed that an abnormally high level of circulating MG was a determinant of cognitive decline in older humans, mentally normal at baseline. Serum levels of MG, a marker associated positively with high dietary AGE intake, and negatively with SIRT1 levels, also predicted impaired insulin sensitivity over time in this population. Thus, these findings point to AGEs as a new environmental risk factor for the combined dementia and metabolic syndrome increasingly recognized in older adults.

Brain dysfunction, as well as insulin resistance, is associated with dietary factors and it has been suggested that the benefits derived from calorie restriction on cognition are related to the increase in SIRT1 expression in the brain. However, modern diets are replete with prooxidant AGEs in addition to calories or specific nutrients. The MG$^+$ diet in our recent studies was shown to reproduce age-related metabolic changes, insulin receptor defects, and inflammation. These changes, however, were absent in MG$^-$ mice, despite identical caloric intake by both groups, providing evidence that age-related changes, which had previously been attributed to calories, could partly be caused by AGEs. We have shown that the SIRT1 pathway is regulated by AGEs and AGE receptor levels. AGE receptors are expressed in brain neurons, microglia, and endothelium, and are differentially regulated by chronically increased levels of AGEs. In recent studies, AGER1, an anti-AGE receptor, was found to be downregulated, but RAGE, a signaling receptor linked to neurotoxicity, was enhanced in brains from MG$^+$-fed mice. Furthermore, AGER1 depletion could lead to a delay in the clearance of AGE-modified proteins, such as AGE-Aβ, accounting for the higher AGE deposits, SIRT1 suppression, and glial activation found in the brains of MG$^+$ but not MG$^-$ mice. The chronic and sustained nature of these effects was reflected in behavioral changes in MG$^+$ mice, which mirrored the early cognitive changes seen in older humans. These changes were absent in mice on the low-AGE diet (MG$^-$ mice) and are not related to calories. A critical and novel finding afforded by the animal studies is that a reduced exposure to oral AGEs preserved key brain gene function, and thus averted cognitive decline, as well as metabolic changes. These data must be further examined in larger clinical trials. However, together with the animal data, the clinical evidence indicates that chronic exposure to exogenous AGEs can result in a gradual depletion of host defenses before evidence of cognitive or metabolic disturbances. It is possible that serum MG levels may be used as an early predictor of these conditions.

AGEs are also involved in abnormalities of peripheral nerves in diabetes; macrophages were found to ingest glycated myelin from the peripheral nerves of diabetic animals,[60] which may contribute to the peripheral neuropathy in diabetes. This area deserves further investigation.

As discussed later, estrogen has been shown to have protective effects against the development of Alzheimer disease in both men and women.[61] Studies in mice reveal that estradiol protects against postischemic hippocampal neurodegeneration.[2] Because estrogen is derived from testosterone by the action of aromatase, several investigators have examined the levels and expression of aromatase in brain and brain injury.[61,62] Although aromatase is not expressed in neurons, it is expressed in astrocytes in the presence of oxidative stress, and this is associated with neuroprotection in animals.[62] Studies of the hippocampus of both men and women have documented estradiol-mediated neuroprotection,[63] and a recent study of single nucleotide polymorphism in the gene coding for aromatase shows that the genotype associated with the greatest levels of estradiol was associated with greater hippocampal gray matter in men.[61] Thus, estrogen may have a neuroprotective effects in both men and women, and could be important in the development of Alzheimer disease. This is a critical point, because estrogen receptor levels are decreased in the presence of chronic oxidative stress, such as in diabetes.[64]

In summary, AGE-induced reductions in estrogen receptor function and estradiol production may be associated with cognitive and peripheral nerve dysfunction. In this context, both MG and Glo-1 have both been shown to play significant roles in the function of brain cell types and the blood-brain barrier.

Kidney

AGE metabolism

The kidneys are a major site for the disposal of oxidants from the circulation, especially AGEs. The kidneys receive a disproportionate amount of the cardiac output on a size/weight basis. In addition, other than the brain and heart, they are the only organs in which blood flow is determined by cardiac output, rather than vascular contraction. After passing the glomerulus, this large amount of blood enters a rich capillary bed around the tubules. Thus, the tubules are directly exposed to AGEs in the blood, and can remove AGEs from the capillaries and place them into the tubular lumen for disposal. Because of their large exposure to circulating AGEs and their role in the removal of AGEs, the kidneys are a target for AGE-induced oxidative stress. The exact mechanism for the disposal of AGEs in the kidneys remains incompletely understood, but because reactive AGEs (such as MG) are highly charged, they are unlikely to be filtered in large amounts at the glomerular barrier. Thus, if AGEs are to be removed by the kidneys, they must be actively excreted. This conclusion is supported by the observation that when the levels of AGEs in the circulation are reduced by either dietary restriction or drugs, the kidneys excrete an increased amount of AGEs.[6,15] This suggests that the kidneys are injured by high circulating levels of oxidants, such as those present in T2D. On the other hand, relatively inactive AGEs (such as CML-modified peptides) are not highly charged and may pass more easily through the glomerular filter and would be less dependent on intact tubular function.

AGE renal toxicity (animal studies)

Direct evidence of the toxicity of AGEs for normal kidney structure and function was obtained in normal mice who received AGEs intravenously for 4 weeks.[65] These animals developed deposits of AGEs in the kidneys and both glomerular and interstitial fibrosis, suggesting that circulating AGEs can be deposited in the kidneys and cause kidney disease. Specifically, it was found that AGEs induced an increase in glomerular extracellular matrix alpha 1(IV) collagen, laminin B1, and transforming growth factor (TGF) β1 mRNA levels, as well as glomerular hypertrophy. The AGE response was specific because the coadministration of an AGE inhibitor, aminoguanidine, reduced all these changes. Recently, it was found that TGFβ induced changes in mir-192 and p53 that resulted in a fibrotic response in glomerular mesangial cells.[66]

AGE removal (clinical studies)

The importance of the excretion of circulating AGEs could be inferred from a study of nearly 1500 participants without cardiovascular disease or T2D.[67] The investigators found that increased cystatin C (a marker of decreased kidney function) carried a 3-fold increased risk of progression from normoglycemia to prediabetes. This suggests that abnormalities in kidney function, possibly because of an inability to excrete large amounts of ingested oxidants (AGEs, ALEs), result in the initiation of a series of events that carry a high risk of developing diabetes.

AGEs and the induction diabetic kidney disease

High levels of AGEs and chronic inflammation in T2D have been suggested to predispose to the development of diabetic kidney disease (DKD). AGEs induce inflammation (especially TNFα) in patients and in animal models.[4,15,68] The association between high levels of MG and progression of DKD was confirmed in T1D in a longitudinal study of children with T1D whose follow-up included a kidney biopsy.[69] Another study of long-term survivors of T1D followed at the Joslin Clinic revealed that DKD was present only in those with high levels of AGEs.[70] Another group of investigators at the Joslin Clinic found that increased TNF receptors predicted progressive chronic kidney disease in both T1D and T2D in the United States.[71,72] These data were confirmed in a study of 106 nonobese Japanese individuals with T2D; it was found that circulating TNF receptor 2 was associated with the development of stage 3 chronic kidney disease (glomerular filtration rate $\sim$30). Because AGEs enhance the expression of TNF receptors[73] and AGEs are increased in T2D, these studies suggest that AGEs could be a significant contributor to the progression of DKD in patients with either T1D or T2D.

AGE toxicity in hemodialysis patients

AGE levels are often several-fold higher in hemodialysis patients than in normal controls.[74] These patients have a high incidence of complications, and a high mortality rate, especially those who also have diabetes (US Renal Data System). Reduction of AGEs by a drug that sequesters AGEs in the gut, thereby preventing them from being taken into the body, led to a substantial reduction in both AGEs and other risk factors for cardiovascular disease.[45] These changes were apparent after only 3 weeks of treatment. In a cross-sectional study of 139 patients on hemodialysis and 50 patients on peritoneal dialysis[75]; the investigators found that serum CML level correlated significantly with dietary AGE intake, based on 3-day food records ($P = .003$). Although no correlation was observed with protein, fat, saturated fat, or carbohydrate intake, both serum CML and MG levels correlated with blood urea nitrogen ($P = .03$ and $P = .02$, respectively) and serum albumin levels ($P = .04$ and $P = .02$, respectively). The investigators confirmed that dietary AGE content, independent of other diet constituents, is an important contributor to the high serum AGE levels in patients with renal failure. Moreover, the lack of correlation between serum AGE levels and dietary protein, fat, and carbohydrate intake indicates that a reduction in dietary AGE content can be obtained safely without compromising the content of obligatory nutrients in these very ill patients who are generally malnourished.

Toxicity of AGEs in patients on peritoneal dialysis

The fact that reduction of AGEs by dialysis is independent of dialysis method was shown in an intervention trial conducted on 26 patients with renal failure on maintenance peritoneal dialysis who were randomized to either a high-AGE or a low-AGE diet for 4 weeks. Those on the low dietary AGE intake had decreased serum CML ($P<.002$) and serum MG ($P<.008$) levels and lower levels of 2 glycated lipid molecules that induce inflammatory responses, CML-LDL ($P<.011$) and CML-apoB ($P<.028$). On the other hand, patients on the regular diet were found to have increased levels of serum CML ($P<.028$), serum MG ($P<.09$), CML-LDL ($P<.011$), and CML-apoB ($P<.028$). Other findings related to metabolic changes that are directly correlated with cardiovascular risk were as follows: serum AGE correlated with blood urea nitrogen (CML, $P<.002$, MG, $P<.05$), serum creatinine (CML, $P<.05$; MG, $P<.004$), total serum protein (CML, $P<.05$, MG, $P<.05$ for MG), serum albumin ($P<.02$ for CML; $r = 0.4$; $P<.05$ for MG), and serum phosphorus (CML; $P<.006$; MG, $P<.01$). The investigators concluded that dietary glycotoxins contribute significantly to the increased AGE levels in patients with renal failure, and that dietary AGE restriction is an effective and feasible method to reduce excess toxic AGEs and mortality associated with cardiovascular disease, and to favorably alter several metabolic parameters.

Mortality in patients with T2D admitted to the intensive case unit and the effects of the levels of AGEs and DKD on outcome in acute trauma patients
The presence of T2D has been associated with increased 1-year mortality in patients who had been admitted to an intensive care unit (36%) compared with 29.1% in nondiabetic patients.[76] However, the presence of kidney disease was associated with a 1-year mortality of 54.6%, again emphasizing the importance of kidney function in controlling oxidative stress. Another study of AGEs in patients with acute trauma admitted to the intensive care unit revealed that those with the most severe trauma had increased levels of AGEs that persisted, whereas the levels decreased within 1 week in those with less severe injuries.

In summary, these data show that restricted exposure to AGEs is important for the prevention of DKD and progression of established nephropathy.

AGEs in Cardiovascular Disease

General comments
Although there have been many animal studies showing that chronic high levels of AGEs promote the induction and progression of cardiovascular disease,[12] a recent study of 7447 individuals from the Mediterranean region showed that a low-AGE diet reduced the incidence of major cardiovascular events in persons at high cardiovascular risk.[77] This study was a randomized prospective trial of 3 diets, 2 Mediterranean diets (1 supplemented with virgin olive oil and 1 supplemented with nuts) and a regular diet. This study confirms the results of several previous trials, and suggests that a low-AGE diet is cardioprotective in a European population. Small studies in more diverse populations[3] suggest that these data may apply more broadly. The latter study points out that it is not only the amount and type of food ingested but that the method of food preparation plays a major role.[3] Namely, food that is rich in animal protein and is cooked at high temperature for prolonged periods contains many cytotoxic AGEs.

Studies on rat models of hypertension revealed that MG-mediated changes in arterial wall medial/intimal thickness was associated with hypertension.[11] These changes were attenuated by metformin.

The question of the effects of AGE cross-linking on large blood vessels was studied in rats with streptozotocin-induced diabetes treated with the AGE breaker, alagebrium for 1 to 3 weeks.[65] The diabetes-induced increase in large artery stiffness was reversed as measured by systemic arterial compliance, aortic impedance, and carotid artery compliance and distensibility. These findings could be important in the treatment of patients with diabetes-related complications.

Estrogen in men with diabetes and the risk of peripheral vascular disease
Our recent unpublished data show that monocytes of aged men with T2D have suppressed levels of estrogen receptor α mRNA, which is reversed by removal of AGEs. Thus, AGEs may play a role in the effects of estradiol on peripheral vascular disease. Although there have been few studies of estrogen and the risk of aging-related diseases in men, a recent cross-sectional study of Framingham Heart Study participants revealed that there was a 62% increased risk of incident diabetes per cross-sectional doubling of estradiol levels.[78] This risk was 40% for estrone, which was associated with impaired fasting glucose at visit 7. In follow-up over a period of 6.8 years, there was an increasing risk of diabetes with increasing quartiles of both estradiol and estrone and an increased incidence of diabetes with increasing quartiles of estrone. Thus, at the last visit, in those with a 2-fold increase in total estrone at visit 7, there was a 77% increase in the risk of incident diabetes. An analysis of the same study

subjects showed that the age-related increase in total estrone was greater than that in total estradiol. Estrone was positively associated with smoking, body mass index (BMI, calculated as weight in kilograms divided by the square of height in meters), and testosterone, and total and free estradiol were associated with diabetes, BMI, testosterone, and comorbid conditions; in addition, free estradiol was associated negatively with smoking. An investigation of a middle-aged community-based sample suggests that lower free testosterone and higher estrone concentrations may be associated with peripheral vascular disease and ankle brachial index change in men, but sex hormones did not affect these parameters in women. Peripheral vascular disease may also be related to AGEs and their influence on estrogen levels.

In summary, there is now considerable evidence that the amount of AGEs provided in the food environment can have a profound effect on cardiovascular disease. However, AGEs can be controlled by modifying the diet or by introducing drugs that modify uptake or inhibit AGEs.

Liver

Nonalcoholic fatty liver disease
Visceral fat is a risk factor for both T2D and nonalcoholic fatty liver disease (NAFLD) and the 2 diseases are often seen together.[14] Both diseases may be preceded by the metabolic syndrome, and both have been associated with increased AGE levels (JCEM/Plos1).[3,13] A recent study in animals to address the relationship between high AGE intake and NAFLD[79] showed that chronically increased levels of dietary AGEs were associated with the initiation of inflammation, in the absence of steatosis. The investigators concluded that high levels of dietary AGEs could be a precipitating factor for the initiation and progression of NAFLD.

Estrogen and liver disease
Because estrogen receptor alpha (the major estrogen receptor isoform in the liver) is downregulated in high oxidative stress conditions, such as T2D, and estrogen has been shown to be protective against the induction of inflammation in the liver, an investigation of models of steatosis in mice was conducted.[80] Both estradiol and tamoxiphen (which mimics estradiol effects in the liver) had hepatoprotective effects against steatosis and NAFLD. These data were confirmed in men with obesity and NAFLD.[81] In a study of 251 postmenopausal women, of whom 37% had NAFLD, those on hormone replacement therapy had a low frequency of metabolic syndrome and insulin resistance compared with those who were not on hormone replacement therapy.[82] The investigators suggested that hormone replacement therapy could be a protective factor against liver disease, but cautioned that this remains as an area of investigation.

In summary, these studies in mice and humans suggest that AGEs can be hepatotoxic and that restriction of AGEs can have positive effects on NAFLD.

AGEs at Different Chronologic Ages

Gestation and infants
Because maternal diabetes has been associated with an increased risk of diabetes and obesity in the offspring, and the transmission of AGEs from mother to fetus is unknown, AGEs were examined in the sera of healthy mothers in labor (n = 60), their infants, and in infant foods.[83] Significant correlations were found between newborn and maternal serum CML levels ($P = .001$) serum MG derivatives ($P = .001$), and 8-isoprostanes ($P = .001$). High maternal serum MGs predicted higher infant insulin or homeostasis model assessment ($P = .027$), and CML and adiponectin levels in

infants negatively correlated with maternal serum CML ($P = .011$). The levels of serum AGEs significantly increased with the initiation of processed infant food intake, increasing daily AGE consumption by ~7.5-fold in a year, suggesting that the high content of AGEs in processed food could not be handled by the infants' kidneys. These data are consistent with the observations that processed food commercially available for infants often has a high content of AGEs and suggest that AGE exposure in infants may predispose them to the later development of diabetes.[84]

Adults

Although it has generally been believed that oxidative stress inevitably increases with aging and underlies the increased incidence of cardiovascular or kidney disease in this period, it is now a subject of active debate as to whether unopposed oxidative stress is an obligatory process of normal aging in humans. Furthermore, with the rapid increase in the number of aging persons, it is of concern whether oxidative stress is principally the cause or the result of chronic diseases of late adulthood, and whether it can be modified. It is critical to understand if increased oxidative stress is an inevitable component of normal aging, whether it affects the age of onset of aging-related changes, whether it can be reduced in healthy adults, and whether increased oxidative stress in patients with chronic diseases can be reduced. AGEs play a significant role in the pathogenesis of many chronic diseases in the middle-aged and the aged, including cardiovascular disease, chronic kidney disease, and diabetes. In a recent study, the levels of AGEs and oxidative stress in 345 healthy urban adults aged 18 to 45 years or more than 60 years of age were examined to determine if they were correlated with dietary AGEs, if AGEs and oxidative stress could be modified by restricting the amount of AGEs in the diet, and if the levels of AGEs correlated with changes in AGER1 levels.[3] Both serum CML and MG levels were higher on average in healthy participants older than 60 years than in those aged 18 to 45 years and as a group independently correlated with dietary AGEs ($P = .0001$). Somewhat surprisingly, some of the participants aged 18 to 45 years of age had serum CML values in the range found in participants older than 60 years. These findings clearly established that the intake of dietary AGEs strongly affects the levels of circulating AGEs, oxidative stress, and proinflammatory markers at all ages. In addition, the levels of AGER1 in peripheral blood mononuclear cells positively correlated with serum and urine AGEs and oxidant stress markers in healthy participants. One of the most important findings in this study was that reducing dietary AGE intake significantly decreased oxidative stress in healthy adults. This suggests that increased oxidative stress is not an obligate correlate of aging, that reduction of AGEs in the diet could be a safe and efficient intervention in normal aging, and that it may improve outcomes in age-related diseases.

DRUGS THAT INFLUENCE AGES
General Comments

There are at least 3 classes of drugs that may reduce the amount of AGEs presented to the gastrointestinal tract. One is to bind AGEs in the gut and eliminate them in the stool. Sevelamer carbonate fits into this category.[45] This effectively reduces circulating and cellular AGEs in patients with DKD, increases antioxidant defenses and decreases prooxidant molecules. The second group of oral drugs include those that bind or chelate AGEs in food and after they have been absorbed into the body. They are soluble and pass the intestinal barrier and enter most cells. There are several drugs in this category (listed in the ascending order of efficacy of binding AGEs): metformin, vitamin B analogues such as pyridoxamine and benfotiamine, and aminoguanidine. In addition to these drugs, there is a drug that breaks AGE complexes formed in tissues, making them more available for degradation. A third category is an injectable form of soluble RAGE, which has become available for experimental use. There are animal study reports on this drug, but none in humans.

Oral Drugs Directly Influencing the Degradation of AGEs

Metformin
In a study of 57 individuals with T2D, of whom 30 were treated with metformin, MG levels were increased in all patients with T2D, compared with 28 controls.[10] MG levels correlated with increasing HbA1c levels in the patients who were not treated with metformin and patients on low-dose metformin (<1000 mg/d), but not those on the high dosage (1500–2000 mg/d). The investigators concluded that metformin reduces MG levels in a dose-dependent fashion and that this effect is independent of its effects on glycemic levels.

Aminoguanidine
There is a rich literature showing that aminoguanidine decreases nephropathy, cardiac hypertrophy, and aortic lesions in various animal models. Age-related cardiac hypertrophy has been prevented in both Sprague-Dawley and Fischer 344 rats by aminoguanidine treatment. Although AGE clearance declined in untreated aged rats, this was blunted by aminoguanidine treatment, and loss of renal mass with aging was prevented in Sprague-Dawley rats. Aminoguanidine treatment was also shown to reduce aortic accumulation of injected AGEs, reduce mononuclear cell infiltration, and improve vasodilatory responses to acetylcholine and nitroglycerin. The metabolic turnover of food-derived reactive orally absorbed AGEs or glycotoxins may be delayed in patients with diabetes and kidney disease. Another study[6] asked whether pharmacologic inhibition of dietary AGE bioreactivity by aminoguanidine improved the turnover and renal excretion of radiolabeled AGEs in normal Sprague-Dawley rats. The radiolabeled AGE diet produced serum absorption and urinary excretion peaks kinetically distinct from those of free [^{14}C]glucose or ^{125}I-labelled ovalbumin. Twenty-six percent of the orally absorbed AGE-ovalbumin was excreted in the urine, whereas after aminoguanidine treatment, urinary excretion of dietary AGEs increased markedly (to >50% of that absorbed). More than 60% of tissue-bound radioactivity was found to be covalently deposited in kidneys and liver, whereas after treatment with aminoguanidine, tissue AGE deposits were reduced to less than 15% of the amount found in untreated AGE-fed controls. Thus, reduction of dietary bioreactive AGEs by aminoguanidine improves their renal elimination and prevents tissue deposition of AGEs derived from the food. The investigators concluded that this may protect against excessive tissue AGE toxicity in diabetic patients, especially those with renal disease. A clinical trial was conducted using 2 doses of aminoguanidine in 317 patients with T1D with nephropathy and retinopathy.[85] The primary end point was doubling of serum creatinine, and secondary end points included proteinuria, retinopathy, and kidney function. After a follow-up of 2 to 4 years, the primary end point was not reached. However, in the aminoguanidine group, the estimated glomerular filtration rate decreased more slowly, proteinuria was decreased, and fewer participants reached a 3-step or greater progression of retinopathy.

Pyridoxamine
Hudson and colleagues have shown that pyridoxamine scavenges methylglyoxal, and related pathogenic reactive carbonyl species from interacting with proteins.[86] Because pyridoxamine is an oral drug with a good safety profile, it has been the subject of clinical trials in DKD, none of which reached the study goal of reducing the

doubling of serum creatinine. However, one trial showed that those with the lowest serum creatinine level at study entry seemed to gain more benefit than either the middle or upper third, suggesting there might be some benefit in the early stages of DKD.[87]

Benfotiamine

In a study of 20 inpatients with T2DM in a randomized crossover design,[88] the effects of a low-AGE and high-AGE meal on flow-mediated dilatation (FMD) and laser-Doppler flowmetry, serum E-selectin, intracellular adhesion molecule 1, and vascular cell adhesion molecule 1, oxidative stress, and serum AGE were assessed at baseline and 2, 4, and 6 hours after each meal. Although the meals had identical ingredients, they had different amounts of AGEs (15,100 compared with 2.750 kU AGE in the high-AGE and low-AGE meals, respectively). The differences were obtained by varying the cooking temperature and time. Flow-mediated dilation decreased by 36.2% (P<.01 for all compared with baseline) after the high-AGE meal, After the low-AGE meal, FMD decreased by 20.9% (P<.001 for all compared with the high-AGE meal). After the high-AGE meal, both macrovascular function and microvascular function were impaired (−67.2%), and serum AGE and markers of endothelial dysfunction and oxidative stress were increased. The investigators concluded that a high-AGE meal in patients with T2DM can induce a more pronounced acute impairment of vascular function than a low-AGE meal that is otherwise identical. They suggested that chemical modifications of food during cooking may play a major role in influencing the extent of acute postprandial vascular dysfunction. This study was followed by an analysis of the effect of benfotiamine on the same parameters in this population in 13 patients with T2D given a meal with a high AGE content before and after a 3-day therapy with benfotiamine (1050 mg/d).[89] The same measures as in the first study were repeated. The investigators found that the effects of high AGE on both FMD and reactive hyperemia were completely prevented by benfotiamine. Although serum markers of endothelial dysfunction and oxidative stress, as well as AGE, increased after high AGE, these effects were significantly reduced by benfotiamine treatment.

ALAGEBRIUM

Alagebrium was developed as a compound that had the capability of breaking preformed AGE links with proteins.[90] A large number of animal studies have been published, but there are no clinical trials showing efficacy.

REFERENCES

1. Ward RA, McLeish KR. Methylglyoxal: a stimulus to neutrophil oxygen radical production in chronic renal failure? Nephrol Dial Transplant 2004;19(7):1702–7.
2. Kim KM, Kim YS, Jung DH, et al. Increased glyoxalase I levels inhibit accumulation of oxidative stress and an advanced glycation end product in mouse mesangial cells cultured in high glucose. Exp Cell Res 2012;318(2):152–9.
3. Vlassara H, Cai W, Goodman S, et al. Protection against loss of innate defenses in adulthood by low advanced glycation end products (AGE) intake: role of the anti-inflammatory AGE receptor-1. J Clin Endocrinol Metab 2009;94(11):4483–91.
4. Vlassara H, Cai W, Crandall J, et al. Inflammatory mediators are induced by dietary glycotoxins, a major risk factor for diabetic angiopathy. Proc Natl Acad Sci U S A 2002;99(24):15596–601.
5. Koschinsky T, He CJ, Mitsuhashi T, et al. Orally absorbed reactive glycation products (glycotoxins): an environmental risk factor in diabetic nephropathy. Proc Natl Acad Sci U S A 1997;94(12):6474–9.

6. He C, Sabol J, Mitsuhashi T, et al. Dietary glycotoxins: inhibition of reactive products by aminoguanidine facilitates renal clearance and reduces tissue sequestration. Diabetes 1999;48(6):1308–15.

7. Brownlee M. Biochemistry and molecular cell biology of diabetic complications. Nature 2001;414(6865):813–20.

8. Vlassara H, Brownlee M, Cerami A. Nonenzymatic glycosylation: role in the pathogenesis of diabetic complications. Clin Chem 1986;32(Suppl 10):B37–41.

9. Cai W, He JC, Zhu L, et al. Oral glycotoxins determine the effects of calorie restriction on oxidant stress, age-related diseases, and lifespan. Am J Pathol 2008;173(2):327–36.

10. Lind M, Garcia-Rodriguez LA, Booth GL, et al. Mortality trends in patients with and without diabetes in Ontario, Canada and the UK from 1996 to 2009: a population-based study. Diabetologia 2013. [Epub ahead of print].

11. Linder BL, Fradkin JE, Rodgers GP. The TODAY study: an NIH perspective on its implications for research. Diabetes Care 2013;36(6):1775–6.

12. Vlassara H, Striker GE. AGE restriction in diabetes mellitus: a paradigm shift. Nat Rev Endocrinol 2011;7(9):526–39.

13. Zhao Z, Zhao C, Zhang XH, et al. Advanced glycation end products inhibit glucose-stimulated insulin secretion through nitric oxide-dependent inhibition of cytochrome c oxidase and adenosine triphosphate synthesis. Endocrinology 2009;150(6):2569–76.

14. Hawa MI, Kolb H, Schloot N, et al. Adult-onset autoimmune diabetes in Europe is prevalent with a broad clinical phenotype: Action LADA 7. Diabetes Care 2013;36(4):908–13.

15. Uribarri J, Cai W, Ramdas M, et al. Restriction of advanced glycation end products improves insulin resistance in human type 2 diabetes: potential role of AGER1 and SIRT1. Diabetes Care 2011;34(7):1610–6.

16. Peppa M, Brem H, Cai W, et al. Prevention and reversal of diabetic nephropathy in db/db mice treated with alagebrium (ALT-711). Am J Nephrol 2006;26(5): 430–6.

17. Everard A, Belzer C, Geurts L, et al. Cross-talk between *Akkermansia muciniphila* and intestinal epithelium controls diet-induced obesity. Proc Natl Acad Sci U S A 2013;110(22):9066–71.

18. Karlsson FH, Tremaroli V, Nookaew I, et al. Gut metagenome in European women with normal, impaired and diabetic glucose control. Nature 2013; 498(7452):99–103.

19. Cai W, He JC, Zhu L, et al. High levels of dietary advanced glycation end products transform low-density lipoprotein into a potent redox-sensitive mitogen-activated protein kinase stimulant in diabetic patients. Circulation 2004;110(3): 285–91.

20. Staprans I, Pan XM, Rapp JH, et al. Oxidized cholesterol in the diet is a source of oxidized lipoproteins in human serum. J Lipid Res 2003;44(4):705–15.

21. Vistoli G, Maddis D, De Maddis D, et al. Advanced glycoxidation and lipoxidation end products (AGEs and ALEs): an overview of their mechanisms of formation. Free Radic Res 2013;47(Suppl 1):3–27.

22. Cai W, He C, Zhu L, et al. Dietary-AGE-modified LDL is a potent redox-sensitive MAPk stimulant in diabetic patients. Circulation 2004;110:285–91.

23. Hodgkinson CP, Laxton RC, Patel K, et al. Advanced glycation end-product of low density lipoprotein activates the toll-like 4 receptor pathway implications for diabetic atherosclerosis. Arterioscler Thromb Vasc Biol 2008;28(12): 2275–81.

24. Shi H, Kokoeva MV, Inouye K, et al. TLR4 links innate immunity and fatty acid-induced insulin resistance. J Clin Invest 2006;116(11):3015–25.
25. Thornalley PJ. Glyoxalase I–structure, function and a critical role in the enzymatic defence against glycation. Biochem Soc Trans 2003;31(Pt 6):1343–8.
26. Vlassara H. The AGE-receptor in the pathogenesis of diabetic complications. Diabetes Metab Res Rev 2001;17(6):436–43.
27. Makita Z, Bucala R, Rayfield EJ, et al. Reactive glycosylation endproducts in diabetic uraemia and treatment of renal failure. Lancet 1994;343(8912):1519–22.
28. Makita Z, Radoff S, Rayfield EJ, et al. Advanced glycosylation end products in patients with diabetic nephropathy. N Engl J Med 1991;325(12):836–42.
29. Schmidt AM, Yan SD, Yan SF, et al. The multiligand receptor RAGE as a progression factor amplifying immune and inflammatory responses. J Clin Invest 2001; 108(7):949–55.
30. Brownlee M. Biochemistry and molecular cell biology of diabetic complications. Nature 2001;414(6865):813–20.
31. Bucala R, Makita Z, Koschinsky T, et al. Lipid advanced glycosylation: pathway for lipid oxidation in vivo. Proc Natl Acad Sci U S A 1993;90(14):6434–8.
32. Baynes JW, Thorpe SR. Role of oxidative stress in diabetic complications: a new perspective on an old paradigm. Diabetes 1999;48(1):1–9.
33. Fu MX, Requena JR, Jenkins AJ, et al. The advanced glycation end product, Nepsilon-(carboxymethyl)lysine, is a product of both lipid peroxidation and glycoxidation reactions. J Biol Chem 1996;271(17):9982–6.
34. Monnier VM, Bautista O, Kenny D, et al. Skin collagen glycation, glycoxidation, and crosslinking are lower in subjects with long-term intensive versus conventional therapy of type 1 diabetes: relevance of glycated collagen products versus HbA1c as markers of diabetic complications. DCCT Skin Collagen Ancillary Study Group. Diabetes Control and Complications Trial. Diabetes 1999;48(4):870–80.
35. Finot PA. The absorption and metabolism of modified amino acids in processed foods. J AOAC Int 2005;88(3):894–903.
36. Brands CM, Alink GM, van Boekel MA, et al. Mutagenicity of heated sugar-casein systems: effect of the Maillard reaction. J Agric Food Chem 2000;48:2271–5.
37. Ahmed N, Thornalley PJ. Advanced glycation endproducts: what is their relevance to diabetic complications? Diabetes Obes Metab 2007;9(3):233–45.
38. Xue M, Rabbani N, Momiji H, et al. Transcriptional control of glyoxalase 1 by Nrf2 provides a stress-responsive defence against dicarbonyl glycation. Biochem J 2012;443(1):213–22.
39. Vlassara H, Brownlee M, Cerami A. High-affinity-receptor-mediated uptake and degradation of glucose-modified proteins: a potential mechanism for the removal of senescent macromolecules. Proc Natl Acad Sci U S A 1985; 82(17):5588–92.
40. Li YM, Mitsuhashi T, Wojciechowicz D, et al. Molecular identity and cellular distribution of advanced glycation endproduct receptors: Relationship of p60 to OST-48 and p90 to 80K-H membrane proteins. Proc Natl Acad Sci USA 1996; 93(20):11047–52.
41. He CJ, Koschinsky T, Buenting C, et al. Presence of diabetic complications in type 1 diabetic patients correlates with low expression of mononuclear cell AGE-receptor-1 and elevated serum AGE. Mol Med 2001;7(3):159–68.
42. Cai W, Torreggiani M, Zhu L, et al. AGER1 regulates endothelial cell NADPH oxidase-dependent oxidant stress via PKC-delta: implications for vascular disease. Am J Physiol Cell Physiol 2009;298(3):C624–34.

43. Cai W, He JC, Zhu L, et al. Advanced glycation end product (AGE) receptor 1 suppresses cell oxidant stress and activation signaling via EGF receptor. Proc Natl Acad Sci U S A 2006;103(37):13801–6.
44. Torreggiani M, Liu H, Wu J, et al. Advanced glycation end product receptor-1 transgenic mice are resistant to inflammation, oxidative stress, and post-injury intimal hyperplasia. Am J Pathol 2009;175(4):1722–32.
45. Vlassara H, Uribarri J, Cai W, et al. Effects of sevelamer on HbA1c, inflammation, and advanced glycation end products in diabetic kidney disease. Clin J Am Soc Nephrol 2012;7(6):934–42.
46. Romero R, Espinoza J, Hassan S, et al. Soluble receptor for advanced glycation end products (sRAGE) and endogenous secretory RAGE (esRAGE) in amniotic fluid: modulation by infection and inflammation. J Perinat Med 2008;36(5): 388–98.
47. Yan SF, D'Agati V, Schmidt AM, et al. Receptor for Advanced Glycation End-products (RAGE): a formidable force in the pathogenesis of the cardiovascular complications of diabetes & aging. Curr Mol Med 2007;7(8):699–710.
48. Cai W, He JC, Zhu L, et al. Reduced oxidant stress and extended lifespan in mice exposed to a low glycotoxin diet: association with increased AGER1 expression. Am J Pathol 2007;170(6):1893–902.
49. Vlassara H, Li YM, Imani F, et al. Identification of galectin-3 as a high-affinity binding protein for advanced glycation end products (AGE): a new member of the AGE-receptor complex. Mol Med 1995;1(6):634–46.
50. Gale EA. The rise of childhood type 1 diabetes in the 20th century. Diabetes 2002;51(12):3353–61.
51. Beyan H, Riese H, Hawa MI, et al. Glycotoxin and autoantibodies are additive environmentally determined predictors of type 1 diabetes: a twin and population study. Diabetes 2012;61(5):1192–8.
52. Cai W, Ramdas M, Zhu L, et al. Oral advanced glycation endproducts (AGEs) promote insulin resistance and diabetes by depleting the antioxidant defenses AGE receptor-1 and sirtuin 1. Proc Natl Acad Sci U S A 2012;109(39):15888–93.
53. Liang F, Kume S, Koya D. SIRT1 and insulin resistance. Nat Rev Endocrinol 2009;5(7):367–73.
54. Olefsky JM, Glass CK. Macrophages, inflammation, and insulin resistance. Annu Rev Physiol 2010;72:219–46.
55. Krautwald M, Munch G. Advanced glycation end products as biomarkers and gerontotoxins - a basis to explore methylglyoxal-lowering agents for Alzheimer's disease? Exp Gerontol 2010;45(10):744–51.
56. Willette AA, Xu G, Johnson SC, et al. Insulin resistance, brain atrophy, and cognitive performance in late middle-aged adults. Diabetes Care 2013;36(2):443–9.
57. Beeri MS, Moshier E, Schmeidler J, et al. Serum concentration of an inflammatory glycotoxin, methylglyoxal, is associated with increased cognitive decline in elderly individuals. Mech Ageing Dev 2011;132(11–12):583–7.
58. Belanger M, Yang J, Petit JM, et al. Role of the glyoxalase system in astrocyte-mediated neuroprotection. J Neurosci 2011;31(50):18338–52.
59. Li W, Maloney RE, Circu ML, et al. Acute carbonyl stress induces occludin glycation and brain microvascular endothelial barrier dysfunction: role for glutathione-dependent metabolism of methylglyoxal. Free Radic Biol Med 2013;54:51–61.
60. Vlassara H, Brownlee M, Cerami A. Accumulation of diabetic rat peripheral nerve myelin by macrophages increases with the presence of advanced glycosylation endproducts. J Exp Med 1984;160(1):197–207.

61. Bayer J, Rune G, Kutsche K, et al. Estrogen and the male hippocampus: genetic variation in the aromatase gene predicting serum estrogen is associated with hippocampal gray matter volume in men. Hippocampus 2013;23(2):117–21.

62. Lepore G, Gadau S, Peruffo A, et al. Aromatase expression in cultured fetal sheep astrocytes after nitrosative/oxidative damage. Cell Tissue Res 2011; 344(3):407–13.

63. Azcoitia I, Sierra A, Veiga S, et al. Brain aromatase is neuroprotective. J Neurobiol 2001;47(4):318–29.

64. Doublier S, Lupia E, Catanuto P, et al. Estrogens and progression of diabetic kidney damage. Curr Diabetes Rev 2011;7(1):28–34.

65. Vlassara H, Striker LJ, Teichberg S, et al. Advanced glycation end products induce glomerular sclerosis and albuminuria in normal rats. Proc Natl Acad Sci U S A 1994;91(24):11704–8.

66. Kato M, Dang V, Wang M, et al. TGF-beta induces acetylation of chromatin and of Ets-1 to alleviate repression of miR-192 in diabetic nephropathy. Sci Signal 2013;6(278):ra43.

67. Richard P, Donahue RP, Stranges S, et al. Elevated cystatin concentration and progression to pre-diabetes. Diabetes Care 2007;30:1724–9.

68. Zheng F, He C, Cai W, et al. Prevention of diabetic nephropathy in mice by a diet low in glycoxidation products. Diabetes Metab Res Rev 2002;18(3):224–37.

69. Beisswenger PJ, Howell SK, Russell GB, et al. Early progression of diabetic nephropathy correlates with methylglyoxal-derived advanced glycation end products. Diabetes Care 2013. [Epub ahead of print].

70. Sun JK, Keenan HA, Cavallerano JD, et al. Protection from retinopathy and other complications in patients with type 1 diabetes of extreme duration: the Joslin 50-Year Medalist Study. Diabetes Care 2011;34(4):968–74.

71. Gohda T, Niewczas MA, Ficociello LH, et al. Circulating TNF receptors 1 and 2 predict stage 3 CKD in type 1 diabetes. J Am Soc Nephrol 2012; 23(3):516–24.

72. Niewczas MA, Gohda T, Skupien J, et al. Circulating TNF receptors 1 and 2 predict ESRD in type 2 diabetes. J Am Soc Nephrol 2012;23(3):507–15.

73. Wu J, Zhang R, Torreggiani M, et al. Induction of diabetes in aged C57B6 mice results in severe nephropathy: an association with oxidative stress, endoplasmic reticulum stress, and inflammation. Am J Pathol 2010;176(5):2163–76.

74. Peppa M, Uribarri J, Cai W, et al. Glycoxidation and inflammation in renal failure patients. Am J Kidney Dis 2004;43(4):690–5.

75. Vlassara H, Cai W, Chen X, et al. Managing chronic inflammation in the aging diabetic patient with CKD by diet or sevelamer carbonate: a modern paradigm shift. J Gerontol A Biol Sci Med Sci 2012;67(12):1410–6.

76. Christiansen CF, Johansen MB, Christensen S, et al. Type 2 diabetes and 1-year mortality in intensive care unit patients. Eur J Clin Invest 2013;43(3):238–47.

77. Estruch R, Ros E, Salas-Salvado J, et al. Primary prevention of cardiovascular disease with a Mediterranean diet. N Engl J Med 2013;368(14):1279–90.

78. Jasuja GK, Travison TG, Davda M, et al. Circulating estrone levels are associated prospectively with diabetes risk in men of the Framingham Heart Study. Diabetes Care 2013;36:2591–6.

79. Patel R, Baker SS, Liu W, et al. Effect of dietary advanced glycation end products on mouse liver. PLoS One 2012;7(4):e35143.

80. Miyashita T, Toyoda Y, Tsuneyama K, et al. Hepatoprotective effect of tamoxifen on steatosis and non-alcoholic steatohepatitis in mouse models. J Toxicol Sci 2012;37(5):931–42.

81. Tian GX, Sun Y, Pang CJ, et al. Oestradiol is a protective factor for non-alcoholic fatty liver disease in healthy men. Obes Rev 2012;13(4):381–7.
82. Florentino G, Cotrim HP, Florentino A, et al. Hormone replacement therapy in menopausal women: risk factor or protection to nonalcoholic fatty liver disease? Ann Hepatol 2012;11(1):147–9.
83. Mericq V, Piccardo C, Cai W, et al. Maternally transmitted and food-derived glycotoxins: a factor preconditioning the young to diabetes? Diabetes Care 2010; 33(10):2232–7.
84. Sebekova K, Saavedra G, Zumpe C, et al. Plasma concentration and urinary excretion of N epsilon-(carboxymethyl)lysine in breast milk- and formula-fed infants. Ann N Y Acad Sci 2008;1126:177–80.
85. Vasan S, Foiles P, Founds H. Therapeutic potential of breakers of advanced glycation end product-protein crosslinks. Archives of biochemistry and biophysics. Arch Biochem Biophys 2003;419(1):89–96.
86. Voziyan P, Brown KL, Chetyrkin S, et al. Site-specific AGE modifications in the extracellular matrix: a role for glyoxal in protein damage in diabetes. Clin Chem Lab Med 2013;13:1–7.
87. Lewis EJ, Greene T, Spitalewiz S, et al. For the Collaborative Study Group. Pyridorin in type 2 diabetic nephropathy. J Am Soc Nephrol 2012;23:131–6.
88. Negrean M, Stirban A, Stratmann B, et al. Effects of low- and high-advanced glycation endproduct meals on macro- and microvascular endothelial function and oxidative stress in patients with type 2 diabetes mellitus. Am J Clin Nutr 2007;85(5):1236–43.
89. Stirban A, Pop A, Tschoepe D. A randomized, double-blind, crossover, placebo-controlled trial of 6 weeks benfotiamine treatment on postprandial vascular function and variables of autonomic nerve function in Type 2 diabetes. Diabet Med 2013. [Epub ahead of print].
90. Asif M, Egan J, Vasan S, et al. An advanced glycation endproduct cross-link breaker can reverse age-related increases in myocardial stiffness. Proc Natl Acad Sci USA 2000;97(6):2809–13.

Diabetic Retinopathy
Current Concepts and Emerging Therapy

Daniel F. Rosberger, MD, PhD, MPH[a,b]

KEYWORDS

- Diabetic retinopathy • Anti-VEGF therapy • Intravitreal medications
- Microvascular complications of diabetes • Laser photocoagulation

KEY POINTS

- The epidemiology of diabetic retinopathy indicates that although diabetes remains the leading cause of blindness among Americans, tight glucose control and lifestyle modification can reduce its prevalence.
- Although laser photocoagulation remains the mainstay of treatment of both proliferative diabetic retinopathy and clinically significant macular edema, the paradigm is shifting toward treatment with intravitreal medications.
- Emerging therapy with anti–vascular endothelial growth factor agents, long-acting corticosteroids, protein kinase C inhibitors, tumor necrosis factor modulators, and other medications may dramatically improve the treatment of diabetic retinopathy in the coming years.
- The Diabetes Retinopathy Clinical Research Network is a National Institutes of Health–funded collaborative network of more than 300 physicians dedicated to multicenter clinical research of diabetic retinopathy, diabetic macular edema, and associated conditions.

INTRODUCTION

Diabetic retinopathy is a disease that eventually affects nearly all patients with long-standing diabetes mellitus. The earliest visualized lesions are generally intraretinal hemorrhages and microaneurysms. With progression, fibrovascular proliferation and neovascularization can occur. Visual loss eventually results from macular edema, macular ischemia from capillary nonperfusion, vitreous hemorrhage, fibrous distortion of the macula, neovascular glaucoma, and tractional or rhegmatogenous retinal detachments (RD). The Diabetes Control and Complications Trial (DCCT) and the United Kingdom Prospective Diabetes Study (UKPDS) have clearly demonstrated that tight glucose control in both type 1 and type 2 diabetes can significantly delay the onset and progression of retinopathy. (**Table 1** lists the commonly used abbreviations in diabetic retinopathy.) For both diabetic macular edema (DME) and proliferative diabetic

[a] Weill-Cornell Medical College of Cornell University, 1300 York Avenue, New York, NY 10021, USA; [b] MaculaCare, PLLC, 52 East 72nd Street, New York, NY 10021, USA
E-mail address: drosberger@gmail.com

Endocrinol Metab Clin N Am 42 (2013) 721–745
http://dx.doi.org/10.1016/j.ecl.2013.08.001
0889-8529/13/$ – see front matter © 2013 Elsevier Inc. All rights reserved.

Table 1	
Commonly used abbreviations in diabetic retinopathy	
CSME	Clinically significant diabetic retinopathy
CWS	Cotton wool spot
DCCT	Diabetes Control and Complications Trial
DME	Diabetic macular edema
DRCR net	Diabetic Retinopathy Clinical Research network
DRS	Diabetic Retinopathy Study
ETDRS	Early Treatment Diabetic Retinopathy Study
FA	Fluorescein angiography
FVP	Fibrovascular proliferation
HR	High risk
IRH	Intraretinal hemorrhage
IVTA	Intravitreal triamcinolone acetonide
ma	Microaneurysm
NHR	Non–high risk
NPDR	Nonproliferative diabetic retinopathy
NVA	Neovascularization of the trabecular angle
NVD	Neovascularization of the optic disk
NVE	Neovascularization elsewhere (other than the optic disk)
NVG	Neovascular glaucoma
NVI	Neovascularization of the iris
OCT	Optical coherence tomography
POAG	Primary open angle glaucoma
PDR	Proliferative diabetic retinopathy
RD	Retinal detachment
SLE	Slit lamp examination
UKPDS	United Kingdom Prospective Diabetes Study
VH	Vitreous hemorrhage
WESDR	Wisconsin Epidemiologic Study of Diabetic Retinopathy

retinopathy (PDR), the mainstay of treatment has been laser photocoagulation. However, in the past few years, new agents and new delivery systems have been developed that are fundamentally changing the treatment paradigm.

EPIDEMIOLOGY

Diabetic retinopathy remains one of the most common complications of chronic diabetes mellitus and the leading cause of new cases of blindness (defined by central visual acuity worse than 20/200) in the United States in people aged 20 to 74 years. An estimated 50 000 new cases of retinal neovascularization and macular edema occur yearly.[1–3] Despite this, as many as half of the patients who would benefit from treatment remain untreated.[4] The DCCT demonstrated a marked reduction in the development and progression of diabetic retinopathy in intensively treated type 1 diabetes compared with those treated conventionally.[5–7] The UKPDS showed similar results in patients with type 2 diabetes.[8]

Much of what we know about the epidemiology of diabetic retinopathy in the United States comes from the Wisconsin Epidemiologic Study of Diabetic Retinopathy

(WESDR), which received its initial funding from the National Institutes of Health (NIH) in 1979. The primary aims of this study were to (1) describe the prevalence and severity of retinopathy and visual loss in people with diabetes and their relationship to other systemic complications and mortality, (2) quantitate the association of risk factors with retinopathy, and (3) provide information on health care delivery and quality of life in people with diabetes.

Table 2 summarizes the baseline prevalence and disease severity in WESDR. In an 11-county region of southwestern Wisconsin, 452 of the 457 physicians who provided primary medical care to patients with diabetes participated by collecting lists of all the patients with diabetes they saw during the 1-year period from July 1, 1979 through June 30, 1980.[9,10] A total of 10 135 patients were identified, and an initial sample of 2990 patients was selected for a baseline examination. The sample was divided into 2 groups. The first, type 1 diabetes, was referred to as *younger onset* and consisted of 1210 patients diagnosed with diabetes before 30 years of age who were taking insulin. The second group, referred to as *older onset*, consisted of a probability sample of 1780 patients taken from all eligible patients who were diagnosed with diabetes at 30 years of age or older with a postprandial serum glucose measurement of 11.1 mmol/L or more or a fasting serum glucose measurement of 7.8 mmol/L or more on at least 2 separate occasions. The older-onset group was further stratified by (1) the duration of diabetes (less than 5 years [576 patients], 5 to 14 years [579 patients], and greater than 15 years [625 patients]) and (2) insulin usage (824 patients were taking insulin and 956 were not).

At the study initiation visit, approximately 70% of the younger-onset patients had some degree of diabetic retinopathy and 23% had PDR.[11] In the older-onset arm, 70% of the patients taking insulin had some degree of retinopathy, whereas only 39% of the patients not taking insulin did. Moreover, 14% of the older-onset patients taking insulin and 3% of the patients who were not on insulin had PDR.[12] Clinically significant macular edema (CSME) was present in approximately 6% of the younger-onset patients, 12% of the older-onset patients taking insulin, and 4% of the older-onset patients not taking insulin.[13]

A recent study analyzed a cross-sectional, nationally representative sample of the National Health and Nutrition Examination Survey 2005–2008 (n = 1006).[14] Among US adults with diabetes, the estimated prevalence of diabetic retinopathy and vision-threatening diabetic retinopathy was 28.5%. Retinopathy was slightly more

Table 2
Baseline prevalence and disease severity in the WESDR

Retinopathy Status	Younger Onset, (N = 996)	Older Onset, Taking Insulin (N = 673)	Older Onset, Not Taking Insulin (N = 673)
None (%)	29.3	29.9	61.3
Mild NPDR (%)	30.4	30.6	27.3
Moderate and severe NPDR (%)	17.6	25.7	8.5
PDR without HR characteristics (%)	13.2	9.1	1.4
Proliferative with HR characteristics or worse (%)	9.5	4.8	1.4
CSME (%)	5.9	11.6	3.7

Abbreviations: CSME, clinically significant diabetic retinopathy; HR, high risk; NPDR, nonproliferative diabetic retinopathy.

prevalent among men than women. Non-Hispanic blacks with diabetes had a higher crude prevalence than non-Hispanic whites of diabetic retinopathy (38.8% vs 26.4%) and vision-threatening diabetic retinopathy (9.3% vs 3.2%). Independent risk factors for the presence of diabetic retinopathy included male sex, higher hemoglobin A1c measurement, longer duration of diabetes insulin use, and higher systolic blood pressure.

However, microvascular changes consistent with diabetic retinopathy can occur even before the diagnosis of diabetic retinopathy using current definitions. The Diabetes Prevention Program was a multicentered, randomized, controlled clinical trial that enrolled 3234 overweight participants that had elevated blood glucose levels but had not yet met the definitional criteria for diabetes. The study demonstrated that intensive lifestyle changes including a low-fat diet, weight loss, and increased physical activity could reduce the development of type 2 diabetes by 58% compared with placebo and that metformin (850 mg twice daily) lowered diabetes incidence by 31% compared with placebo. It also demonstrated that approximately 8% of these patients who were prediabetic already had diabetic retinopathy.[15]

PATHOGENESIS

The precise processes by which diabetes results in retinopathy are not completely understood; however, damage to the retinal microvasculature is clearly paramount. The molecular mechanism of microvasculature damage is likely multifactorial, with roles for hyperglycemia-induced polyol pathway activation, production of advanced glycation end products, oxidative stress, and activation of the diacylglycerol–protein kinase C (PKC) transcription pathway.

Fig. 1 demonstrates the layers of the retina and the relationship of the retina to the overlying vitreous and the underlying retinal pigment epithelium (RPE). Abnormalities in most of these layers can be seen in diabetic retinopathy.

Vasculature abnormalities are a prominent finding in diabetic retinopathy and can occur anywhere between the nerve fiber layer (NFL) and the outer plexiform layer. Early damage in diabetic retinopathy can be seen by light microscopic evaluation of retinal vessels as a reduction in the number of pericytes surrounding retinal capillary endothelial cells.[16] Microaneurysms are the outpouching of these damaged capillaries. Microaneurysmal leakage likely plays a significant role in DME. Endothelial cell proliferation, deposition of excess basement membrane material, closing of the microaneurysm lumen, and loss of endothelial cells may lead to capillary dropout and ischemia. With progressive damage and capillary nonperfusion, arteriovenous shunts can form. Intraretinal microvascular abnormalities (IRMA) arise in areas of ischemia and can sometimes appear similar to neovascularization except that IRMA does not leak on fluorescein angiography, generally occur deeper in the retina, and are not present on the optic disk.

Cotton wool spots (CWS) are seen in the NFL and under the internal limiting membrane (ILM). They are cytoid bodies and represent stasis of axoplasmic flow in the axons of ganglion cells in the NFL.

Hard exudates are fat-filled, lipoidal histiocytes occurring in the outer plexiform layer. This exudation surrounds damaged retinal vasculature and microaneurysms and may appear in a circinate pattern.

Venous dilatations are the result of abnormalities in the walls of retinal veins. Thickening of the capillary basement membranes and increased constriction at crossing points of retinal arteries and veins are also commonly seen. As the severity of the

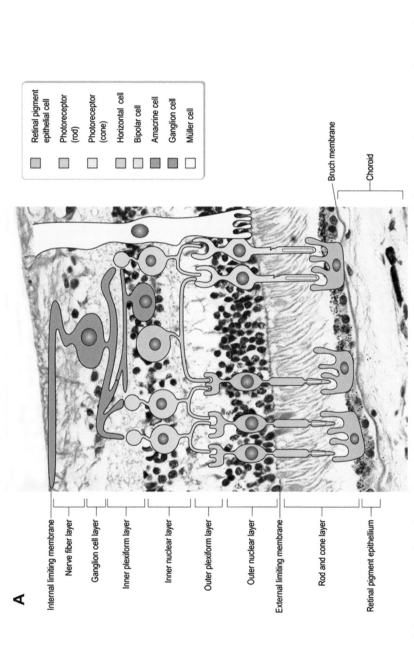

Fig. 1. Layers of the retina and the relationship of the retina to the overlying vitreous and the underlying retinal pigment epithelium. *(From [A]* Herzlich AA, Patel M, Sauer TC, et al. Chapter 2: retinal anatomy and pathology. Retinal pharmacotherapy. Copyright Elsevier 2010; *[B]* The eye. Potter's pathology of the fetus, infant and child. Copyright Elsevier 2007.)

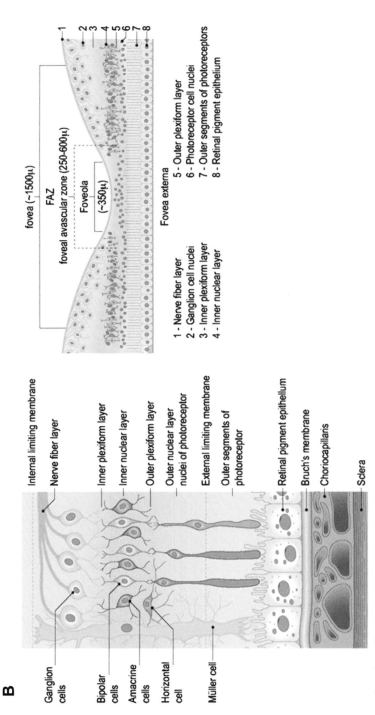

Fig. 1. (continued)

retinopathy progresses, beading of the retinal veins resulting from dilated venous walls and saccular aneurysmal dilatation occurs. The appearance of hemorrhages in the retina depends on the layer where the hemorrhage occurs. Intraretinal dot or blot hemorrhages occur in the inner retinal layer but can spread to the outer plexiform layer. They appear as dots because they are contained between the perpendicularly oriented cellular elements. Flame-shaped or splinter intraretinal hemorrhages spread out within the parallel elements of the NFL. Large confluent hemorrhages can involve all of the retinal layers and even break through the ILM into the vitreous space and into the subretinal space.[7]

Thickening of the ILM and posterior vitreous face can be seen in early retinopathy with progressive fibrotic attachment of the ILM to the vitreous as retinopathy advances with fibroblasts, fibrous astrocytes, myofibroblasts, and macrophages present in the ILM and the vitreous in patients with DME.[17]

Retinal neovascularization arises in regions of hypoxia, and it is thought to be mediated by the elaboration of vascular endothelial growth factor (VEGF). New blood vessels commonly arise from retinal venues at the margin of an area of capillary nonperfusion. Fibrovascular proliferation can break through the ILM and onto the surface of the retina and extend into the vitreous space. Rupture of these fragile neovascular vessels can cause extensive hemorrhage into the vitreous. As the fibrovascular process matures, fibrosis can occur on the surface of the retina causing macular distortion. With sufficient contraction, the neurosensory retina can be pulled up of the RPE creating a tractional RD. In extreme cases, the retina can rip, leading to a rhegmatogenous RD.

DIAGNOSIS AND CLASSIFICATION

Despite the fact that the paradigm for treating diabetic retinopathy is moving away from laser photocoagulation (see discussion elsewhere in this article), the classification of retinopathy and, therefore, the timing of treatment and follow-up are still largely based on clinical trials of focal and panretinal laser photocoagulation.

In general, diabetic retinopathy is classified as either nonproliferative (NPDR) or proliferative (PDR) based on the absence or presence of retinal vascular neovascularization. Macular edema can be present independently in either NPDR or PDR and is classified as absent, present, and clinically significant (CSME) or nonclinically significant. Correct classification is important because it gives us information about the preferred intervention and the risk of progression that will determine the appropriate follow-up. Immediate treatment is almost always recommended for macular edema once the threshold for clinical significance has been reached and for PDR once high-risk criteria are met. No treatment is generally recommended for NPDR in the absence of CSME. Classification is based on standard fundus photographs used in the Early Treatment Diabetic Retinopathy Study (ETDRS).[18]

NPDR

Mild NPDR

Patients with mild NPDR have at least one microaneurysm; however, there are fewer intraretinal dot or blot hemorrhages than in the ETDRS standard photograph 2A (**Fig. 2**), and no other retinal abnormalities associated with diabetes are present. Patients with mild NPDR have only a 5% risk of progressing to PDR within 1 year and only a 15% risk of progressing to high-risk PDR necessitating panretinal laser photocoagulation within 5 years.[7]

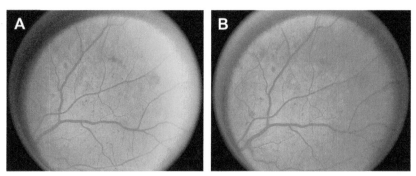

Fig. 2. Stereoscopic pairs of standard photograph 2A of the modified Airlie House classification of diabetic retinopathy illustrates a moderate degree of hemorrhages and microaneurysms. (*From* Aiello LM. Perspectives on diabetic retinopathy. Am J Ophthalmol 2003;136(1):131; with permission.)

Moderate NPDR

Patients with moderate NPDR have more microaneurysms or intraretinal hemorrhages than in the ETDRS standard photograph 2A (see **Fig. 2**) in one field; however, they are present in fewer than 4 quadrants of the retina. NFL infarctions (commonly referred to as CWS or soft exudates), undulations in the caliber of retinal veins (referred to as venous beading [VB]), and IRMA are present but less prominent than in the ETDRS standard photograph 8A (**Fig. 3**). Patients with moderate NPDR have a 12% to 27% risk of progressing to PDR within 1 year and a 33% 5-year risk of reaching the criteria for high-risk PDR.[7]

Severe NPDR

Patients with severe NPDR are defined by having one of the elements of the 4-2-1 rule. They have either 4 quadrants of intraretinal hemorrhages or microaneurysms greater than the ETDRS standard photograph 2A (see **Fig. 2**), 2 quadrants of significant VB, or 1 quadrant of IRMA greater than the ETDRS standard photograph 8A (see **Fig. 3**) and no retinal vascular neovascularization. Patients with severe NPDR have a 52% risk of progressing to PDR within 1 year and a 60% 5-year risk of reaching the criteria for high-risk PDR.[7]

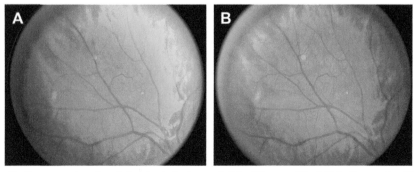

Fig. 3. Stereoscopic pairs of standard photograph 8A of the modified Airlie House classification of diabetic retinopathy illustrates a moderate degree of IRMA. (*From* Aiello LM. Perspectives on diabetic retinopathy. Am J Ophthalmol 2003;136(1):131; with permission.)

Very severe NPDR

Patients with very severe NPDR have at least 2 of the elements of the 4-2-1 rule (defined earlier for severe NPDR) but have no retinal vascular neovascularization. They have a 75% risk of progressing to PDR within 1 year.[7]

PDR

PDR is characterized by neovascularization on the optic disk (NVD) or elsewhere (NVE) on the retina, hemorrhage present within the vitreous or trapped between the interface of the surface of the retina and the posterior margin of the vitreous body (subhyaloid hemorrhage), or fibrovascular proliferation, which can cause pulling on the retina sometimes leading to tractional or rhegmatogenous RD. PDR is defined as either early or high risk. Eyes with early PDR have a 75% 5-year risk of developing high-risk PDR. High-risk PDR is defined by the presence of NVD greater than approximately one-third of the area of the optic disk as defined by the ETDRS reference photograph 10 A (**Fig. 4**), or any NVD associated with vitreous or subhyaloid hemorrhage, or an area of NVE greater than one-half of the area of the optic disk with concomitant vitreous or subhyaloid hemorrhage. Early PDR includes all eyes that meet the criteria for PDR but do not meet the criteria for high risk.[7]

Macular Edema

Damage to the macula can occur at any level of NPDR or PDR. It may involve leakage of serosanguinous fluid from retinal vasculature damaged by diabetes or microaneurysms and result in a collection of intraretinal fluid within the macula causing the macula to become thickened or edematous. This damage may occur in a cystoid (not true cysts because there is no endothelial lining) pattern and may be associated with precipitated lipids sometimes referred to as hard exudates. Macular edema is usually defined as retinal thickening within 2 disk diameters (approximately 3 mm) of the center of the macula. Alternatively, macular damage can be the result of parafoveal capillary nonperfusion and ischemia with or without edema; fibrovascular traction on the macula causing wrinkling, distortion, or detachment of the macula; intraretinal or subhyaloid hemorrhage, which can cause a physical barrier to images reaching the macula; or the formation of macular holes.

CSME

CSME is defined by the ETDRS as macular edema meeting one or more of the following 3 criteria: (1) retinal thickening occurring at or within 500 μm of the center

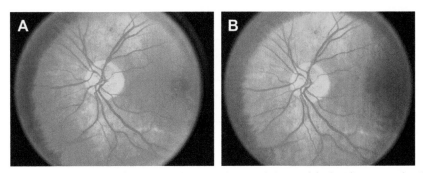

Fig. 4. Stereoscopic pairs of standard photograph 10A of the modified Airlie House classification of diabetic retinopathy illustrates a moderate degree of NVD. (*From* Aiello LM. Perspectives on diabetic retinopathy. Am J Ophthalmol 2003;136(1):131; with permission.)

of the macula; (2) lipid precipitate deposition (hard exudates) with adjacent, associated retinal thickening at or within 500 μm of the center of the macula; or (3) a zone of retinal thickening of at least 1 disk area in size, any part of which is at or within 1 disk diameter (approximately 1.5 mm) of the center of the macula. Identifying CSME is important because patients with CSME were shown to benefit from focal laser photocoagulation in the ETDRS. Visual acuity was not a criterion for defining CSME.

Although recommendations are evolving because of the increased use of intravitreal medications in the treatment of the neovascular and macular edema complications of diabetic retinopathy, recommendations for follow-up are still largely defined by the ETDRS findings regarding the progression of disease. **Table 3** (progression and follow-up recommendations) summarizes the current standard recommendations regarding the appropriate follow-up of patients with various levels of retinopathy.

DIAGNOSTIC MODALITIES FOR EVALUATION OF RETINOPATHY

The mainstay for diagnosis of diabetic retinopathy remains the clinical examination by a qualified examiner; however, additional diagnostic testing may often be helpful. The American Academy of Ophthalmology has developed preferred practice patterns related to the appropriate diagnosis and management of diabetic retinopathy.[19]

Visual acuity measurement with a standard Snellen or ETDRS chart is an easy, low-cost, and useful method of assessing visual function.[20] But visual acuity was not a criterion for determining the need for laser photocoagulation in the ETDRS, and patients with extensive and sight-threatening retinopathy might maintain excellent visual acuity for periods of time.

Slit lamp biomicroscopy of the anterior segment including the cornea, lens, and iris should be performed. In addition, the measurement of the intraocular pressure by any

Table 3
Risk and timing of progression of diabetic retinopathy

Retinopathy Classification	Risk of Progression to		Recommended Follow-up	Treatment
	PDR in 1 y (%)	High-Risk PDR in 5 y (%)		
Mild NPDR	5	15		
(−) CSME			Yearly	No
(+) CSME			3 mo	Yes
Moderate NPDR	12–27	33		
(−) CSME			6 mo	No
(+) CSME			3 mo	Yes
Severe NPDR	52	60		
(−) CSME			4 mo	Rarely
(+) CSME			3 mo	Yes
Very Severe NPDR	75	75		
(−) CSME			3 mo	Occasionally
(+) CSME			3 mo	Yes
Early PDR	—	75		
(−) CSME			2–3 mo	Occasionally
(+) CSME			2–3 mo	Yes
High-Risk PDR	—	—		
(−) CSME			2–3 mo	Yes
(+) CSME			1–2 mo	Yes

of several methods and gonioscopic evaluation of the iris and trabecular structures looking for signs of neovascularization of the iris and angle are necessary to diagnose primary open angle glaucoma, which may be more prevalent in patients with diabetes, and neovascular glaucoma, which is one of the most feared complications of PDR leading, in some cases, to uncontrollable increases in intraocular pressure and blindness. Stereoscopic slit lamp biomicroscopy, with the use of accessory lenses, is the preferred method for evaluating retinopathy of the posterior pole, including the optic disk and macula, as well as the retinal midperiphery.[16] This technique allows for careful evaluation for the presence of macular edema, intraretinal hemorrhages, IRMA, CWS, VB, NVD, and NVE as well as epiretinal membranes and fibrovascular proliferation that can lead to tractional and rhegmatogenous RD. Binocular indirect ophthalmoscopy is used to examine the peripheral retina for NVE, vitreous hemorrhage, and RD. Alternatively, the peripheral retina can be examined with wide-angle or angled-mirror lenses at the slit lamp. Dilation of the pupil is required to adequately assess the retina for the presence of retinopathy because only 50% of eyes have been shown to be accurately graded for retinopathy through undilated pupils.[21] New scanning laser ophthalmoscopic imaging systems may improve visualization of the peripheral retina in undilated eyes.

Ancillary testing, if used appropriately, can enhance the accuracy of diagnosis and improve patient care.[14] Color fundus photography, often with stereoscopic imaging, may be a more reproducible technique than examination at the slit lamp for detecting retinopathy; but clinical examination is frequently superior for detecting macular edema and fine-caliber NVD and NVE. Photographic documentation of a previous examination, however, can be helpful in ascertaining disease progression, response to treatment, and can influence the decision as to whether or not to treat.[22]

Although it is not part of the routine evaluation of patients with diabetes, fluorescein angiography, in which 10% or 25% fluorescein sodium solution is rapidly injected intravenously, can be useful in identifying areas of macular and peripheral capillary nonperfusion; sources of capillary leakage, such as microaneurysms responsible for macular edema; and sometimes in visualizing subtle foci of IRMA and neovascularization. Fluorescein angiography is not needed to diagnose CSME or PDR because both of these are clinical diagnoses[14]; however, it is frequently used as a guide for the treatment CSME.[19] Fluorescein angiography is a very safe procedure; but mild side effects, including nausea and vomiting, are not infrequent, and severe medical complications, including death (approximately 1 per 200 000 patients) can occur.[23] Although adverse effects on the fetus have never been documented, fluorescein angiography is not generally recommended, other than in exceptional circumstances, during pregnancy because fluorescein dye can cross the placental barrier and enter the fetal circulation.[24]

B-scan ultrasonography can be very helpful in diagnosing RD in diabetic eyes with media opacities secondary to corneal clouding, cataracts, and most frequently vitreous hemorrhage.

Ocular coherence tomography (OCT) provides cross-sectional imaging of the retina and macula, the vitreoretinal interface and epiretina, and the subretinal space.[25] Time domain and, more recently, spectral domain instruments allow for high-resolution imaging (<10 μm) and quantification of retinal thickness. OCT's ability to qualitatively and quantitatively assess retinal thickening can frequently be useful in monitoring macular edema and response to treatment as well as identifying areas of vitreoretinal traction that might not be evident by standard clinical examination. OCT is frequently used as a secondary measure during clinical trials; however, OCT measurements of retinal thickness do not always correlate with visual acuity.[26]

CURRENT TREATMENT

Laser photocoagulation for diabetic retinopathy was proposed by Meyer-Schwickerath in 1954 and has remained the mainstay of treatment of both DME and PDR.[27] In 1985, the ETDRS demonstrated that in patients with mild or moderate NPDR, focal laser photocoagulation, either directly to microaneurysms thought to be responsible for the edema or in a grid pattern in the case of more diffuse vascular leakage, could reduce the likelihood of further vision loss in patients with CSME.[28,29] Patients with initial visual acuity worse than 20/40 had twice the likelihood of improvement in vision with laser treatment.

PDR can be treated with panretinal photocoagulation (PRP). The Diabetic Retinopathy Study showed that PRP could reduce the risk of severe vision loss (visual acuity less than 5/200 at 2 consecutive visits) in patients with high-risk PDR.[10,30] Whenever both focal laser treatment of CSME and PRP for neovascularization are needed simultaneously, focal laser is applied first to reduce the likelihood of worsening macular edema caused by the heavier scatter laser. In a recent investigation, no difference in the rate of occurrence or worsening of macular edema was noted whether the PRP was administered in one session or divided into 4 sessions.[31]

Side effects and complications are not rare with laser photocoagulation; however, in most cases, they are not particularly serious, especially when compared with the risk of blindness present without treatment.[32] The most feared complication of focal laser treatment is inadvertent photocoagulation of the fovea. This complication can lead to immediate loss of central vision leaving patients unable to read. This risk can be minimized by properly identifying macular landmarks before the initiation of treatment, but it may also result from accidental movement of either the surgeon or patients. In addition to the usually mild discomfort felt by patients, PRP can cause decreases in peripheral vision, especially when heavy confluent or fill-in laser is needed. Decreases in color and night vision may also be seen following PRP. Transient impairment of central reading vision may also occur but generally resolves over several hours. Persistent loss of acuity may usually resolve over several weeks; but when associated with ischemia or refractory macular edema, it may be permanent. Exudative RD can infrequently occur following PRP, presumably from damage to choroidal vessels causing exudation of fluid through the retinal pigment epithelial barrier into the subretinal space. Vitreous hemorrhage can result from direct photocoagulation treatment of retinal neovascularization.

EMERGING TREATMENTS

Table 4 summarizes the pharmacologic agents used for DME.

Table 4 Pharmacologic agents used for DME		
Drug	FDA Approved for Intravitreal Use	FDA Approved for DME
Aflibercept	Yes	No
Bevacizumab	No	No
Dexamethasone (Ozurdex)	Yes	No
Fluocinolone (Retisert, Iluvien)	Yes (Retisert)	No
Infliximab	No	No
Pegaptanib	Yes	No
Ranibizumab	Yes	Yes
Triamcinolone (Triessence)	Yes	No

Diabetic Retinopathy and Inflammatory Modulators

It has become clear over the past several years that inflammation may play a significant role in the progression of diabetic retinopathy and that modulating inflammation may have a role in its treatment. Steroids, nonsteroidal antiinflammatory drugs (NSAIDs), anti-VEGF agents, and anti–tumor necrosis factor (TNF) agents have all been shown to influence the progression of diabetic retinopathy; it is proposed that at least some of this effect is through their antiinflammatory properties. NSAIDs have been demonstrated to prevent progression of retinopathy by inhibiting TNF-alpha.[33]

CORTICOSTEROIDS
Triamcinolone Acetonide

Several studies have demonstrated a benefit to intravitreal triamcinolone acetonide (IVTA) in the treatment of DME.[34–36] Laser photocoagulation was recently compared with1-mg and 4-mg doses of IVTA. Superior visual and anatomic outcomes with laser photocoagulation were reported at both 2[37] and 3[38] years following randomization. However, 4 mg IVTA was associated with better visual outcomes than laser treatment in patients with poor initial visual acuity (20/200 to 20/320) and a reduced risk for progression of retinopathy.[39] Moreover, IVTA may have short-term benefits in patients with PDR in conjunction with panretinal laser photocoagulation[40,41] and may be associated with decreased risks of vitreous hemorrhage following pars plans vitrectomy.[42]

In the United States, there are at least 4 commercially available preparations of IVTA: Kenalog-40, Triesence, Trivaris, and preservative-free triamcinolone acetonide from compounding pharmacies.

Treatment of DME, which is a chronic condition, may require repeated injections, exposing patients to cumulative risks for complications and side effects, such as endophthalmitis, increased intraocular pressure, and cataracts. Additionally, there may be clinically relevant differences between intermittent high-dose administration of corticosteroids and sustained, lose-dose elution. Several extended-release delivery systems have been investigated: Retisert (Bausch & Lomb, Rochester, NY), a surgically implanted device containing fluocinolone acetonide, which received approval by the Food and Drug Administration (FDA) in 2005 for the treatment of chronic, noninfectious posterior uveitis; Iluvien (Alimera Sciences, Alpharetta, GA), an injectable delivery system for fluocinolone acetonide; and Ozurdex (Allergan Inc, Irvine, CA), an injectable sustained delivery system for dexamethasone.

Dexamethasone (Ozurdex)

A novel biodegradable, sustained-released dexamethasone delivery system (Ozurdex) has recently been approved by the FDA for use in macular edema associated with retinal vein occlusions and for noninfectious intermediate and posterior uveitis. A specially designed 22-gauge applicator is used to deliver the implant in a sutureless office-based procedure. Ozurdex (700 μg) has been shown to reduce central retinal thickness as measured by OCT, reduce retinal vascular leakage seen on fluorescein angiography, and improve best-corrected visual acuity (BCVA) in patients with persistent macular edema compared with untreated eyes.[43,44] The beneficial effects may be present within a few days of implantation[45] and were sustained at the 180-day protocol visit.[28] Complications, such as increased intraocular pressure and cataract, may be less frequent with the Ozurdex implant than with repeated intravitreal injections of triamcinolone acetonide.[28,29] In difficult-to-treat eyes that had previous vitrectomy surgery, treatment with Ozurdex led to statistically and clinically significant improvements in both vision and vascular leakage from DME. At present, Ozurdex is approved by the FDA for intravitreal use in noninfectious uveitis and macular edema secondary to retinal vein occlusions. An approval for use in diabetic retinopathy has not been granted yet.

Fluocinolone Acetonide (Retisert, Iluvien)

The Fluocinolone Acetonide in Diabetic Macular Edema (FAME) study investigated the safety and efficacy of a sustained-release fluocinolone acetonide intravitreal implant (Retisert, Iluvien) for the treatment of DME. Fluocinolone acetonide is a soluble, potent steroid and more lipophilic than triamcinolone acetonide or dexamethasone. The FDA has previously approved Retisert for persistent noninfectious posterior uveitis. Retisert is implanted through a pars plana surgical incision and sutured into the sclera in the operating room. It releases fluocinolone for up to 3 years. Iluvien also releases fluocinolone for nearly 3 years, but it is a nonerodible, intravitreal implant that is small enough to be injected through a 25-gauge needle creating a self-sealing wound in an in-office procedure. In a study comparing the 0.59-mg Retisert implant versus standard-of-care laser photocoagulation in patients with persistent or recurrent DME, the fluocinolone implant demonstrated superiority with regard to improved visual acuity and decreased macular edema.[46] Visual acuity improved 3 or more lines in 16.8% of the fluocinolone-implanted eyes at 6 months compared with 1.4% of the standard-of-care eyes (P = .0012). At 1 year, there was an improvement of 3 or more lines in 16.4% in the fluocinolone-implanted eyes compared with 8.1% of the standard-of-care eyes (P = .1191). By year 2, 31.8% of the fluocinolone-implanted eyes had an improvement of 3 or more lines compared with 9.3% of the standard-of-care eyes (P = .0016); and at 3 years, 31.1% of the fluocinolone-implanted eyes had an improvement of 3 or more lines compared with 20.0% of the standard-of-care laser-treated eyes (P = .1566). Moreover, the number of Retisert-implanted eyes with no evidence of retinal thickening at the center of the macula was higher than the standard-of-care laser-treated eyes at all time points through 3 years.

However, the side effects were significant. Intraocular pressure of 30 mm Hg or more was recorded in 61.4% of the implanted eyes compared with only 5.8% of the standard-of-care eyes; 33.8% of the Retisert-implanted eyes required surgery for ocular hypertension by 4 years. In addition, more than 90% of Retisert-implanted eyes that had not previously had cataract surgery required cataract extraction by 4 years.

Iluvien is an 0.18-mg fluocinolone acetonide delivery system being evaluated for the treatment of DME in addition to other indications.[47] At present, neither Iluvien nor Retisert is approved for the indication of DME.

PROTEIN KINASE C (PKC) INHIBITION

Ruboxistaurin (RBX) is an orally administered, isoform-selective inhibitor of PKC β that has been shown to have a positive effect in animal models of diabetic retinopathy[48] and improve diabetes-induced retinal hemodynamic abnormalities in patients with diabetes.[49] Two randomized controlled studies and a combined analysis of 2 additional studies have suggested a benefit to oral RBX in terms of reducing the rate of sustained moderate vision loss in patients with diabetes.[50–52] However, these studies did not achieve statistical significance in their primary end points and morphologic analysis of macular anatomy, including occurrence of significant center of macula involvement, OCT-determined center of macula thickness, and need for application of focal photocoagulation did not show a consistent trend in favor of or against

RBX. Additional studies are underway with other oral PKC inhibitors, and there may be a benefit to PKC inhibitors delivered intravitreally.

ANTI-VEGF AGENTS

There are currently 4 major anti-VEGF agents that are available in the United States and have been evaluated in treating DME: pegaptanib sodium (Macugen), ranibizumab (Lucentis), bevacizumab (Avastin), and aflibercept (Eylea)[53]; however, at present, only ranibizumab is approved by the FDA for this indication. Ranibizumab is the Fab fragment of the bevacizumab antibody.

The FDA approved pegaptanib sodium, an aptamer that binds selectively to the 165 isoform of VEGF, in 2004 for the treatment of all subtypes of neovascular age-related macular degeneration.[54] A phase 3, multicenter, randomized study (n = 260) has compared 0.3 mg of intravitreal pegaptanib every 6 weeks with a sham injection for DME. Patients in the study were permitted to receive focal macular laser treatment after study week 18 based on the ETDRS criteria. No significant safety issues were identified, and pegaptanib was found to be superior to sham injection with respect to 2-line visual acuity gains at 1 year (37% [pegaptanib] vs 20% [sham; P = .0047]). The mean BCVA at month 12 was +5.1 letters (pegaptanib) compared with +1.2 letters (sham; P<.05). Mean and BCVA at month 24 was +6.1 letters (pegaptanib) compared with 1.3 letters (sham; P<.01).[55]

Intravitreal bevacizumab is used off label to treat DME. A short-term level II study by Soheilian and colleagues[56,57] evaluating the visual acuity results of intravitreal bevacizumab alone or combined with intravitreal triamcinolone versus laser photocoagulation for DME found that patients who received bevacizumab injections had significantly better visual acuity outcomes at the 12- and 24-week follow-up compared with patients who received laser photocoagulation.

The Diabetic Retinopathy Clinical Research network (DRCR net) reported a phase II randomized exploratory clinical trial of the short-term effect of intravitreal bevacizumab for DME.[58] Patients in the study who received either 1.25 mg or 2.5 mg of intravitreal bevacizumab at baseline and again at 6 weeks had a greater reduction in retinal thickness measured by OCT at 3 weeks and an approximately 1-line improvement in vision at 12 weeks when compared with patients who had received focal laser photocoagulation. The study failed to demonstrate any short-term benefit by combining bevacizumab with laser photocoagulation.

Several additional studies have also demonstrated anatomic improvement in the morphology of the macula with decreased central retinal thickness in patients receiving 1.25 mg or 2.5 mg of intravitreal bevacizumab compared with laser treatment.[59–61] Most recently, the Bevacizumab or Laser Therapy study has provided support for longer-term usage of bevacizumab for DME.[62] This study (n = 80) compared 2-year results of intravitreal bevacizumab 1.25 mg versus focal macular laser treatment. The median improvement in BCVA was greater for intravitreal bevacizumab (+9 letters; median, 13 treatments) compared with macular laser treatment (+2.5 letters; median, 4 laser treatments; P = .005); however, although mean central macular thickness reduction was slightly greater in the intravitreal bevacizumab group at 24 months (−146 μm) compared with the macular laser treatment group (−118 μm), it was not statistically significant (P = .62).

A phase II prospective, double-masked clinical trial of intravitreal aflibercept demonstrated its benefit compared with macular laser for the treatment of DME.[63] In this study, 221 patients with clinically significant DME involving the central macula were randomized to 1 of 5 treatment protocols: group A, 0.5 mg aflibercept every

4 weeks; group B, 2 mg aflibercept every 4 weeks; group C, 2 mg aflibercept every 4 weeks for 3 months, then every 8 weeks; group D, 2 mg aflibercept every 4 weeks for 3 months, then as needed; and group E, focal/grid laser. At 24 weeks, aflibercept treatment groups had visual acuity improvements between +8.5 and +11.4 ETDRS letters compared with +2.5 letters in the laser group ($P \leq .0085$ for each treatment group vs laser). The OCT-measured mean central macular thickness was also reduced significantly in the groups treated with aflibercept. Adverse events were no different than with other intravitreal treatment agents.

Multiple studies have demonstrated the safety and efficacy of intravitreal ranibizumab for the treatment of DME. The DRCR net reported that patients treated with 0.5 mg intravitreal ranibizumab with prompt laser (n = 187, +9 ± 12 letters; $P<.001$) or deferred laser ($\geq$24 weeks; n = 188, +9 ± 12 letters; $P<.001$) had significantly superior visual acuity outcomes at the 1-year mark than those treated with sham injection plus prompt laser (n = 293, +3 ± 13 letters).[64] These positive effects were maintained at the 2-year follow-up.[65]

The ranibizumab monotherapy or combined with laser versus laser monotherapy for diabetic macular edema (RESTORE) trial[64] (345 patients) reported a 12-month visual acuity improvement of 6.1 ETDRS letters with intravitreal 0.5 mg ranibizumab monthly for 3 months then as needed (group A), a 5.9-letter improvement with 0.5 mg ranibizumab monthly for 3 months then as needed combined with focal laser photocoagulation (group B), compared with a 0.8-letter improvement with focal laser alone (group C). There was a statistically significant difference between both groups A and B compared with group C ($P<.0001$). In addition, the mean central retinal thickness also decreased significantly in both ranibizumab groups compared with laser alone (group A, -118.7 μm; group B, -128.3 μm; group C, $+61.3$ μm; $P<.001$ for both group A and group B).

The RISE (377 patients) and RIDE (382 patients) trials[65] are identical, parallel studies comparing monthly injections of 0.3 mg ranibizumab (group A), 0.5 mg ranibizumab (group B), or sham injection (group C) for the treatment of DME. At 3 months, rescue laser was made available to all patients. In the RISE trial at 24 months, 44.8% of patients (56 of 125) who received 0.3 mg ranibizumab and 39.2% of patients (49 of 125) who received 0.5 mg ranibizumab were able to read at least 15 more letters than at baseline compared with 18.1% of patients (23 of 127) who received sham injections. In the RIDE trial, at 24 months, 33.6% of patients (42 of 125) who received 0.3 mg ranibizumab and 45.7% of patients (58 of 127) who received 0.5 mg ranibizumab were able to read at least 15 more letters than at baseline compared with 12.3% of patients (16 of 130) who received sham injections. The 3-year follow-up results from RISE and RIDE have recently been published.[66] Visual acuity outcomes seen at month 24 were consistent through month 36; the proportions of patients who gained 15 or more letters from baseline at month 36 in the sham, 0.3-mg, and 0.5-mg ranibizumab groups were 19.2%, 36.8%, and 40.2%, respectively, in RIDE and 22.0%, 51.2%, and 41.6%, respectively, in RISE. Central retinal thickness reductions remained stable through 36 months. Patients originally in the sham injection group who ultimately crossed over to 0.5 mg ranibizumab did not achieve the visual acuity improvements seen in the groups originally randomized to intravitreal ranibizumab suggesting that early intervention is preferable to delayed treatment.

The short-term 6-month Ranibizumab for Edema of the Macula in Diabetes (READ-2) study[67] (126 patients) demonstrated that at 6 months patients who had received 0.5 mg of intravitreal ranibizumab at baseline and again at months 1, 3, and 5 had a significantly improved BCVA (+7.24 ETDRS letters; $P = .01$) compared with patients who had received focal/grid laser at baseline and month 3 if needed or a combination of 0.5 mg ranibizumab and focal/grid laser at baseline and month 3 (group 3). Improvement in visual acuity of 3 lines or more (>15 ETDRS letters) was observed in 22% in the intravitreal ranibizumab–alone group compared with 0% in the laser treatment–alone group (P = .002).

The Safety and Efficacy of Ranibizumab in Diabetic Macular Edema (RESOLVE) trial[68] (151 patients) compared 0.3 mg or 0.5 mg intravitreal ranibizumab monthly for 3 months, with dose-doubling allowed after 1 month (group A), with sham injection monthly for 3 months then as needed (group B). All patients were eligible to receive rescue grid laser at 1 year. The BCVA in the ranibizumab group was significantly superior (+10.3 ± 9.1 letters) versus the sham group (−1.4 ± 14.2 letters) (P<.0001). A total of 60.8% of the ranibizumab group had 10-letter gains compared with only 18.4% in the sham group (P<.0001). A corresponding reduction in central retinal thickness of −194.2 μm was seen in the ranibizumab group versus an increase of 48.4 μm (P<.0001) in the sham group. Moreover, a larger proportion of patients in the sham group (34.7) required rescue laser photocoagulation compared with the ranibizumab group (34.7%).

Based on these accumulated data, the FDA has approved the indication of treatment of DME for intravitreal bevacizumab (0.3 mg). The American Diabetes Association has now included intravitreal ranibizumab in its standards of care.[69]

However, treatment with intravitreal bevacizumab is not without significant expense. An analysis of the relative costs and treatment benefits of the various intravitreal anti-VEGF agents as well as other treatment methods for DME has been performed.[70] The cost per line of vision saved at 1 year was $11 372 to $11 609 for ranibizumab compared with $1329 to $2246 for bevacizumab, $3287 for vitrectomy surgery, $3749 for intravitreal triamcinolone, $5099 for laser photocoagulation, $5666 for dexamethasone implant, and $10 500 for pegaptanib. These costs translated to quality-adjusted life-years are $19 251 to $23 119 for ranibizumab compared with $2013 to $4160 for bevacizumab, $5862 for grid photocoagulation, $6246 for intravitreal triamcinolone, $8706 for vitrectomy surgery, $9446 for the dexamethasone implant, and $16 667 for pegaptanib. These costs will clearly increase as treatment and follow-up extend past 1 year.

TUMOR NECROSIS FACTOR (TNF)

TNF is a pleiotropic cytokine that has central importance to the development and homeostasis of the immune system and is a key regulator of cell activation, differentiation, and death.[38] Infliximab (Remicade) is a chimeric monoclonal antibody specific for human TNF that has been demonstrated to be of benefit in the treatment of chronic inflammatory diseases involving the joints, skin, and gut. It has been proposed that abnormal local expression of TNF may be important in the pathogenesis of diabetic vascular damage leading to macular edema and neovascularization[71,72] and that mild subclinical inflammation may influence many of the typical pathologic vascular changes of diabetic retinopathy.[73] It is also possible that high-dose NSAIDs delay the onset of diabetic retinopathy via TNF-alpha suppression. Furthermore, studies in patients with arthritis have shown that anti-TNF therapy decreases vascular permeability and angiogenesis by downregulating VEGF,[74] a key factor in the development and progression of diabetic retinopathy.

A small, randomized, double-blind, placebo-controlled, crossover study has recently shown that short-term intravenous treatment with infliximab could significantly improve BCVA in eyes with advanced-stage sight-threatening DME refractory to standard focal laser treatment with no noted systemic complications.[75] However, because of concerns about systemic toxicity and recent experience with the administration of several drugs intravitreally, a larger, retrospective, multicentered study from the Pan-American Collaborative Retina Study Group reviewing their experience with intravitreal infliximab and adalimumab for the treatment of refractory DME was recently published. This study did not find any visual benefit with intravitreally administered 1 mg or 2 mg of infliximab or 2 mg of adalimumab in eyes with DME that had not responded to focal laser photocoagulation but noted a high rate of severe inflammatory reactions elicited with the 2-mg dose of infliximab.[76] This finding has prompted a call for a moratorium on additional studies of intravitreal anti-TNF agents outside of a well-designed clinical trial.[77]

VITRECTOMY

Vitrectomy surgery has long been the treatment of patients with PDR who have lost vision from tractional and rhegmatogenous RD, epiretinal membranes, and nonclearing vitreous hemorrhages. Vitrectomy for DME was proposed more than 20 years ago. However, because of the high costs of the use of ongoing intravitreal pharmacologic agents, the need for close follow-up when these drugs are used, as well as long-term safety concerns (endophthalmitis, glaucoma, cataract, and so forth) vitrectomy and even peeling of the ILM for DME is being given closer scrutiny.

Vitrectomy for DME was initially described in a series of 10 patients with taut and thickened posterior vitreous hyaloid membranes, with 9 patients having improved vision postoperatively.[78] Studies in animals have shown that vitrectomy surgery to remove the formed vitreous gel and replace it with saline markedly improved the diffusion of oxygen throughout the vitreous cavity.[79] Reports that DME is present in 55% of the eyes of patients with diabetic retinopathy without posterior vitreous separation from the retina (PVD) but only in 20% with PVD[80] and that resolution of DME occurred in 55% of eyes experiencing spontaneous PVDs but in only 25% of eyes that did not develop PVD provide additional rationale to explain the benefit of vitrectomy surgery.[81] Although these studies did not provide proof of the exact mechanisms responsible for these differences, removal of the preretinal vitreous with its low partial pressure of oxygen and substituting the relatively highly oxygenated aqueous that fills the void is a reasonable explanation.

At present, there are no level 1 data proving the benefit of vitrectomy for DME, but a meta-analysis[82] of 37 studies (1881 patients) published since 2002 describing vitrectomy for DME suggests excellent reduction in OCT-measured central macular thickness (weighted average change of -187 μm), following vitrectomy comparing favorably with that achieved by intravitreal injections of anti-VEGF drugs with or without laser photocoagulation (range: -80 μm to -194 μm). These studies also demonstrate that macular edema resolves quickly after vitrectomy and that the effect is long lasting.[83] Studies of eyes that had previously undergone focal laser photocoagulation also demonstrated significant macular thinning after vitrectomy.[84] This finding was true for both retrospective (-242 μm) and prospective (-198 μm) studies.

Unfortunately, although vitrectomy surgery seems to cause rapid and long-lasting resolution of diabetic macular thickening, it is not at all clear whether it produces improvement in visual acuity. This ambiguity may be because in most series, vitrectomy was performed as a salvage procedure on eyes that had persistent and long-lasting edema resistant to other forms of treatment. Permanent and significant structural damage to the macula may have already occurred before undertaking vitrectomy. It is possible that vitrectomy performed earlier in the course of disease, maybe even as first-line therapy, would lead to better visual acuity results.[85]

It is also possible that in the future enzymatic vitreolysis may replace mechanical vitrectomy in some patients. Ocriplasmin (Jetrea, Thrombogenics, Iselin, NJ) has recently been approved by the FDA for enzymatic lysis of symptomatic vitreo-macular adhesions[86]; although there is no specific indication for patients with diabetic macular traction, with or without macular edema (patients with diabetes were excluded from the study), ocriplasmin may have a therapeutic role for selected patients. Vitreosolve (Vitreoretinal Technologies, Inc) is another vitreolytic agent currently in clinical trials for DME and the inhibition of progression of diabetic retinopathy.

DRCR NET

The DRCR net was initiated in 2002 with funding from the National Eye Institute of the NIH as a collaborative network dedicated to facilitating multicenter clinical research of diabetic retinopathy, DME, and associated conditions. The network currently includes more than 100 participating institutions and more than 300 physician investigators.

DRCR Protocol A compared the standard ETDRS technique of focal laser photocoagulation with a new mild macular grid (MMG) strategy for the treatment of clinically significant macular edema. This alternative approach involved the application of mild, widely spaced burns throughout the macula, avoiding the central foveal region. By protocol design, some of the MMG treatment burns were placed in areas of clinically normal retina if the entire retina was not abnormally thickened. These areas could include areas within the macula that were relatively distant from the area of clinically observed thickening. At 12 months after treatment, the MMG technique was found to be less effective at reducing retinal thickening than the standard ETDRS photocoagulation protocol. However, no statistically significant difference was seen in visual acuity outcomes between the two methods of treatment.[87]

DRCR Protocol B evaluated the efficacy and safety of 1-mg and 4-mg doses of intravitreal triamcinolone compared with focal/grid photocoagulation for the treatment of DME. Small previous studies had suggested a role for intravitreal steroids in refractory DME.[88,89] At the 4-month follow-up, the mean visual acuity was better in the 4-mg triamcinolone group than in either the laser group or the 1-mg triamcinolone group. However, by 1 year, no significant differences among groups in the mean visual acuity were seen; from the 16-month through 2-year follow-up, the mean visual acuity was better in the laser group than in the other two groups.[37] Intravitreal triamcinolone acetonide (4 mg) did seem to slightly reduce the risk of progression to PDR but not sufficiently to recommend its use given the cataract and glaucoma side effects.[39] In a separate DRCR protocol (Protocol E), no benefit was seen with peribulbar (adjacent to the eye but not directly into it) triamcinolone with or without laser photocoagulation in patients with DME and relatively good visual acuity (20/40 or better).[90]

DRCR Protocol H, a phase 2 study, suggested that in some patients anti-VEGF treatment with intravitreal bevacizumab (Avastin) may be of benefit in DME. DRCR Protocol T, which is currently underway, is comparing the 3 available anti-VEGF medications bevacizumab, ranibizumab, and aflibercept for DME.

DRCR Protocol I demonstrated that intravitreal ranibizumab (Lucentis) with prompt or deferred laser is more effective compared with prompt laser alone for the treatment of DME involving the central macula. In eyes that have already undergone cataract surgery, intravitreal triamcinolone with prompt laser seems more effective than laser alone; however, it frequently increases the risk of intraocular pressure elevation.[91,92]

DRCR Protocol J showed that one intravitreal triamcinolone injection or 2 ranibizumab injections in conjunction with focal/grid laser for DME and PRP is associated with better visual acuity and decreased macular edema than with laser treatment alone.[93]

Other current DRCR investigations include the following:

Protocol M: Effect of Diabetes Education During Retinal Ophthalmology Visits on Diabetes Control

Protocol N: An Evaluation of Intravitreal Ranibizumab for Vitreous Hemorrhage Due to Proliferative Diabetic Retinopathy

Protocol O: Comparison of Time Domain OCT and Spectral Domain OCT Retinal Thickness Measurement in Diabetic Macular Edema

Protocol P: A Pilot Study in Individuals with Center-Involved DME Undergoing Cataract Surgery

Protocol Q: An Observational Study in Individuals with Diabetic Retinopathy without Center-Involved DME Undergoing Cataract Surgery

Protocol R: A Phase II Evaluation of Topical Non-steroidal Antiinflammatory Agents in Eyes With Non-Central Involved Diabetic Macular Edema

Protocol S: Prompt PRP Compared With Ranibizumab With Deferred PRP for Proliferative Diabetic Retinopathy

Protocol T: A Comparative Effectiveness Study of Intravitreal Aflibercept, Bevacizumab, and Ranibizumab for Diabetic Macular Edema

Protocol V: Treatment (prompt anti-VEGF or prompt focal laser) versus observation for center involved DME in eye with very good visual acuity

The current understanding of all facets of diabetic retinopathy is still imperfect; however, the last several years have shown a tremendous increase in our knowledge of the pathogenesis of the damage that occurs in both NPDR and PDR as well as in our ability to treat their complications. New intravitreal medical treatments are gradually replacing standard laser photocoagulation for the treatment of all forms of diabetic retinopathy; both government- and industry-supported research is yielding exciting new insights. The challenge will be to deliver these new treatments in a cost-effective manner to the increasing number of patients who will need them.

REFERENCES

1. National Society to Prevent Blindness. Operational research department. Vision problems in the US: a statistical analysis. New York: National Society to Prevent Blindness; 1980. p. 146.
2. Patz A, Smith RE. The ETDRS and diabetes 2000. Ophthalmology 1991;98:739–40.
3. Kahn HA, Hiller R. Blindness caused by diabetic retinopathy. Am J Ophthalmol 1974;78(1):58.
4. Klein R, Klein BE, Moss SE, et al. The Wisconsin epidemiologic study of diabetic retinopathy. VI. Retinal photocoagulation. Ophthalmology 1987;94(7):747.
5. The Diabetes Control and Complications Trial Research Group: The effect of intensive treatment of diabetes on the development and progression of long-term complications in insulin-dependent diabetes mellitus. N Engl J Med 1993;329:977–86.
6. The DCCT Research Group: Effect of intensive diabetes management on macrovascular events and risk factors in the Diabetes Control and Complication Trial. Am J Cardiol 1995;75:894–903.

7. The DCCT Research Group: The relationship of glycemic exposure (HbA1c) to the risk of development and progression of retinopathy in the Diabetes Control and Complications Trial. Diabetes 1995;44:968–83.
8. UK Prospective Diabetes Study Group. Intensive blood-glucose control with sulphonylureas or insulin compared with conventional treatment and risk of complications in patients with type 2 diabetes. UKPDS 33. Lancet 1998;352(9131): 837–53.
9. Klein R, Klein BE, Syrjala SE, et al. Wisconsin Epidemiologic Study of Diabetic Retinopathy. 1. Relationship of diabetic retinopathy to management of diabetes. Preliminary report. In: Friedman EA, L'Esperance FA, editors. Diabetic renal-retinal syndrome. New York: Grune & Stratton; 1982. p. 21–40.
10. Klein R, Klein BE, Davis MD. Is cigarette smoking associated with diabetic retinopathy? Am J Epidemiol 1983;118:228–38.
11. Klein R, Klein BE, Moss SE, et al. The Wisconsin Epidemiologic Study of Diabetic Retinopathy. II. Prevalence and risk of diabetic retinopathy when age at diagnosis is less than 30 years. Arch Ophthalmol 1984;102:520–6.
12. Klein R, Klein BE, Moss SE, et al. The Wisconsin Epidemiologic Study of Diabetic Retinopathy. III. Prevalence and risk of diabetic retinopathy when age at diagnosis is 30 or more years. Arch Ophthalmol 1984;102:527–32.
13. Klein R, Klein BE, Moss SE, et al. The Wisconsin Epidemiologic Study of Diabetic Retinopathy. IV. Diabetic macular edema. Ophthalmology 1984;91:1464–74.
14. Zhang X, Saaddine JB, Chou C, et al. Prevalence of diabetic retinopathy in the United States, 2005-2008. JAMA 2010;304(6):649–56.
15. Diabetes Prevention Program Research Group. The prevalence of retinopathy in impaired glucose tolerance and recent-onset diabetes in the Diabetes Prevention Program. Diabet Med 2007;24:137–44.
16. Yanoff M, Fine BS. Ocular pathology: a text and atlas. Philadelphia: Harper and Row; 1982.
17. Gandorfer A, Rohleder M, Kampik A. Epiretinal pathology of vitreomacular traction syndrome. Br J Ophthalmol 2002;86:902–9.
18. Early treatment diabetic retinopathy study. Report number 12. Fundus photographic risk factors for progression of diabetic retinopathy. Ophthalmology 1991;98:823–33.
19. American Academy of Ophthalmology Retina Panel. Preferred practice pattern guidelines. Diabetic retinopathy. San Francisco (CA): American Academy of Ophthalmology; 2008 (4th printing 2012). Available at: www.aao.org/ppp.
20. Early Treatment Diabetic Retinopathy Study Research Group. Early photocoagulation for diabetic retinopathy. ETDRS report number 9. Ophthalmology 1991; 98:766–85.
21. Klein R, Klein BE, Neider MW, et al. Diabetic retinopathy as detected using ophthalmoscopy, a nonmydriatic camera and a standard fundus camera. Ophthalmology 1985;92:485–91.
22. Rosberger DF, Schachat AP, Bressler SB, et al. Availability of color fundus photographs from previous visit affects practice patterns for patients with diabetes mellitus. Arch Ophthalmol 1998;116(12):1607.
23. Yannuzzi LA, Rohrer KT, Tindel LJ, et al. Fluorescein angiography complication survey. Ophthalmology 1986;93:611–7.
24. Sunness JS. The pregnant woman's eye. Surv Ophthalmol 1988;32:219–39.
25. McDonald HR, Williams GA, Scott IU, et al. Laser scanning imaging for macular disease: a report by the American Academy of Ophthalmology. Ophthalmology 2001;114:1221–8.

26. Browning DJ, Glassman AR, Aiello LP, et al. Relationship between ocular coherence tomography-measured central retinal thickness and visual acuity in diabetic macular edema. Ophthalmology 2007;114:525–36.

27. Röttinger EM, Heckemann R, Scherer E, et al. Radiation therapy of choroidal metastases from breast cancer. Albrecht Von Graefes Arch Klin Exp Ophthalmol 1976;200(3):243–50.

28. ETDRS Research Group. Photocoagulation for diabetic macular edema. Arch Ophthalmol 1985;103:1796–806.

29. Bressler NM, Rosberger DF. Photocoagulation for diabetic retinopathy and other causes of retinal neovascularization. In: Gottsch J, Stark W, Goldberg M, editors. Ophthalmic surgery. London: Oxford University Press; 1999. p. 361–73.

30. Diabetic Retinopathy Study Research Group. Indications for photocoagulation treatment of diabetic retinopathy: diabetic retinopathy study report number 14. Int Ophthalmol Clin 1987;27:239–53.

31. Diabetic Retinopathy Clinical Research Network, Brucker AJ, Qin H, et al. Observational study of the development of diabetic macular edema following panretinal (scatter) photocoagulation given in 1 or 4 sittings. Arch Ophthalmol 2009;127(2):132–40.

32. Bressler NB, Rosberger D. Complications of photocoagulation. In: Gottsch J, Stark W, Goldberg M, editors. Ophthalmic surgery. Oxford University Press; 1999. p. 361–73 p. 390–3.

33. Joussen AM. Nonsteroidal anti-inflammatory drugs prevent early diabetic retinopathy via TNF-a suppression. FASEB J 2002;16:438.

34. Gillies MC, Simpson JM, Gaston C, et al. Five-year results of a randomized trial with open label extension of triamcinolone acetonide for refractory diabetic macular edema. Ophthalmology 2009;116(11):2182–7.

35. Lam DS, Chan CK, Mohamed S, et al. Prospective randomized trial of different doses of intravitreal triamcinolone for diabetic macular edema. Br J Ophthalmol 2007;91(2):199–203.

36. Kim JE, Pollack JS, Miller DG, et al, ISIS Study Group. ISIS-DME: a prospective, randomized, dose escalation intravitreal steroid injection study for refractory diabetic macular edema. Retina 2008;28(5):735–40.

37. Diabetic Retinopathy Clinical Research Network. A randomized trial comparing intravitreal triamcinolone acetonide and focal/grid photocoagulation for diabetic macular edema. Ophthalmology 2008;115(9):1447–9, 1449.e1–10.

38. Beck RW, Edwards AR, Aiello LP, et al, Diabetic Retinopathy Clinical Research Network (DRCR.net). Three-year follow-up of a randomized trial comparing focal/grid photocoagulation and intravitreal triamcinolone for diabetic macular edema. Arch Ophthalmol 2009;127(3):245–51.

39. Bressler NM, Edwards AR, Beck RW, et al, for the Diabetic Retinopathy Clinical Research Network. Exploratory analysis of diabetic retinopathy progression through 3 years in a randomized clinical trial that compares intravitreal triamcinolone acetonide with focal/grid photocoagulation. Arch Ophthalmol 2009;127(12):1566–71.

40. Zacks DN, Johnson MW. Combined intravitreal injection of triamcinolone acetonide and panretinal photocoagulation for concomitant diabetic macular edema and proliferative diabetic retinopathy. Retina 2005;25(2):135–40.

41. Margolis R, Singh RP, Bhatnagar P, et al. Intravitreal triamcinolone as adjunctive treatment to laser panretinal photocoagulation for concomitant proliferative diabetic retinopathy and clinically significant macular oedema. Acta Ophthalmol 2008;86(1):105–10.

42. Faghihi H, Taheri A, Farahvash MS, et al. Intravitreal triamcinolone acetonide injection at the end of vitrectomy for diabetic vitreous hemorrhage: a randomized, clinical trial. Retina 2008;28(9):1241–6.
43. Haller JA, Kuppermann BD, Blumenkranz MS, et al. Randomized controlled trial of an intravitreous dexamethasone drug delivery system in patients with diabetic macular edema. Arch Ophthalmol 2010;128(3):289–96.
44. Kuppermann BD, Blumenkranz MS, Haller JA, et al, Dexamethasone DDS Phase II Study Group. Randomized controlled study of an intravitreous dexamethasone drug delivery system in patients with persistent macular edema. Arch Ophthalmol 2007;125(3):309–17.
45. Zucchiatti I, Lattanzio R, Querques G, Querques L, Del Turco C, Cascavilla ML, Bandello F. Intravitreal dexamethasone implant in patients with persistent diabetic macular edema. Ophthalmologica 2012;228:117–22.
46. Pearson PA, Comstock TL, Ip M, et al. Fluocinolone acetonide intravitreal implant for diabetic macular edema: a 3-year multicenter, randomized, controlled clinical trial. Ophthalmology 2011;118:1580–7.
47. Kane FE, Burdan J, Cutino A. Iluvien: a new sustained delivery technology for posterior eye disease. Expert Opin Drug Deliv 2008;5(9):1039–46.
48. Aiello LP, Bursell SE, Clermont A, et al. Vascular endothelial growth factor-induced retinal permeability is mediated by protein kinase C in vivo and suppressed by an orally effective beta-isoform-selective inhibitor. Diabetes 1997; 46:1473–80.
49. Aiello LP, Clermont A, Arora V, et al. Inhibition of PKC beta by oral administration of ruboxistaurin is well tolerated and ameliorates diabetes-induced retinal hemodynamic abnormalities in patients. Invest Ophthalmol Vis Sci 2006;47:86–92.
50. The PKC-DRS Study Group. The effect of ruboxistaurin on visual loss in patients with moderately severe to very severe nonproliferative diabetic retinopathy: initial results of the Protein Kinase C beta Inhibitor Diabetic Retinopathy Study (PKC-DRS) multicenter, randomized clinical trial. Diabetes 2005;54:2188–97.
51. The PKC-DRS2 Study Group. The effect of ruboxistaurin on visual loss in patients with diabetic retinopathy. Ophthalmology 2006;113:2221–30.
52. Sheetz MJ, Aiello LP, Davis MD, et al. The effect of oral PKC beta inhibitor ruboxistaurin on vision loss in two phase 3 studies. Invest Ophthalmol Vis Sci 2013;54: 1750–7.
53. Ho AC, Scott IU, Kim SJ, et al. Anti–vascular endothelial growth factor pharmacotherapy for diabetic macular edema: a report by the American Academy of Ophthalmology. Ophthalmology 2012;119:2179–88.
54. U.S. Food and Drug Administration new drug application (NDA) number: 21–756. Approved labeling. Macugen (pegaptanib sodium injection).
55. Sultan MB, Zhou D, Macugen 1013 Study Group, et al. A phase 2/3, multicenter, randomized, double-masked, 2-year trial of pegaptanib sodium for the treatment of diabetic macular edema. Ophthalmology 2011;118:1107–18.
56. Soheilian M, Ramezani A, Bijanzadeh B, et al. Intravitreal bevacizumab (Avastin) injection alone or combined with triamcinolone versus macular photocoagulation as primary treatment of diabetic macular edema. Retina 2007;27:1187–95.
57. Soheilian M, Ramezani A, Obudi A, et al. Randomized trial of intravitreal bevacizumab alone or combined with triamcinolone versus macular photocoagulation in diabetic macular edema. Ophthalmology 2009;116:1142–50.
58. Diabetic Retinopathy Clinical Research Network. A phase II randomized clinical trial of intravitreal bevacizumab for diabetic macular edema. Ophthalmology 2007;114:1860–7.

59. Solaiman KA, Diab MM, Abo-Elenin M. Intravitreal bevacizumab and/or macular photocoagulation as a primary treatment for diffuse diabetic macular edema. Retina 2011;30:1638–45.
60. Arevalo JF, Sanchez JG, Pan-American Collaborative Retina Study Group (PACORES), et al. Primary intravitreal bevacizumab for diffuse diabetic macular edema: the Pan-American Collaborative Retina Study Group at 24 months. Ophthalmology 2009;116:1488–97.
61. Haritoglou C, Kook D, Neubauer A, et al. Intravitreal bevacizumab (Avastin) therapy for persistent diffuse diabetic macular edema. Retina 2006;26:999–1005.
62. Rajendram R, Fraser-Bell S, Kaines A, et al. A 2-year prospective randomized controlled trial of intravitreal bevacizumab or laser therapy (BOLT) in the management of diabetic macular edema: 24-month data: report 3. Arch Ophthalmol 2012;130(8):972–9.
63. Do DV, Schmidt-Erfurth U, Gonzalez VH, et al. The DA VINCI Study: phase 2 primary results of VEGF Trap-Eye in patients with diabetic macular edema. Ophthalmology 2011;118:1819–26.
64. Mitchell P, Bandello F, RESTORE Study Group, et al. The RESTORE Study: ranibizumab monotherapy or combined with laser versus laser monotherapy for diabetic macular edema. Ophthalmology 2011;118:615–25.
65. Nguyen QD, Brown DM, Marcus DM, et al, RISE and RIDE Research Group. Ranibizumab for diabetic macular edema: results from 2 phase III randomized trials: RISE and RIDE. Ophthalmology 2012;119:789–801.
66. Brown DM, Nguyen QD, Marcus DM. Long-term outcomes of ranibizumab therapy for diabetic macular edema: the 36-month results from two phase III trials: RISE and RIDE. Ophthalmology 2013;120(10):2013–22.
67. Nguyen QD, Shah SM, READ-2 Study Group, et al. Primary end point (six months) results of the Ranibizumab for Edema of the mAcula in Diabetes (READ-2) study. Ophthalmology 2009;116:2175–81.
68. Massin P, Bandello F, Garweg JG, et al. Safety and efficacy of ranibizumab in diabetic macular edema (RESOLVE Study): a 12-month, randomized, controlled, double-masked, multicenter phase II study. Diabetes Care 2010;33:2399–405.
69. American Diabetes Association. Standards of medical care in diabetes—2013. Diabetes Care 2013;36:S11–66.
70. Smiddy WE. Economic considerations of macular edema therapies. Ophthalmology 2011;118:1827–33.
71. Limb GA, Webster L, Soomro H, et al. Platelet expression of tumour necrosis factor-α (TNF-α), TNF receptors and intercellular adhesion molecule-1 (ICAM-1) in patients with proliferative diabetic retinopathy. Clin Exp Immunol 1999;118: 213–8.
72. Limb GA, Hollifield RD, Webster L, et al. Soluble TNF receptors in vitreoretinal proliferative disease. Invest Ophthalmol Vis Sci 2001;42:1586–91.
73. Adamis AP, Berman AJ. Immunological mechanisms in the pathogenesis of diabetic retinopathy. Semin Immunopathol 2008;30:65–84.
74. Cañete JD, Pablos JL, Sanmartí R, et al. Antiangiogenic effects of anti-tumor necrosis factor α therapy with infliximab in psoriatic arthritis. Arthritis Rheum 2004; 50:1636–41.
75. Sfikakis PP, Grigoropolous V, Emfietzoglou I, et al. Infliximab for diabetic macular edema refractory to laser photocoagulation: a randomized, double-blind, placebo-controlled, crossover, 32-week study. Diabetes Care 2010;33:1523–8.
76. Wu L, Hernandez-Bogantes E, Roca J, et al. Intravitreal tumor necrosis factor inhibitors in the treatment of refractory diabetic macular edema: a pilot study

from the Pan American Collaborative Retina Study Group. Retina 2011;31: 298–303.

77. Pulido JS, Pulido JE, Michet CJ, et al. More questions than answers: a call for a moratorium on the use of intravitreal infliximab outside of a well-designed trial. Retina 2010;30:1–5.

78. Lewis H, Abrams GW, Blumenkranz MS, et al. Vitrectomy for diabetic macular traction and edema associated with posterior hyaloidal traction. Ophthalmology 1992;99:753–9.

79. Gisladottir S, Loftsson T, Stefansson E. Diffusion characteristics of vitreous humour and saline solution follow the Stokes Einstein equation. Graefes Arch Clin Exp Ophthalmol 2009;247:1677–84.

80. Nasrallah FP, Jalkh AE, VanCoppenrolle F, et al. The role of the vitreous in diabetic macular edema. Ophthalmology 1988;95:1335–9.

81. Hikichi T, Fujio N, Akiba Y, et al. Association between the short-term natural history of diabetic macular edema and the vitreomacular relationship in type 2 diabetes mellitus. Ophthalmology 1997;104:473–8.

82. Landers MB, Kon Graveren VA, Stewart MW. Early vitrectomy for DME: does it have a roll? Retin Physician 2013;10:46–53.

83. Kumagai K, Furukawa M, Ogino N, et al. Long-term follow-up of vitrectomy for diffuse nontractional diabetic macular edema. Retina 2009;29:464–72.

84. Browning DJ, Fraser CM, Powers ME. Comparison of the magnitude and time course of macular thinning induced by different interventions for diabetic macular edema: implications for sequence of application. Ophthalmology 2006;113: 1713–9.

85. Kimura T, Kiryu J, Nishiwaki H, et al. Efficacy of surgical removal of the internal limiting membrane in diabetic cystoid macular edema. Retina 2005;25: 454–61.

86. Stalmans P, Benz MS, Gandorfer A, et al. Enzymatic vitreolysis with ocriplasmin for vitreomacular traction and macular holes. N Engl J Med 2012;367:606–15.

87. Writing Committee for the Diabetic Retinopathy Clinical Research Network, Fong DS, Strauber SF, et al. Comparison of the modified Early Treatment Diabetic Retinopathy Study and mild macular grid laser photocoagulation strategies for diabetic macular edema. Arch Ophthalmol 2007;125(4):469–80.

88. Jonas JB, Sofker A. Intraocular injection of crystalline cortisone as adjunctive treatment of diabetic macular edema. Am J Ophthalmol 2001;132:425–7.

89. Martidis A, Duker JS, Greenberg PB, et al. Intravitreal triamcinolone for refractory diabetic macular edema. Ophthalmology 2002;109:920–7.

90. Diabetic Retinopathy Clinical Research Network, Chew E, Strauber S, et al. Randomized trial of peribulbar triamcinolone acetonide with and without focal photocoagulation for mild diabetic macular edema: a pilot study. Ophthalmology 2007;114(6):1190–6.

91. Diabetic Retinopathy Clinical Research Network. Randomized trial evaluating ranibizumab plus prompt or deferred laser or triamcinolone plus prompt laser for diabetic macular edema. Ophthalmology 2010;117(6):1064–77.e35.

92. Diabetic Retinopathy Clinical Research Network. Expanded 2-year follow-up of ranibizumab plus prompt or deferred laser or triamcinolone plus prompt laser for diabetic macular edema. Ophthalmology 2011;118(4):609–14.

93. Diabetic Retinopathy Clinical Research Network. Randomized trial evaluating short-term effects of intravitreal ranibizumab or triamcinolone acetonide on macular edema following focal/grid laser for diabetic macular edema in eyes also receiving panretinal photocoagulation. Retina 2011;31(6):1009–27.

Diabetic Neuropathy

Aaron I. Vinik, MD, PhD*, Marie-Laure Nevoret, MD,
Carolina Casellini, MD, Henri Parson, PhD

KEYWORDS

- Diabetic nephropathy • Painful neuropathy • Diabetes mellitus • Pregabalin

KEY POINTS

- Diabetic neuropathy (DN) is the most common and troublesome complication of diabetes mellitus, leading to the greatest morbidity and mortality and resulting in a huge economic burden for diabetes care.
- Diabetic peripheral neuropathy has been recently defined as a symmetric, length-dependent sensorimotor polyneuropathy attributable to metabolic and microvascular alterations as a result of chronic hyperglycemia exposure (diabetes) and cardiovascular risk covariates.
- Both the clinical assessment and treatment options are multifactorial. Patients with DN should be screened for autonomic neuropathy, as there is a high degree of coexistence of the 2 complications.
- Two drugs have been approved for neuropathic pain in the United States, pregabalin and duloxetine, but neither of these has afforded complete relief, even when used in combination.

INTRODUCTION

Diabetic neuropathy (DN) is the most common and troublesome complication of diabetes mellitus (DM), leading to the greatest morbidity and mortality and resulting in a huge economic burden for diabetes care.[1,2] It is the most common form of neuropathy in the developed countries of the world, accounts for more hospitalizations than all the other diabetic complications combined, and is responsible for 50% to 75% of nontraumatic amputations.[2,3] DN is a set of clinical syndromes that affect distinct regions of the nervous system, singly or combined. It may be silent and go undetected while exercising its ravages; or it may present with clinical symptoms and signs that, although nonspecific and insidious with slow progression, also mimic those seen in many other diseases. DN is, therefore, diagnosed by exclusion. Unfortunately both endocrinologists and nonendocrinologists have not been trained to recognize the condition, and even when DN is symptomatic, less than one-third of physicians recognize the cause or discuss this with their patients.[4]

Internal Medicine, Strelitz Diabetes Center, Eastern Virginia Medical School, 855 West Brambleton Avenue, Norfolk, VA 23510, USA
* Corresponding author.
E-mail address: VinikAI@evms.edu

Endocrinol Metab Clin N Am 42 (2013) 747–787
http://dx.doi.org/10.1016/j.ecl.2013.06.001
0889-8529/13/$ – see front matter © 2013 Elsevier Inc. All rights reserved.

The true prevalence is not known, and reports vary from 10% to 90% in diabetic patients, depending on the criteria and methods used to define neuropathy.[2,3,5,6] Twenty-five percent of patients attending a diabetes clinic volunteered symptoms; 50% were found to have neuropathy after a simple clinical test such as the ankle jerk or vibration perception test; and almost 90% tested positive to sophisticated tests of autonomic function or peripheral sensation.[7] Neurologic complications occur equally in type 1 and type 2 DM and additionally in various forms of acquired diabetes.[6] The major morbidity associated with somatic neuropathy is foot ulceration, the precursor of gangrene and limb loss. Neuropathy increases the risk of amputation 1.7-fold, 12-fold if there is deformity (itself a consequence of neuropathy), and 36-fold if there is a history of previous ulceration.[8] Each year 96,000 amputations are performed on diabetic patients in the United States, yet up to 75% of them are preventable.[3] Globally there is an amputation every 30 seconds. DN also has a tremendous impact on patients' quality of life (QOL) predominantly by causing weakness, ataxia, and incoordination, predisposing to falls and fractures.[9] Once autonomic neuropathy sets in, life can become dismal and the mortality rate can approximate 25% to 50% within 5 to 10 years.[10,11]

SCOPE OF THE PROBLEM

Diabetic peripheral neuropathy (DPN) is a common late complication of diabetes. It results in a variety of syndromes for which there is no universally accepted classification. Such neuropathies are generally subdivided into focal/multifocal neuropathies, including diabetic amyotrophy, and symmetric polyneuropathies, including sensorimotor polyneuropathy (DSPN). The latter is the most common type, affecting about 30% of diabetic patients in hospital care and 25% of those in the community.[12,13] DPN has been recently defined as a symmetric, length-dependent sensorimotor polyneuropathy attributable to metabolic and microvascular alterations as a result of chronic hyperglycemia exposure (diabetes) and cardiovascular risk covariates.[14] Its onset is generally insidious, and without treatment the course is chronic and progressive. The loss of small-fiber–mediated sensation results in the loss of thermal and pain perception, whereas large-fiber impairment results in loss of touch and vibration perception. Sensory-fiber involvement may also result in "positive" symptoms, such as paresthesias and pain. Nonetheless, up to 50% of neuropathic patients can be asymptomatic. DPN can be associated with the involvement of the autonomic nervous system (ie, diabetic autonomic neuropathy that rarely causes severe symptoms),[15,16] but in its cardiovascular form is definitely associated with at least a 3-fold increased risk for mortality.[17–19] More recently, diabetic autonomic neuropathy or even autonomic imbalance between the sympathetic and the parasympathetic nervous systems has been implicated as a predictor of cardiovascular risk.[18,19]

EPIDEMIOLOGY OF NEUROPATHIC PAIN

Neuropathic pain is not uncommon, but may be correctable in some instances. Perhaps a little recognized fact is that mononeuritis and entrapments are 3 times as common as DPN, and fully one-third of the diabetic population has some form of entrapment[20] which, when recognized, is readily amenable to intervention.[21] Even more impressive is the mounting evidence that even with impaired glucose tolerance (IGT), patients may experience pain.[22–24] In the general population (region of Augsburg, Southern Germany), the prevalence of painful peripheral neuropathy was 13.3% in the diabetic subjects, 8.7% in those with IGT, 4.2% in those with impaired fasting glucose (IFG), and 1.2% in those with normal glucose tolerance (NGT).[25] Among survivors of myocardial infarction (MI) from the Augsburg MI Registry, the prevalence of neuropathic pain was 21% in the patients with diabetes, 14.8% in those with IGT, 5.7% in those with IFG, and 3.7% in those with NGT.[24] Thus, subjects with macrovascular disease appear to be prone to neuropathic pain. The most important risk factors of DSPN and neuropathic pain in these surveys were age, obesity, and low physical activity while the predominant comorbidity was peripheral arterial disease, highlighting the paramount role of cardiovascular risk factors and diseases in prevalent DSPN.

CLASSIFICATION OF DIABETIC NEUROPATHIES

Fig. 1 and **Table 1** describe the different forms of diabetic neuropathies. It is important to be aware that different forms of DN often coexist in the same patient (eg, distal polyneuropathy and carpal tunnel syndrome).

PATHOGENESIS OF DIABETIC NEUROPATHIES

Causative factors include persistent hyperglycemia, microvascular insufficiency, oxidative and nitrosative stress, defective neurotropism, and autoimmune-mediated nerve destruction. **Fig. 2** summarizes the current view of the pathogenesis of DN.[12] Detailed discussion of the different theories is beyond the scope of this article, and there are several excellent recent reviews. However, DN is a heterogeneous group of conditions with widely varying pathology, suggesting differences in pathogenic mechanisms for the different clinical syndromes. Recognition of the clinical homolog of these pathologic processes is the first step in achieving the appropriate form of intervention.

CLINICAL PRESENTATION

The spectrum of clinical neuropathic syndromes described in patients with DM includes dysfunction of almost every segment of the somatic peripheral and autonomic nervous system.[26] Each syndrome can be distinguished by its pathophysiologic, therapeutic, and prognostic features.

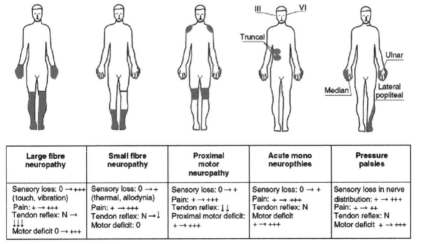

Large fibre neuropathy	Small fibre neuropathy	Proximal motor neuropathy	Acute mono neuropthies	Pressure palsies
Sensory loss: 0 →+++ (touch, vibration) Pain: + → +++ Tendon reflex: N → ↓↓↓ Motor deficit 0 → +++	Sensory loss: 0 →+ (thermal, allodynia) Pain: + →+++ Tendon reflex: N→↓ Motor deficit: 0	Sensory loss: 0→+ Pain: +→+++ Tendon reflex: ↓↓ Proximal motor deficit: + → +++	Sensory loss: 0 → + Pain: + → +++ Tendon reflex: N Motor deficit + →+++	Sensory loss in nerve distribution: + → +++ Pain: + → ++ Tendon reflex: N Motor deficit + → +++

Fig. 1. Clinical manifestations of small-fiber and large-fiber neuropathies. N, normal. (*From* Vinik AI, Mehrabyan A. Diabetic neuropathies. Med Clin N Am 2004;88:947–99; with permission.)

Table 1
Distinguishing characteristics of mononeuropathies, entrapment syndromes, and distal symmetric polyneuropathy

Feature	Mononeuropathy	Entrapment Syndrome	Neuropathy
Onset	Sudden	Gradual	Gradual
Pattern	Single nerve but may be multiple	Single nerve exposed to trauma	Distal symmetric poly neuropathy
Nerves involved	CN III, VI, VII, ulnar, median, peroneal	Median, ulnar, peroneal, medial, and lateral plantar	Mixed, motor, sensory, autonomic
Natural history	Resolves spontaneously	Progressive	Progressive
Distribution of sensory loss	Area supplied by the nerve	Area supplied beyond the site of entrapment	Distal and symmetric. "Glove and stocking" distribution

Abbreviation: CN, cranial nerves.

Focal and Multifocal Neuropathies

Focal neuropathies comprise focal-limb neuropathies and cranial neuropathies. Focal-limb neuropathies are usually due to entrapment, and mononeuropathies must be distinguished from these entrapment syndromes (see **Fig. 1**).[27,28] Mononeuropathies often occur in the older population; they have an acute onset, are associated with pain, and have a self-limiting course resolving in 6 to 8 weeks. Mononeuropathies

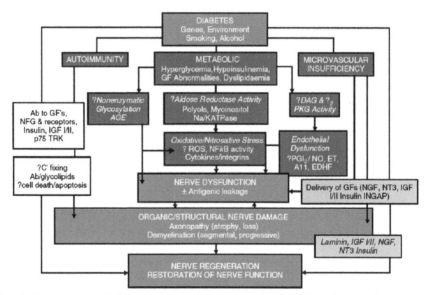

Fig. 2. Pathogenesis of diabetic neuropathies. Ab, antibody; AGE, advance glycation end products; ATPase, adenosine triphosphatase; C', complement; DAG, diacylglycerol; EDHF, endothelium-derived hyperpolarizing factor; ET, endothelin; GF, growth factor; IGF, insulin-like growth factor; NFkB, nuclear factor κB; NGF, nerve growth factor; NO, nitric oxide; NT3, neurotropin 3; PGI₂, prostaglandin I₂; PKC, protein kinase C; ROS, reactive oxygen species; TRK, tyrosine kinase. (*From* Vinik A, Ullal J, Parson HK, et al. Diabetic neuropathies: clinical manifestations and current treatment options. Nat Clin Pract Endocrinol Metab 2006;2:269–81; with permission.)

can involve the median (5.8% of all diabetic neuropathies), ulnar (2.1%), radial (0.6%), and common peroneal nerves.[29] Cranial neuropathies in diabetic patients are extremely rare (0.05%) and occur in older individuals with a long duration of diabetes.[30] Entrapment syndromes start slowly, and will progress and persist without intervention. Carpal tunnel syndrome occurs 3 times as frequently in diabetics as in healthy populations,[31] and is found in up to one-third of patients with diabetes. Its increased prevalence in diabetes may be related to repeated undetected trauma, metabolic changes, and/or accumulation of fluid or edema within the confined space of the carpal tunnel.[28] The diagnosis is confirmed by electrophysiologic studies. Treatment consists of rest, aided by placement of a wrist splint in a neutral position to avoid repetitive trauma. Anti-inflammatory medications and steroid injections are sometimes useful. Surgery should be considered if weakness appears and medical treatment fails.[16,27]

Proximal Motor Neuropathy (Diabetic Amyotrophy) and Chronic Demyelinating Neuropathies

For many years proximal neuropathy has been considered a component of DN. Its pathogenesis was ill understood,[32] and its treatment was neglected with the anticipation that the patient would eventually recover, albeit over a period of some 1 to 2 years and after suffering considerable pain, weakness, and disability. The condition has several synonyms including diabetic amyotrophy and femoral neuropathy. It can be clinically identified based on the occurrence of these common features: (1) it primarily affects the elderly (50–60 years old) with type 2 DM; (2) onset can be gradual or abrupt; (3) it presents with severe pain in the thighs, hips, and buttocks, followed by significant weakness of the proximal muscles of the lower limbs with inability to rise from the sitting position (positive Gower maneuver); (4) it can start unilaterally and then spread bilaterally; (5) it often coexists with distal symmetric polyneuropathy; and (6) it is characterized by muscle fasciculation, either spontaneous or provoked by percussion. Pathogenesis is not yet clearly understood, although immune-mediated epineurial microvasculitis has been demonstrated in some cases. The condition is now recognized as being secondary to a variety of causes unrelated to diabetes, but which have a greater frequency in patients with diabetes than in the general population. It includes patients with chronic inflammatory demyelinating polyneuropathy (CIDP), monoclonal gammopathy, circulating GM1 antibodies, and inflammatory vasculitis.[30,31,33,34]

Treatment options include: intravenous immunoglobulin for CIDP,[35] plasma exchange for monoclonal gammopathy of unknown significance, steroids and azathioprine for vasculitis, and withdrawal of drugs or other agents that may have caused vasculitis. It is important to divide proximal syndromes into these 2 subcategories, because the CIDP variant responds dramatically to intervention,[36,37] whereas amyotrophy runs its own course over months to years. Until more evidence is available, they should be considered separate syndromes.

Diabetic Truncal Radiculoneuropathy

Diabetic truncal radiculoneuropathy affects middle-aged to elderly patients and has a predilection for males. Pain is the most important symptom, and occurs in a girdle-like distribution over the lower thoracic or abdominal wall. It can be unilaterally or bilaterally distributed. Motor weakness is rare. Resolution generally occurs within 4 to 6 months.

Rapidly Reversible Hyperglycemic Neuropathy

Reversible abnormalities of nerve function may occur in patients with recently diagnosed or poorly controlled diabetes. These disorders are unlikely to be caused by structural abnormalities, as recovery soon follows restoration of euglycemia. Rapidly reversible hyperglycemic neuropathy usually presents with distal sensory symptoms, and whether these abnormalities result in an increased risk of developing chronic neuropathies in the future remains unknown.[16,38]

Generalized Symmetric Polyneuropathy

Acute sensory neuropathy

Acute sensory (painful) neuropathy is considered by some investigators a distinctive variant of distal symmetric polyneuropathy. The syndrome is characterized by severe pain, cachexia, weight loss, depression, and, in males, erectile dysfunction. It occurs predominantly in male patients and may appear at any time in the course of both type 1 and type 2 DM. Conditions such as Fabry disease, amyloidosis, human immunodeficiency virus (HIV) infection, heavy-metal poisoning (such as arsenic), and excess alcohol consumption should be excluded.[39]

Acute sensory neuropathy is usually associated with poor glycemic control, but may also appear after sudden improvement of glycemia, and has been associated with the onset of insulin therapy, being termed insulin neuritis on occasions.[40] Although the pathologic basis has not been determined, one hypothesis suggests that changes in blood glucose flux produce alterations in epineurial blood flow, leading to ischemia. Other investigators relate this syndrome to diabetic lumbosacral radiculoplexus neuropathy (DLRPN) and propose an immune-mediated mechanism.[41]

The key in the management of this syndrome is achieving stability of blood glucose.[40] Most patients also require medication for neuropathic pain.[42] The natural history of this disease is resolution of symptoms within 1 year.[43]

Chronic Sensorimotor Neuropathy or Distal Symmetric Polyneuropathy

Clinical presentation and pain characteristics

DPN is probably the most common form of the diabetic neuropathies.[16,41] It is seen in both type 1 and type 2 DM with similar frequency, and may be already present at the time of diagnosis of type 2 DM.[44] A population survey reported that 30% of type 1 and 36% to 40% of type 2 diabetic patients experienced neuropathic symptoms.[45] Several studies have also suggested that IGT may lead to polyneuropathy, reporting rates of IGT in patients with chronic idiopathic polyneuropathies between 30% and 50%.[46–49] Studies using skin and nerve biopsies have shown progressive reduction in peripheral nerve fibers from the time of the diagnosis of diabetes or even in earlier prediabetic stages (IGT and metabolic syndrome).[50,51] Sensory symptoms are more prominent than motor symptoms and usually involve the lower limbs; these include pain, paresthesias, hyperesthesias, deep aching, burning, and sharp stabbing sensations similar to but less severe than those described in acute sensory neuropathy. In addition, patients may experience negative symptoms such as numbness in the feet and legs, leading in time to painless foot ulcers and subsequent amputations if the neuropathy is not promptly recognized and treated. Unsteadiness is also frequently seen, owing to abnormal proprioception and muscle sensory function.[52,53] Alternatively, some patients may be completely asymptomatic, and signs may be only discovered by a detailed neurologic examination.

On physical examination a symmetric stocking-like distribution of sensory abnormalities in both lower limbs is usually seen. In more severe cases the hands may be involved. All sensory modalities can be affected, particularly vibration, touch, and position perceptions (large Aα/β fiber damage); and pain, with abnormal heat and cold temperature perception (small thinly myelinated Aδ and unmyelinated C fiber damage) (**Fig. 3**). Deep tendon reflexes may be absent or reduced, especially in the lower

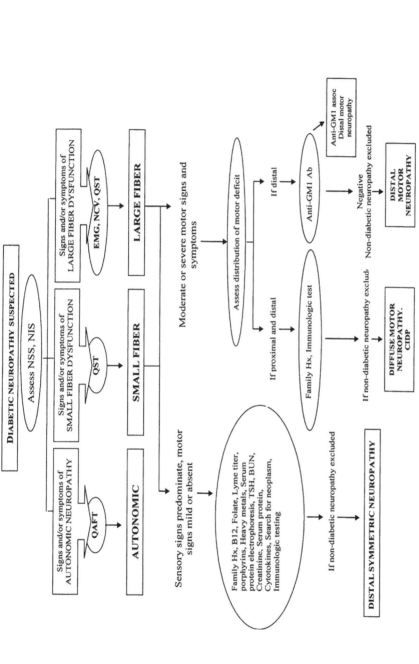

Fig. 3. Evaluation of the patient suspected of having DPN. A diagnostic algorithm for assessment of neurologic deficit and classification of neuropathic syndromes. B12, vitamin B$_{12}$; BUN, blood urea nitrogen; CIDP, chronic inflammatory demyelinating polyneuropathy; EMG, electromyogram; Hx, history; MGUS, monoclonal gammopathy of unknown significance; NCV, nerve conduction velocity studies; NIS, neurologic impairment score (sensory and motor evaluation); NSS, neurologic symptom score; QAFT, quantitative autonomic function tests; QST, quantitative sensory tests.

extremities. Mild muscle wasting may be seen, but severe weakness is rare and should raise the question of a possible nondiabetic origin of the neuropathy.[6,16,41] DPN is frequently accompanied by autonomic neuropathy (see later discussion). It is important to remember that all patients with DPN are at increased risk of neuropathic complications such as foot ulceration and Charcot neuroarthropathy.

Pain associated with a peripheral nerve injury has several distinct clinical characteristics. Some describe bees stinging through the socks, whereas others talk of walking on hot coals. The pain, worse at night, keeps the patient awake and is associated with sleep deprivation.[9] Patients volunteer allodynia (pain due to a stimulus that does not normally cause pain, eg, stroking) or pain from normal stimuli, such as the touch of bedclothes, and may have hyperesthesias (increased sensitivity to touch) or hyperalgesia (increased sensitivity to painful stimuli). These symptoms may be paradoxic, with differences in sensation to one or other modality of stimulation. Unlike animal models of DPN, the pain is spontaneous and does not need provocation. It has a glove-and-stocking distribution. Pain usually occurs at rest and improves with ambulation, in contrast to osteoarthritic pain, which is worsened with ambulation and decreased with rest. Pain may persist over several years, causing considerable disability and impaired QOL in some patients, whereas it remits partially or completely in others despite further deterioration in small-fiber function. Pain exacerbation or even acute onset of pain tends to be associated with sudden metabolic changes, insulin neuritis, short duration of pain or diabetes, or preceding weight loss, and has less severe or no sensory loss, and normal strength and reflexes.

By contrast, the nociceptive pain of inflammatory arthritis does not have these qualities. It is localized to the joints, starts with morning stiffness, and improves as the day wears on.[54] Fasciitis pain is localized to the fascia; entrapment produces pain in a dermatome; and claudication is made worse by walking.

Clinical manifestations of small-fiber neuropathies (see **Fig. 1**):

- Small thinly myelinated Aδ and unmyelinated C fibers are affected
- Prominent symptoms with burning, superficial, or lancinating pain often accompanied by hyperalgesia, dysesthesia, and allodynia
- Progression to numbness and hypoalgesia (disappearance of pain may not necessarily reflect nerve recovery but rather nerve death, and progression of neuropathy must be excluded by careful examination)
- Abnormal cold and warm thermal sensation
- Abnormal autonomic function with decreased sweating, dry skin, impaired vasomotion and skin blood flow, with cold feet
- Intact motor strength and deep tendon reflexes
- Negative findings from nerve conduction velocity (NCV) studies
- Loss of cutaneous nerve fibers on skin biopsies
- Can be diagnosed clinically by reduced sensitivity to 1.0 g Semmes-Weinstein monofilament and prickling pain perception using the Wartenberg wheel or similar instrument
- Patients are at higher risk of foot ulceration and subsequent gangrene and amputations

Clinical manifestations of large-fiber neuropathies (see **Fig. 1**):

- Large myelinated, rapidly conducting Aα/β fibers are affected and may involve sensory and/or motor nerves
- Prominent signs with sensory ataxia (waddling like a duck), wasting of small intrinsic muscles of feet and hands, with hammertoe deformities and weakness of hands and feet

- Abnormal deep tendon reflexes
- Impaired vibration perception (often the first objective evidence), light touch, and joint position perception
- Shortening of the Achilles tendon with pes equinus
- Symptoms may be minimal: sensation of walking on cotton, pain is deep-seated and gnawing in quality, "like a toothache" in the foot, floors feeling "strange," inability to turn the pages of a book, or inability to discriminate among coins; in some patients with severe distal muscle weakness, inability to stand on the toes or heels
- Abnormal NCV findings
- Increased skin blood flow with hot feet
- Patients are at higher risk of falls, fractures, and development of Charcot neuroarthropathy
- Most patients with DPN, however, have a "mixed" variety of neuropathy with both large and small nerve-fiber damage

Diagnostic assessment of DPN

Because of the lack of agreement on the definition and diagnostic assessment of neuropathy, several consensus conferences were convened to overcome the current problems, the most recent of which has redefined the minimal criteria for the diagnosis of typical DSPN as summarized here.[14] **Tables 2** and **3** provide information on the appropriate testing for each nerve fiber type and its function.

Toronto classification of distal symmetric diabetic polyneuropathies[14]:

1. *Possible DSPN*. The presence of symptoms or signs of DSPN may include the following: symptoms—decreased sensation, positive neuropathic sensory symptoms (eg, "asleep numbness," prickling or stabbing, burning or aching pain) predominantly in the toes, feet, or legs; or signs—symmetric decrease of distal sensation or unequivocally decreased or absent ankle reflexes.
2. *Probable DSPN*. The presence of a combination of symptoms and signs of neuropathy including any 2 or more of the following: neuropathic symptoms, decreased distal sensation, or unequivocally decreased or absent ankle reflexes.
3. *Confirmed DSPN*: The presence of an abnormality of nerve conduction and a symptom or symptoms, or a sign or signs, of neuropathy confirm DSPN. If nerve conduction is normal, a validated measure of small-fiber neuropathy (SFN) (with class 1 evidence) may be used. To assess for the severity of DSPN, several approaches can be recommended: for example, the graded approach outlined

Table 2			
Examination: bedside sensory tests			
Sensory Modality	**Nerve Fiber**	**Instrument**	**Associated Sensory Receptors**
Vibration	Aβ (large)	128 Hz tuning fork	Ruffini corpuscle mechanoreceptors
Pain (pinprick)	C (small)	Neuro-tips	Nociceptors for pain and warmth
Pressure	Aβ, Aα (large)	1 g and 10 g monofilament	Pacinian corpuscle
Light touch	Aβ, Aα (large)	Wisp of cotton	Meissner corpuscle
Cold	Aδ (small)	Cold tuning fork	Cold thermoreceptors

Table 3
Advanced objective testing for diabetic neuropathy

Neurologic Test	Type of Neuropathy	Measurement	Advantages
Quantitative sensory testing	Small- and large-fiber neuropathies	Assessment of sensory deficits	Uses controlled quantifiable stimuli with standard procedures
Skin biopsy and intraepidermal nerve fiber (IENF) density	Small-fiber neuropathy	Small-caliber sensory nerves including somatic unmyelinated IENFs, dermal myelinated nerve fibers, and autonomic nerve fibers	Quantitates small epidermal nerve fibers through various antibody staining
Corneal confocal microscopy	Small-fiber neuropathy	Detects small nerve fiber loss in the cornea	Noninvasive technique that correlates with neuropathy severity
Contact heat evoked potentials	Small-fiber neuropathy	Uses nociceptive heat as a stimulus that is recorded through electroencephalographic readings	Detects small-fiber neuropathy in the absence of other indices
Sudomotor function	Distal small-fiber neuropathy	Assesses the sweat response by analyzing sweat production or sweat chloride concentrations	Detects early neurophysiologic abnormalities in peripheral autonomic function
Nerve conduction studies	Small- and large-fiber neuropathy	Measure the ability of the nerves to conduct an electrical stimulus	Standardized universal technique that is well documented and recommended

above; various continuous measures of sum scores of neurologic signs, symptoms, or nerve test scores; scores of function of activities of daily living; or scores of predetermined tasks or of disability.

4. *Subclinical DSPN.* The presence of no signs or symptoms of neuropathy are confirmed with abnormal nerve conduction or a validated measure of SFN (with class 1 evidence). Definitions 1, 2, or 3 can be used for clinical practice, and definitions 3 or 4 can be used for research studies.

5. *Small-fiber neuropathy (SFN).* SFN should be graded as follows: (1) possible: the presence of length-dependent symptoms and/or clinical signs of small-fiber damage; (2) probable: the presence of length-dependent symptoms, clinical signs of small-fiber damage, and normal sural nerve conduction; and (3) definite: the presence of length-dependent symptoms, clinical signs of small-fiber damage, normal sural nerve conduction, and altered intraepidermal nerve-fiber (IENF) density at the ankle and/or abnormal thermal thresholds at the foot.

The diagnosis of DSPN should rest on the findings of the clinical and neurologic examinations; that is, the presence of neuropathic symptoms (positive and negative, sensory and motor) and signs (sensory deficit, allodynia and hyperalgesia, motor weakness, absence of reflexes).[55]

1. Symptoms alone have poor diagnostic accuracy in predicting the presence of polyneuropathy.
2. Signs are better predictors than symptoms.
3. Multiple signs are better predictors than a single sign.
4. Relatively simple examinations are as accurate as complex scoring systems.

Thus, both symptoms and signs should be assessed. The following findings should alert the physician to consider causes for DSPN other than diabetes and referral for a detailed neurologic workup: (1) pronounced asymmetry of the neurologic deficits, (2) predominant motor deficits, mononeuropathy, or cranial nerve involvement, (3) rapid development or progression of the neuropathic impairments, (4) progression of the neuropathy despite optimal glycemic control, (5) symptoms from the upper limbs, (6) family history of nondiabetic neuropathy, and (7) a diagnosis of DSPN cannot be ascertained by clinical examination.[56]

Conditions Mimicking Diabetic Neuropathy

There are several conditions that can be mistaken for painful DN: intermittent claudication, whereby the pain is exacerbated by walking; Morton neuroma, whereby the pain and tenderness are localized to the intertarsal space and are elicited by applying pressure with the thumb in the appropriate intertarsal space; osteoarthritis, whereby the pain is confined to the joints, made worse with joint movement or exercise, and associated with morning stiffness that improves with ambulation; radiculopathy, whereby the pain originates in the shoulder, arm, thorax, or back, and radiates into the legs and feet; Charcot neuropathy, whereby the pain is localized to the site of the collapse of the bones of the foot, and the foot is hot rather than cold as occurs in neuropathy; plantar fasciitis, whereby there is shooting or burning in the heel with each step and there is exquisite tenderness in the sole of the foot; and tarsal tunnel syndrome, whereby the pain and numbness radiate from beneath the medial malleolus to the sole and are localized to the inner side of the foot. These conditions contrast with the pain of DPN, which is bilateral, symmetric, covers the whole foot and particularly the dorsum, and is worse at night, interfering with sleep.

The most important differential diagnoses from the general medicine perspective include neuropathies caused by alcohol abuse, uremia, hypothyroidism, vitamin B_{12} deficiency, peripheral arterial disease, cancer, inflammatory and infectious diseases, and neurotoxic drugs.[57]

A good medical history is essential to exclude other causes of neuropathy: a history of trauma, cancer, unexplained weight loss, fever, substance abuse, or HIV infection suggests that an alternative source should be sought. As recommended for all patients with distal symmetric polyneuropathy, screening laboratory tests may be considered in selected patients with DSPN, serum B_{12} with its metabolites and serum protein immunofixation electrophoresis being those with the highest yield of abnormalities.[58]

Clinical Assessment Tools for Diabetic Neuropathy

Clinical assessment should be standardized using validated scores for both the severity of symptoms and the degree of neuropathic deficits which are sufficiently reproducible. These assessments would include the Michigan Neuropathy Screening Instrument (MNSI)[59]; the Neuropathy Symptom Score for neuropathic symptoms; and the Neuropathy Disability Score or the Neuropathy Impairment Score (NIS) for neuropathic deficits.[5] The Neurologic Symptom Score has 38 items that capture symptoms of muscle weakness, sensory disturbances, and autonomic dysfunction. The neurologic history and examination should be performed initially and then with all subsequent visits. These questionnaires are useful for patient follow-up and to assess response to treatment. As discussed earlier, the exclusive presence of neuropathic symptoms without deficits is not sufficient to diagnose DSPN. Therefore, early stages of DSPN or painful small-fiber neuropathy with or without minimal deficits can only be verified using more sophisticated tests such as thermal thresholds or skin biopsy.

Objective Devices for the Diagnosis of Neuropathy

The neurologic examination should focus on the lower extremities and should always include an accurate foot inspection for deformities, ulcers, fungal infection, muscle wasting, hair distribution or loss, and the presence or absence of pulses. Sensory modalities should be assessed using simple handheld devices (touch by cotton wool or soft brush; vibration by 128-Hz tuning fork; pressure by the Semmes-Weinstein 1-g and 10-g monofilament; pinprick by Wartenberg wheel, Neurotip, or temperature by cold and warm objects) (level of evidence Ia/A).[60] Finally, the Achilles reflexes should be tested (see **Table 2**).[61,62]

More sophisticated testing of DN can be conducted according to the findings of the clinical neurologic examination. These tests and indications for their use are described in **Table 2**. Some are readily available in the clinical setting, whereas others are still confined to the research environment.

Summary of Clinical Assessment of DPN

A detailed clinical examination is the key to the diagnosis of DPN. The last position statement of the American Diabetes Association recommends that all patients with diabetes be screened for DN at diagnosis in type 2 DM and 5 years after diagnosis in type 1 DM. DN screening should be repeated annually and must include sensory examination of the feet and ankle reflexes.[61] One or more of the following can be used to assess sensory function: pinprick (using the Wartenberg wheel or similar instrument), temperature, vibration perception (using 128-Hz tuning fork), or 1-g and 10-g monofilament pressure perception at the distal halluces. Combinations of more than 1 test have more than 87% sensitivity in detecting DPN.[61,63] Longitudinal studies have shown that these simple tests are good predictors of risk for foot ulcer.[64] Numerous composite scores to evaluate clinical signs of DN, such as the NIS, are currently available. In combination with symptom scores, these are useful in documenting and monitoring neuropathic patients in the clinic.[65] The feet should always be examined in detail to detect ulcers, calluses, and deformities, and footwear must be inspected at every visit.

It is widely recognized that neuropathy per se can affect the QOL of the diabetic patient. Several instruments have been developed and validated to assess QOL in DN. The NeuroQoL measures patients' perceptions of the impact of neuropathy and foot ulcers.[66] The Norfolk QOL questionnaire for DN is a validated tool addressing specific symptoms and the impact of functions of large, small, and autonomic nerve fibers.

The diagnosis of DPN is mainly a clinical one, with the aid of specific diagnostic tests according to the type and severity of the neuropathy. However, other nondiabetic causes of neuropathy must always be excluded, depending on the clinical findings (vitamin B_{12} deficiency, hypothyroidism, uremia, CIDP, and so forth) (see **Fig. 3**).

TREATMENT OF DIABETIC POLYNEUROPATHIES

Treatment of DN should be targeted toward several different aspects: first, treatment of specific underlying pathogenic mechanisms; second, treatment of symptoms and improvement in QOL; and third, prevention of progression and treatment of complications of neuropathy (see **Fig. 1**, **Tables 6** and **7**).[67]

Treatment of Specific Underlying Pathogenic Mechanisms

Glycemic and metabolic control

Several long-term prospective studies have assessed the effects of intensive diabetes therapy on the prevention and progression of chronic diabetic complications. Studies in type 1 diabetic patients show that intensive diabetes therapy retards but does not completely prevent the development of DSPN. In the DCCT/EDIC cohort, the benefits of former intensive insulin treatment persisted for 13 to 14 years after DCCT closeout and provided evidence of a durable effect of prior intensive treatment on polyneuropathy and cardiac autonomic neuropathy ("hyperglycemic memory") (Ia/A).[68,69]

By contrast, in type 2 diabetic patients, who represent the vast majority of people with diabetes, the results were largely negative. The UK Prospective Diabetes Study (UKPDS) showed a lower rate of impaired vibration perception threshold (VPT) (>25 V) after 15 years for intensive therapy (IT) versus conventional therapy (CT) (31% vs 52%). However, the only additional time point at which VPT reached a significant difference between IT and CT was the 9-year follow-up, whereas the rates after 3, 6, and 12 years did not differ between the groups. Likewise, the rates of absent knee and ankle reflexes as well as the heart-rate responses to deep breathing did not differ between the groups.[70] In the ADVANCE study of 11,140 patients with type 2 DM randomly assigned to either standard glucose control or intensive glucose control, the relative risk reduction (95% confidence interval [CI]) for new or worsening neuropathy for intensive versus standard glucose control after a median of 5 years of follow-up was −4 (−10 to 2), without a significant difference between the groups.[71]

In the Steno 2 Study,[72] intensified multifactorial risk intervention including intensive diabetes treatment, angiotensin-converting enzyme inhibitors, antioxidants, statins, aspirin, and smoking cessation in patients with microalbuminuria showed no effect on DSPN after 7.8 (range: 6.9–8.8) years and again at 13.3 years, after the patients were subsequently followed for a mean of 5.5 years. However, the progression of cardiac autonomic neuropathy (CAN) was reduced by 57%. Thus, there is no evidence that intensive diabetes therapy or a target-driven intensified intervention aimed at multiple risk factors favorably influences the development or progression of DSPN as opposed to CAN in type 2 diabetic patients. However, the Steno study used only vibration detection, which measures exclusively the changes in large-fiber function.

Oxidative stress

Several studies have shown that hyperglycemia causes oxidative stress in tissues that are susceptible to complications of diabetes, including peripheral nerves. **Fig. 2** presents our current understanding of the mechanisms and potential therapeutic pathways for oxidative stress–induced nerve damage. Studies show that hyperglycemia induces an increased presence of markers of oxidative stress, such as superoxide and peroxynitrite ions, and that antioxidant defense moieties are reduced in patients with DPN.[73] Advanced glycation end products (AGE) are the result of nonenzymatic addition of glucose or other saccharides to proteins, lipids, and nucleotides. In diabetes, excess glucose accelerates AGE generation, which leads to intracellular and extracellular protein cross-linking and protein aggregation.

Therapies known to reduce oxidative stress are therefore recommended. Therapies that are under investigation include aldose reductase inhibitors, α-lipoic acid, γ-linolenic acid, benfotiamine, and protein kinase C inhibitors (**Table 4**).

Table 4
Oxidative stress therapeutic targets

Therapy	Mechanism	Clinical Improvements
Aldose reductase inhibitors (ARIs)	Reduce the flux of glucose through the polyol pathway, inhibiting tissue accumulation of sorbitol and fructose	Neuropathy symptoms, nerve conduction velocity, and vibration perception
α-Lipoic acid	Antioxidant properties and thiol-replenishing redox-modulating properties	Microcirculation and reversal of neuropathy symptoms
γ-Linolenic acid	—	Clinical and eletrophysiologic tests
Benfotiamine	Transketolase activator that reduces tissue advanced glycation end products	Conduction velocity in peroneal nerve and vibratory perception when combined with vitamin B_6/B_{12}
Protein kinase C inhibitors	Decrease production of vasoconstrictive, angiogenic, and chemotactic cytokines	Neuropathy symptoms and nerve conduction velocity
Methylcobolamin, methylfolate, and pyridoxal phosphate	Reduction of peroxynitrite and superoxide and restoration of glutathione levels to normal. Also restore the coupling of endogenous nitric acid synthase, reducing nitrosative and oxidative stress and therefore improving microvascular function	Reduce nerve damage, may also improve sensory nerve conduction and skin nerve fiber density

Growth factors

There is increasing evidence that there is a deficiency of nerve growth factor (NGF) in diabetes, as well as the dependent neuropeptides substance P and calcitonin gene-related peptide (CGRP), and that this contributes to the clinical perturbations in small-fiber function.[74] Clinical trials with NGF have not been successful but are subject to certain caveats with regard to design; however, NGF still holds promise for sensory and autonomic neuropathies.[75] The pathogenesis of DN includes loss of vasa nervorum, so it is likely that appropriate application of vascular endothelial growth factor (VEGF) would reverse the dysfunction. Introduction of the VEGF gene into the muscle of DM animal models improved nerve function.[76] There are ongoing VEGF gene studies with transfection of the gene into the muscle in humans. INGAP peptide comprises the core active sequence of Islet Neogenesis-Associated Protein (INGAP), a pancreatic cytokine that can induce new islet formation and restore euglycemia in diabetic rodents. Tam and colleagues[77] showed significant improvement in thermal hypoalgesia in diabetic mice after a 2-week treatment with INGAP peptide; humans have shown an increase in C-peptide secretion in type 1 DM patients and improvement in glycemic control in type 2 DM patients.[78] Nonetheless, information about its effect on DPN is still lacking. Finally, human trials are ongoing with human hepatocyte growth factor (HGF), which has been shown to be a potent angiogenic, antiapoptotic, and neurotropic factor. Because of the multiplicity of its actions, HGF is an intriguing candidate for targeting the complex pathogenesis of DN.[79–84]

Immune therapy

Several different autoantibodies in human sera have been reported that can react with epitopes in neuronal cells and have been associated with DN. The authors have reported a 12% incidence of a predominantly motor form of neuropathy in patients with diabetes associated with monosialoganglioside antibodies (anti-GM1 antibodies).[85] Perhaps the clearest link between autoimmunity and neuropathy has been the demonstration of an 11-fold increased likelihood of CIDP, multiple motor polyneuropathy, vasculitis, and monoclonal gammopathies in diabetes.[86] New data, however, support a predictive role of the presence of antineuronal antibodies on the later development of neuropathy, suggesting that these antibodies may not be innocent bystanders but neurotoxins.[87,88] There may be select cases, particularly those with autonomic neuropathy, evidence of antineuronal autoimmunity, and CIDP, that may benefit from intravenous immunoglobulin or large dose steroids.[36]

Treatment of Symptoms and Improvement in QOL

Pain, QOL, and comorbidities in diabetic neuropathy

Pain is the reason for 40% of patient visits in a primary care setting, and about 20% of these have had pain for longer than 6 months.[89] Chronic pain may be nociceptive, which occurs as a result of disease or damage to tissue wherein there is no abnormality in the nervous system. By contrast, experts in the neurology and pain community define neuropathic pain as "pain arising as a direct consequence of a lesion or disease affecting the somatosensory system."[90] Persistent neuropathic pain interferes significantly with QOL, impairing sleep and recreation; it also significantly affects emotional well-being, and is associated with, if not the cause of, depression, anxiety, loss of sleep, and noncompliance with treatment.[91] Painful diabetic peripheral neuropathy (PDPN) is a clinical problem that is difficult to manage, and patients with PDPN are more apt to seek medical attention than those with other types of DN. Two population-based studies showed that neuropathic pain is associated with a greater psychological burden than nociceptive pain,[92] and is considered to be more severe than other pain types. Early recognition of psychological problems is critical to the management of pain, and physicians need to go beyond the management of pain per se if they are to achieve success. Patients may also complain of decreased physical activity and mobility, increased fatigue, and negative effects on their social lives. Providing significant pain relief markedly improves QOL measures, including sleep and vitality.[9,93] Pathway analysis has shown that drugs that relieve pain may do so directly or indirectly via effects on sleep, depression, and anxiety, and an algorithm is provided for appropriate selection based on the comorbidities (**Fig. 4**).[94,95]

Castro and Daltro[96] studied 400 patients with depression, anxiety, and sleep disturbances. Two-thirds of depressed patients and three-quarters of anxious patients had pain, but the most impressive finding was that more than 90% of sleep-deprived patients had experienced pain. As a corollary, Gore and colleagues[97] showed that with increasing pain severity there was a linear increase in Hospital Anxiety and Depression Scales (HADS) pain and depression scores. The impact of depression complicated diabetes management, increased length of hospital stays, and almost doubled the yearly cost of diabetes management from $7000 to $11,000.[98] Moreover, Gupta and colleagues[99] showed that higher scores for anxiety, depression, and sleep disturbances predicted the development of pain.

Several studies have consistently found that neuropathic pain has a negative impact on global health-related QOL. A systematic review of 52 studies in patients with 1 out of 6 different disorders associated with neuropathic pain, including PDPN, established

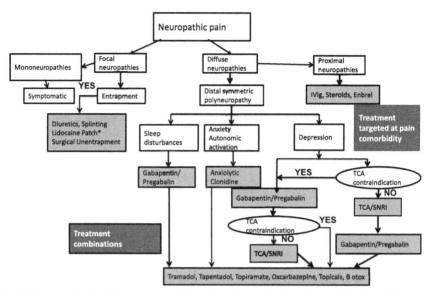

Fig. 4. Treatment algorithm: neuropathic pain after exclusion of nondiabetic etiology and stabilization of glycemic control. (*Adapted from* Vinik A. The approach to the management of the patient with neuropathic pain. J Clin Endocrinol Metab 2010;95:4802–811; and Vinik, A. Management of the Patient with Neuropathic Pain. In: Wartofsky L, editor. A clinical approach to endocrine and metabolic diseases, Vol 2. Chevy Chase (MD): The Endocrine Society, 2012. p. 177–94; with permission.)

that neuropathic pain impairs physical and emotional functioning, role functioning (including participation in gainful employment), sleep, and, to a lesser degree, social functioning. In addition, there is also evidence suggesting an association between neuropathic pain and depression, as for other types of pain.[91,100] The impact of pain on QOL in PDPN has recently been shown in 1111 patients: physical and mental QOL were significantly more impaired in patients with PDPN than in both diabetic patients without neuropathy and those with non-PDPN.[22] The nature of pain may also be important, as Daousi and colleagues[101] have reported significantly poorer QOL in patients with PDPN than in diabetic patients with non-neuropathic pain.

The diagnostic workup
Because of its complexity the presentation of pain poses a diagnostic dilemma for the clinician, who needs to distinguish between neuropathic pain arising as a direct consequence of a lesion or disease of the somatosensory system, and nociceptive pain that is due to trauma, inflammation, or injury. It is imperative to try to establish the nature of any predisposing factor, including the pathogenesis of the pain, if one is to be successful in its management. Management of neuropathic pain requires a sound relationship between patient and physician, with an emphasis on a positive outlook and encouragement that there is a solution, using patience and targeted pain-centered strategies that deal with the underlying disorder rather than the usual Band-Aid prescription of drugs approved for general pain, which do not address the disease process. The inciting injury may be focal or diffuse and may involve single or, more likely, multiple mechanisms such as metabolic disturbances encompassing hyperglycemia, dyslipidemia, glucose fluctuations, or intensification of therapy with insulin. On the other hand, the injury might embrace autoimmune mechanisms, neurovascular insufficiency, deficient neurotropism, oxidative and nitrosative stress, and

inflammation.[12,42] Because pain syndromes in diabetes may be focal or diffuse, proximal or distal, acute or chronic, each has its own pathogenesis, and the treatment must be tailored to the underlying disorder if the outcome is to be successful. The presence of diabetes must be established if this has not already been done.

The diagnosis of neuropathic pain

The diagnosis of neuropathic pain, as opposed to pain from causes other than neuropathy, is first and foremost made by careful history taking. Patients should be queried at the time of an office visit as to whether they are experiencing tingling, burning, or pain at rest in their feet. A positive response warrants further investigation and screening for PDPN. Somatosensory, motor, and autonomic bedside evaluation can be done and is complemented by use of one of the pain screening tools (Douleur Neuropathique en 4 questions [DN4], Pain DETECT, and so forth).[102] The physician should ensure that all the features of pain such as distribution, quality, severity, timing, associated symptoms, and exacerbating and relieving factors (if any) are recorded. In particular, the presence of numbness, burning, tingling, lightning pain, stabbing, and prickling should be recorded, as is done in the Norfolk QOL tool (Ia/A),[9] the Neuropathy Total Symptom Score-6 questionnaire (NTSS-6),[103] and the Pain DETECT.[102] Secondly, pain intensity and quality should be assessed, using pain intensity scales (Visual Analog Scale or NRS) (Ia/A)[104] and pain questionnaires (Brief Pain Inventory [BPI], Neuropathic Pain Symptom Inventory [NPSI]). Several tools and questionnaires have been developed to quantify the impact of pain on sleep, mood, and QOL, mainly to be used in clinical trials. In clinical practice the BPI Interference scale, the Profile of Moods, or the HADS can provide a simple measure of the impact of pain on QOL. Responses to treatment by self-reporting using a diary can record the course of painful symptoms and their impact on daily life (Ia/A).[105] These reports are also most useful for outcomes measures in clinical trials on drugs used for pain relief. Validated scoring systems for symptoms and signs are available in the form of questionnaires or checklists, such as the Neuropathy Symptom Score and the MNSI questionnaire for symptoms, and the MNSI and the Neuropathy Disability Score for signs (Ia/A).[59,106]

Definition of neuropathic pain

A definition of peripheral neuropathic pain in diabetes, adapted from a definition proposed by the International Association for the Study of Pain,[90] is "pain arising as a direct consequence of abnormalities in the peripheral somatosensory system in people with diabetes."[14] A grading system for the degree of certainty of the diagnosis of neuropathic pain has been proposed. It is based on 4 simple criteria, namely:

1. Whether the pain has a distinct neuroanatomical distribution
2. Whether the history of the patient suggests the presence or absence of a lesion or disease of the peripheral or central somatosensory system
3. Whether either of these findings is supported by at least 1 confirmatory test
4. Whether there is an abnormality of nerve conduction[90]

Degree of certainty is defined according to the number of criteria met: 1 to 4 (definite neuropathic pain); 1 and 2 plus 3 or 4 (probable neuropathic pain); or only 1 and 2 (possible neuropathic pain). There is no consensus on their diagnostic validity, because neuropathic pain is a composite of pain and other sensory symptoms associated with nerve injury. For example, sensory deficits, abnormal spontaneous or induced sensations such as paresthesias (eg, tingling), spontaneous attacks of electric shock-like sensations, and allodynia preclude a simple definition (see later discussion).

Distinction between nociceptive and non-nociceptive pain

Several tools have been developed to differentiate non-nociceptive stimuli (allodynia), increased pain sensitivity to stimuli (hyperalgesia),[107] and summation, which is progressive worsening of pain caused by repeated mild noxious stimuli (IIb/B).[102] Several self-administered questionnaires have been developed, validated, translated, and subjected to cross-cultural adaptation to both diagnose and distinguish neuropathic as opposed to non-neuropathic pain (Leeds Assessment of Neuropathic Symptoms and Signs Pain Scale, DN4, Neuropathic Pain Questionnaire, Pain DETECT, and ID-Pain).[102,108–113] Others assess pain quality and intensity (assessment questionnaires such as the Short-Form McGill Pain Questionnaire, the BPI, and the NPSI) (III/B).[108,114,115]

According to IMMPACT (Initiative on Methods, Measurement and Pain Assessment in Clinical Trials), the following pain characteristics should be evaluated to assess the efficacy and effectiveness of chronic pain treatment[116]:

1. Pain intensity measured on a 0 to 10 numerical rating scale (NRS)
2. Physical functioning assessed by the Multidimensional Pain Inventory (MPI) and BPI Interferences scale
3. Emotional functioning, assessed by the Beck Depression Inventory and Profile of Mood states
4. Patient rating of overall improvement, assessed by the Patient Global Impression of Change (PGI-C) (III/B)

Laboratory tests to evaluate neuropathic pain

Because neuropathic pain is subjective there are no tests that can objectively quantify this in humans, meaning that the results of laboratory tests become useful only in the context of a comprehensive clinical examination.

Late laser-evoked potentials (Aδ-LEPs) are the easiest and most reliable neurophysiologic tools for assessing nociceptive Aδ-fiber pathway function, useful in both peripheral and central neuropathic pain, with the limitation of very low availability (IIb/B).[117] The morphologic study of cutaneous nerve fibers using skin biopsy and IENF density assessment is regarded as a reproducible marker of small-fiber sensory pathology, but is still not widely available. Functional neuroimaging techniques, such as positron emission tomography for the central nervous system and functional magnetic resonance (MR) imaging for both central and peripheral nervous systems (MR neurography), have been used mainly for research purposes to evaluate the central mechanisms of pain in chronic pain conditions or to visualize intraneural and extraneural lesions of peripheral nerves (IV/C).[118]

Contact heat-evoked potential stimulation (CHEPS) was introduced to study nociceptive pathways by using a contact thermode that rapidly increases skin temperature. The CHEPS device delivers rapid heat pulses to selectively stimulate Aδ and C fibers while simultaneously recording cerebral evoked potentials. Several groups have established CHEPS as a clinically feasible approach to examine the physiology of thermonociceptive nerves. CHEPS is a noninvasive technique that can objectively evaluate small-fiber dysfunction. It has been shown that patients with sensory neuropathy of differing etiology have lower CHEPS amplitudes, which correlates with IENF densities.[119–121] Chao and colleagues[122] evaluated 32 type 2 diabetic patients with painful neuropathy. CHEP amplitudes were reduced in diabetic patients compared with age- and sex-matched control subjects, and abnormal CHEP patterns (reduced amplitude or prolonged latency) were noted in 81.3% of these patients. The CHEP amplitude was the most significant parameter correlated with IENF density ($P = .003$) and pain perception to contact heat stimuli ($P = .019$) on multiple linear regression models. The authors' group evaluated 31 healthy controls and 30 patients with type 2 DM and DPN using neurologic examination, NCV, autonomic function tests, quantitative sensory tests (QST), and CHEPS. CHEPS amplitudes were significantly reduced in the DPN group at the lower back (44.93 ± 6.5 vs 23.87 ± 3.36 μV; $P<.01$), lower leg (15.87 ± 1.99 vs 11.68 ± 1.21 μV; $P<.05$), and dorsal forearm (29.89 ± 8.86 vs 14.96 ± 1.61 μV; $P<.05$). Pooled data from both groups showed that amplitudes and latencies at different sites significantly correlated with clinical neurologic scores, NCV, QST, and autonomic function.

Evaluation of pain intensity is essential for monitoring response to therapy. There are several symptom-based screening tools such as the NTSS-6, BPI, QOL-DN, SF-36, Visual Analog Scale for Pain Intensity, Neuro-QOL, and Norfolk Neuropathy Symptoms Score (Ia/A). With the visual analog scale the patient marks the intensity of their pain on a scale from 0 to 10, allowing an assessment of the response to intervention. Simultaneously, the patient should complete a QOL tool such as the Norfolk QOL-DN, which needs to include comorbidities such as anxiety, depression, and sleep interference (Ia/A).

PHARMACOLOGIC THERAPEUTIC MODALITIES FOR DIABETIC NEUROPATHIC PAIN
Treatment Based on Pathogenic Concepts of Pain

Painful symptoms in DSPN may constitute a considerable management problem. The efficacy of a single therapeutic agent is not the rule, and simple analgesics are usually inadequate to control the pain. There is agreement that patients should be offered the available therapies in a stepwise fashion (Ia/A).[123–126] Effective pain treatment considers a favorable balance between pain relief and side effects without implying a maximum effect. The following general considerations in the pharmacotherapy of neuropathic pain require attention.

- The appropriate and effective drug has to be tried and identified in each patient by carefully titrating the dose based on efficacy and side effects.
- Lack of efficacy should be judged only after 2 to 4 weeks of treatment using an adequate dose.
- Because the evidence from clinical trials suggests only a maximum response of approximately 50% for any monotherapy, analgesic combinations may be useful.
- Potential drug interactions have to be considered, given the frequent use of polypharmacy in diabetic patients.

The relative benefit of an active treatment over a control in clinical trials is usually expressed as the relative risk, the relative risk reduction, or the odds ratio (OR). However, to estimate the extent of a therapeutic effect (ie, pain relief) that can be translated into clinical practice, it is useful to apply a simple measure that serves the physician to select the appropriate treatment for the individual patient. Such a practical measure is the number needed to treat (NNT); that is, the number of patients that need to be treated with a particular therapy to observe a clinically relevant effect or adverse event in one patient. The OR, NNT, and number needed to harm (NNH) for the individual agents used in the treatment of painful DN are given in **Table 5**. Usually drugs with NNTs exceeding 6 for 50% or greater pain relief are regarded as showing limited efficacy. However, some investigators have cautioned against using NNT estimates because of the lack of homogeneity in treatment therapies, mechanisms of action, pain syndromes, and outcome measures.[127]

The growing knowledge about the neural and pharmacologic basis of neuropathic pain is likely to have important treatment implications, including development and

Table 5
Odds ratios for efficacy and withdrawal, numbers needed to treat (NNT), and numbers needed to harm (NNH)

Drug Class	Odds Ratio: Efficacy	Odds Ratio: Withdrawal (Secondary to Adverse Event)	NNT	NNH
Tricyclics	22.2 (5.8–84.7)	2.3 (0.6–9.7)	1.5–3.5	2.7–17.0
Duloxetine	2.6 (1.6–4.8)	2.4 (1.1–5.4)	5.7–5.8	15.0
Traditional anticonvulsants	5.3 (1.8–16.0)	1.5 (0.3–7.0)	2.1–3.2	2.7–3.0
New-generation anticonvulsants	3.3 (2.3–4.7)	3.0 (1.75–5.1)	2.9–4.3	26.1
Opioids	4.3 (2.3–7.8)	4.1 (1.2–14.2)	2.6–3.9	9.0

Data from Vinik A. The approach to the management of the patient with neuropathic pain. J Clin Endocrinol Metab 2010;95:4802–11.

refinement of a symptom-/mechanism-based approach to neuropathic pain and implementation of novel treatment strategies using the newer antiepileptic agents, which may address the underlying neurophysiologic aberrations in neuropathic pain, allowing the clinician to increase the likelihood of effective management. The neuropharmacology of pain is also becoming better understood. For example, recent data suggest that γ-aminobutyric acid (GABA), voltage-gated sodium channels, and glutamate receptors may be involved in the pathophysiology of neuropathic pain. Many of the newer agents have significant effects on these neurophysiologic mechanisms. Hyperglycemia may be a factor in lowering the pain threshold. Pain is often worse with wide glycemic excursions. Paradoxically, acute onset of pain may appear soon after initiation of therapy with insulin or oral agents.[128] By contrast, it has been reported that a striking amelioration of symptoms can occur with continuous subcutaneous insulin administration, which may reduce the amplitude of excursions of blood glucose.[128] This dichotomy is not well explained. There is a sequence in DN, beginning when Aδ and C nerve fiber function is intact and there is no pain. With damage to C fibers there is sympathetic sensitization, and peripheral autonomic symptoms are interpreted as painful. Topical application of clonidine causes antinociception by blocking emerging pain signals at the peripheral terminals via α2-adrenoceptors,[129] in contrast with the central actions of clonidine on control of blood pressure. With the death of C fibers there is nociceptor sensitization. Aδ fibers conduct all varieties of peripheral stimuli such as touch and these are interpreted as painful (eg, allodynia). With time there is reorganization at the cord level and the patient experiences cold hyperalgesia and, ultimately, even with the death of all fibers, pain is registered in the cerebral cortex whereupon the syndrome becomes chronic without the need for peripheral stimulation. Disappearance of pain may not necessarily reflect nerve recovery but rather nerve death. When patients volunteer the loss of pain, progression of the neuropathy must be excluded by careful examination.

A summary of The Toronto Consensus Panel on Diabetic Neuropathy guidelines,[130] American Academy of Neurology (AAN) recommendations,[131] and treatment options for symptomatic PDPN are shown in **Tables 6–8**.[130–132]

α-Lipoic acid

According to a meta-analysis comprising 1258 patients, infusions of α-lipoic acid (600 mg/d intravenously) ameliorated neuropathic symptoms and deficits after 3 weeks.[133] In a multicenter, randomized, double-masked, parallel-group clinical trial

Table 6
Treatment options for symptomatic diabetic polyneuropathy pain-dosing and side effects

Drug Class	Drug	Dose	Side Effects
Tricyclics (mg)	Amitriptyline	50–150 QHS	Somnolence, dizziness, dry mouth, tachycardia,
	Nortriptyline	50–150 QHS	Constipation, urinary retention, blurred vision
	Imipramine	25–150 QHS	Confusion
	Desipramine	25–150 QHS	
SSRIs (mg)	Paroxetine	40 QD	Somnolence, dizziness, sweating, nausea, anorexia
	Citalopram	40 QD	Diarrhea, impotence, tremor
SNRIs (mg)	Duloxetine	60 QD	Nausea, somnolence, dizziness, anorexia
Anticonvulsants (mg)	Gabapentin	300–1200 TID	Somnolence, dizziness, confusion, ataxia
	Pregabalin	50–150 TID	Somnolence, confusion, edema, weight gain
	Carbamazepine/ oxcarbazepine	Up to 200 QID	Dizziness, somnolence, nausea, leukopenia
	Topiramate	Up to 400 QD	Somnolence, dizziness, ataxia, tremor
Opioids (mg)	Tramadol	50–100 BID	Nausea, constipation, HA, somnolence
	Oxycodone CR	10–30 BID	Somnolence, nausea, constipation, HA
Topical	Capsaicin	0.075% QID	Local irritation
	Lidocaine	0.04% QD	Local irritation
Injection	Botulinum toxin		None

Abbreviations: BID, twice daily; QD, once daily; QHS, every night at bedtime; QID, 4 times daily; TID, 3 times daily.
Data from Vinik A. The approach to the management of the patient with neuropathic pain. J Clin Endocrinol Metab 2010;95:4802–11.

(NATHAN 1), 460 diabetic patients with DSPN were randomly assigned to oral treatment with α-lipoic acid 600 mg (n = 233) or placebo (n = 227). After 4 years of treatment, NIS, but not NCV, was improved, and the drug was well tolerated throughout the trial.[134] A response analysis of clinically meaningful improvement and progression in

Table 7
Treatment algorithm for painful diabetic peripheral neuropathy (The Toronto Consensus Panel on Diabetic Neuropathy)

Painful Diabetic Neuropathy			
First line	α2-δ agonist (pregabalin or gabapentin)	SNRI (duloxetine)	TCA
If pain control is inadequate and considering contraindications			
Second line	TCA or SNRI	TCA or α2-δ agonist (pregabalin or gabapentin)	SNRI or α2-δ agonist (pregabalin or gabapentin)
If pain control is still inadequate			
Third line	Add opioid agonist as combination therapy		

Abbreviations: SNRI, serotonin noradrenaline reuptake inhibitor; TCA, tricyclic antidepressant.
Modified from Tesfaye S, Vileikyte L, Rayman G, et al. Painful diabetic peripheral neuropathy: consensus recommendations on diagnosis, assessment and management. Diabetes Metab Res Rev 2011;27:629–38.

Table 8 Tailoring treatment to the patient (The Toronto Consensus Panel on Diabetic Neuropathy)	
Comorbidities	Contraindication
Glaucoma	TCAs
Orthostatic hypotension	TCAs
Cardiovascular disease	TCAs
Hepatic disease	Duloxetine
Edema	Pregabalin, gabapentin
Unsteadiness and falls	TCAs
Weight gain	TCAs, pregabalin, gabapentin
Other factors: Cost	Duloxetine, pregabalin

Modified from Tesfaye S, Vileikyte L, Rayman G, et al. Painful diabetic peripheral neuropathy: consensus recommendations on diagnosis, assessment and management. Diabetes Metab Res Rev 2011;27:629–38.

the NIS and NIS of the lower limbs (NIS-LL) by at least 2 points showed that the rates of clinical responders were significantly higher and the rates of clinical progressors were lower with α-lipoic acid when compared with placebo for NIS ($P = .013$) and NIS-LL ($P = .025$).

Adrenergic blockers
When there is ongoing damage to the nerves the patient initially experiences pain of the burning, lancinating, dysesthetic type often accompanied by hyperalgesia and allodynia. Because the peripheral sympathetic nerve fibers are also small unmyelinated C fibers, sympathetic blocking agents (clonidine) may improve the pain.

Topical capsaicin
C fibers use the neuropeptide substance P as their neurotransmitter, and depletion of axonal substance P (through the use of capsaicin) will often lead to amelioration of the pain. Prolonged application of capsaicin depletes stores of substance P, and possibly other neurotransmitters, from sensory nerve endings. This process reduces or abolishes the transmission of painful stimuli from the peripheral nerve fibers to the higher centers.[135] Several studies have demonstrated significant pain reduction and improvement in QOL in diabetic patients with painful neuropathy after 8 weeks of treatment with capsaicin cream 0.075%.[136] It has been pointed out that a double-blind design is not feasible for topical capsaicin because of the transient local hyperalgesia (usually mild burning sensation in >50% of the cases) it may produce as a typical adverse event. Treatment should be restricted to a maximum of 8 weeks, as during this period no adverse effect on sensory function (due to the mechanism of action) was noted in diabetic patients. The 8% capsaicin patch (Qutenza), which is effective in post-herpetic neuralgia,[137] is contraindicated in painful DN because of desensitization of nociceptive sensory nerve endings, which may theoretically increase the risk of diabetic foot ulcers (IIb/B).

Lidocaine
A multicenter, randomized, open-label, parallel-group study with a drug washout phase of up to 2 weeks and a comparative phase of 4-week treatment periods of 5% lidocaine (n = 99) versus pregabalin (n = 94) showed that lidocaine was as effective as pregabalin in reducing pain and was free of side effects.[138] This form of therapy

may be most useful in self-limited forms of neuropathy. If successful, therapy can be continued with oral mexiletine. This class of compounds targets the pain caused by hyperexcitability of superficial, free nerve endings.[139]

Opioids and NMDA-receptor antagonists

Tramadol is a centrally acting weak opioid analgesic for treating moderate to severe pain. Tramadol was shown to be better than placebo in a randomized controlled trial[140] of only 6 weeks' duration, but a subsequent follow-up study suggested that symptomatic relief could be maintained for at least 6 months.[141] Side effects are relatively common and similar to other opioid-like drugs, but the development of tolerance and dependence during long-term tramadol treatment is uncommon and its abuse liability appears to be low.[140] Another spinal cord target for pain relief is the excitatory glutaminergic N-methyl-D-aspartate (NMDA) receptor. Blockade of NMDA receptors is believed to be one mechanism by which dextromethorphan exerts analgesic efficacy.[142] The NMDA receptors play an important role in central sensitization of neuropathic pain. Their use, however, has not been widespread, in part because of their dose-limiting side effects (Ia/A).[143]

Severe and refractory pain may require administration of strong opioids such as oxycodone. Although few data are available on combination treatment, combinations of different substance classes have to be used in patients with pain resistant to monotherapy. Several add-on trials have demonstrated significant pain relief and improvement in QOL following treatment with controlled-release oxycodone, a pure μ-agonist in patients with painful DSPN whose pain is not adequately controlled on standard treatment with antidepressants and anticonvulsants.[144,145] Recent recommendations have emphasized the need for clinical skills in risk assessment and management as a prerequisite to the safe and effective prescribing of opioids.[126]

Tapentadol is a novel centrally active analgesic with a dual mode of action: μ-opioid receptor agonist and norepinephrine reuptake inhibitor. The efficacy and tolerability of tapentadol extended release (ER) were evaluated using pooled data from 2 randomized-withdrawal, placebo-controlled, phase 3 trials of similar design in patients with moderate to severe PDPN. With placebo (n = 343) and tapentadol ER (n = 360), respectively, mean (SD) pain intensity scores were 3.48 (2.02) and 3.67 (1.85) at the start of the double-blind maintenance phase and 4.76 (2.52) and 3.77 (2.19) at week 12. Mean (SD) changes from the start to week 12 were 1.28 (2.41) and 0.08 (1.87), indicating that pain intensity worsened with placebo but was relatively unchanged with tapentadol ER. Tapentadol has recently been approved by the Food and Drug Administration for the treatment of PDPN. For the Toronto Consensus Panel on Diabetic Neuropathy recommendations, the reader is referred to **Table 7**.[130] Of note is that the tapentadol publications postdated the AAN and the Toronto Consensus Panel recommendations.

Antidepressants

Antidepressants are now emerging as the first line of agents in the treatment of chronic neuropathic pain.[123] Clinical trials have focused on interrupting pain transmission using antidepressant drugs that inhibit the reuptake of norepinephrine or serotonin. This central action accentuates the effects of these neurotransmitters in activation of endogenous pain-inhibitory systems in the brain that modulate pain-transmission cells in the spinal cord.[146] Putative mechanisms of pain relief by antidepressants include the inhibition of norepinephrine and/or serotonin reuptake at synapses of central descending pain control systems, and the antagonism of NMDA receptors that mediate hyperalgesia and allodynia.

Tricyclic antidepressants

Imipramine, amitriptyline, and clomipramine induce a balanced reuptake inhibition of both norepinephrine and serotonin, whereas desipramine is a relatively selective norepinephrine inhibitor. The NNT (CI) for at least 50% pain relief by tricyclic antidepressants (TCAs) in painful neuropathies is 2.1 (1.9–2.6). The NNH in patients with neuropathic pain for one drop-out of the study due to adverse events is 16 (11–26).[124] The starting dose of amitriptyline should be 25 mg (10 mg in frail patients) taken as a single nighttime dose 1 hour before sleep. It should be increased by 25 mg at weekly intervals until pain relief is achieved or adverse events occur. The maximum dose is usually 150 mg per day.

The use of TCAs is limited by relatively high rates of adverse events and several contraindications (see **Tables 6** and **8**).

Selective serotonin reuptake inhibitors

Because of the relatively high rates of adverse effects and several contraindications of TCAs, it has been reasoned that patients who do not tolerate them because of adverse events could alternatively be treated with selective serotonin reuptake inhibitors (SSRIs). SSRIs specifically inhibit presynaptic reuptake of serotonin but not norepinephrine, and, unlike the tricyclics, they lack the postsynaptic receptor-blocking effects and quinidine-like membrane stabilization. However, only weak effects on neuropathic pain were observed after treatment with fluoxetine, paroxetine, citalopram, and escitalopram. The NNT (CI) for at least 50% pain relief by SSRIs in painful neuropathies is 6.8 (3.9–27).[124] Because of these limited-efficacy data, SSRIs have not been licensed for the treatment of neuropathic pain (IIb/B).

Serotonin noradrenaline reuptake inhibitors

Because SSRIs have been found to be less effective than TCAs, recent interest has focused on antidepressants with dual selective inhibition of serotonin and noradrenaline, such as duloxetine and venlafaxine. Serotonin noradrenaline reuptake inhibitors (SNRIs) relieve pain by increasing the synaptic availability of 5-hydroxytryptamine and noradrenaline in the descending pathways that are inhibitory to pain impulses. A further advantage of duloxetine is that it has antidepressant effects in addition to the analgesic effects in DN. Adverse events are usually mild to moderate, and transient (see **Table 6**). To minimize them the starting dose should be 30 mg/d for 4 to 5 days. Nonetheless, physicians must be aware about the possibility of orthostatic hypotension during the first week of treatment on the 30-mg dose. In contrast to TCAs and some anticonvulsants, duloxetine does not cause weight gain, but a small increase in fasting blood glucose may occur.[147]

Venlafaxine Venlafaxine is another SNRI that has mixed action on catecholamine uptake. At lower doses, it inhibits serotonin uptake and at higher doses it inhibits norepinephrine uptake.[148] The ER version of venlafaxine was found to be superior to placebo in diabetic neuropathic pain in nondepressed patients at doses of 150 to 225 mg daily, and when added to gabapentin there was improved pain, mood, and QOL.[149] Duloxetine, but not venlafaxine, has been licensed in the United States for the treatment of painful DN (Ia/A). See **Table 7** for the Toronto Consensus Panel on Diabetic Neuropathy recommendations.[130]

Antiepileptic Drugs

Antiepileptic drugs (AEDs) have a long history of effectiveness in the treatment of neuropathic pain.[150] Principal mechanisms of action include sodium channel blockade (felbamate, lamotrigine, oxcarbazepine, topiramate, zonisamide), potentiation of

GABA activity (tiagabine, topiramate), calcium channel blockade (felbamate, lamotrigine, topiramate, zonisamide), antagonism of glutamate at NMDA receptors (felbamate) or AMPA (α-amino-3-hydroxy-5-methyl-4-isoxazole propionic acid) receptors (felbamate, topiramate), and mechanisms of action as yet to be fully determined (gabapentin, pregabalin, levetiracetam).[151] An understanding of the mechanisms of action of the various drugs leads to the concept of "rational polytherapy," whereby drugs with complementary mechanisms of action can be combined for synergistic effect. For example, one might choose a sodium-channel blocker such as lamotrigine to be used with a glutamate antagonist such as felbamate. Furthermore, a single drug may possess multiple mechanisms of action, perhaps increasing its likelihood of success (eg, topiramate). If pain is divided according to its derivation from different types of nerve fiber (eg, Aδ vs C fiber), spinal cord or cortical, then different types of pain should respond to different therapies.

The evidence supporting the use of AEDs for the treatment of PDPN continues to evolve.[148] Patients who have failed to respond to 1 AED may respond to another or to 2 or more drugs in combination (Ia/A).[152]

Calcium-channel modulators (gabapentin and pregabalin)

Five types of voltage-gated calcium channels have been identified, and the L and N types of channels have a role to play in the neuromodulation of sensory neurons of the spinal cord. Gabapentin and pregabalin are medications that bind at the α2-δ subunits of the channels. Unlike traditional calcium-channel antagonists, they do not block calcium channels but modulate their activity and sites of expression. The exact mechanism of action of this group of agents on neuromodulation has yet to be clearly defined (IIb/B).

Gabapentin Gabapentin is an anticonvulsant structurally related to GABA, a neurotransmitter that plays a role in pain transmission and modulation. In an 8-week multicenter dose-escalation trial including 165 diabetic patients with painful neuropathy, 60% of the patients on gabapentin (3600 mg/d achieved in 67%) had at least moderate pain relief compared with 33% on placebo. The NNT (CI) for at least 50% pain relief by gabapentin in painful neuropathies is 6.4 (4.3–12). Because of this relatively high NNT and publication bias toward unpublished negative trials,[153] the overall level of evidence in favor of gabapentin in painful DSPN is weak. Gabapentin has the additional benefit of improving sleep.[154] Side effects are listed in **Table 6**; over the long term, it is also known to produce weight gain.[155] Combination therapy has been examined using gabapentin and morphine, indicating slight superiority of the combination (Ia/B).[145]

Pregabalin Pregabalin is a more specific α2-δ ligand with a 6-fold higher binding affinity than gabapentin. Four clinical studies evaluated the efficacy of pregabalin,[156–159] all of which found that it relieved pain, but the effect size was small relative to placebo, reducing pain by 11% to 13% on the 11-point Likert scale in 3 of them. A large dose-dependent effect (24%–50%) reduction in Likert pain scores compared with placebo was observed in the fourth study.[159] The NNT from these studies for a 50% reduction in pain was 4 at 600 mg/d.[156–159] QOL measures, social functioning, mental health, bodily pain, and vitality improved, and sleep interference decreased, and all changes were significant. The most frequent side effects for 150 to 600 mg/d are dizziness (22.0%), somnolence (12.1%), peripheral edema (10.0%), headache (7.2%), and weight gain (5.4%).[160] The evidence supporting a favorable effect in painful DN is more solid, and dose titration is considerably easier for pregabalin than for gabapentin (Ia/A).[131]

Sodium-channel blockers (carbamazepine, oxcarbazepine, lancosamide)

Voltage-gated sodium channels are crucial determinants of neuronal excitability and signaling. After nerve injury, hyperexcitability and spontaneous firing develop at the site of injury and also in the dorsal root ganglion cell bodies. This hyperexcitability results at least partly from accumulation of sodium channels at the site of injury.[161] Carbamazepine and oxcarbazepine are most effective against the "lightning" pain produced by such spontaneous neuronal firing.[162]

Although carbamazepine has been widely used for treating neuropathic pain, it cannot be recommended in painful DN, owing to very limited data. Its successor drug, oxcarbazepine, as well as other sodium-channel blockers such as valproate, mexiletine, topiramate, and lamotrigine, showed only marginal efficacy and have not been licensed for the treatment of painful DN.

Topiramate

Although topiramate failed in 3 clinical trials owing to the use of the wrong end point,[163] it has been shown to successfully reduce pain and induce nerve regeneration.[164,165] Topiramate has the added advantages of causing weight loss and improving the lipoprotein profile, both of which are particularly useful in overweight type 2 diabetic patients.

In summary, 2 drugs have been approved for neuropathic pain in the United States, pregabalin and duloxetine. A recent meta-analysis, in which duloxetine was compared indirectly with pregabalin and gabapentin for the treatment of PDPN, concluded that these 2 agents have comparable efficacy and tolerability.[166] Some studies have analyzed health care costs in patients with PDPN treated with pregabalin, duloxetine, or other commonly used drugs. In general all show similar results, with a good cost-effective profile for both drugs.[167–169]

The response rates to analgesic monotherapy in painful diabetic DSPN are only around 50%. Therefore, combination pharmacotherapy is required in patients who have only partial response or in whom the drug cannot be further titrated because of intolerable side effects. A recent trial showed that the combination of nortriptyline and gabapentin at the maximum tolerated dose was more effective than either monotherapy, despite a lower maximum tolerable dose compared with monotherapy.[170] Appropriate analgesic combinations include antidepressants with anticonvulsants, or each of these with opioids. Some patients may even require a triple combination of these drug classes. The ORs for efficacy and withdrawal from medications are given in **Table 5**.

Based on evidence from clinical trials for the various pharmacologic agents (efficacy and safety) for painful DPN, the Toronto Consensus Panel on Diabetic Neuropathy recommended that a TCA, SNRI, or α2-δ agonist (calcium-channel modulator) should be considered for first-line treatments (see **Table 7**). Based on trial data, duloxetine would be the preferred SNRI and pregabalin would be the preferred α2-δ agonist. If pain is inadequately controlled, depending on contraindications (see **Table 8**) these first-line agents can be combined, although this is not backed by trial evidence. If pain is still inadequately controlled, opioids such as tramadol and oxycodone might be added in a combination treatment.[130]

Natural Products

Metanx

Metanx is a product for management of endothelial dysfunction, containing L-methylfolate, pyridoxal 5′-phosphate, and methylcobalamin. Metanx ingredients counteract endothelial nitric oxide synthase uncoupling and oxidative stress in vascular endothelium and peripheral nerves. A 24-week placebo-controlled trial on the effects of

Metanx on patients with established DN was presented at the American Association of Clinical Endocrinologists annual meeting in 2011. The NTSS-6, which includes numbness, tingling, aching, burning, lancinating pain, and allodynia, improved significantly at week 16 (P = .013 vs placebo) and week 24 (P = .033). Moreover, there were significant improvements in the mental health component of the SF-36 Role Emotional, Social Function, and Vitality. This response occurred with adverse events of less than 2%, mainly rash and gastrointestinal upset, which was no greater than occurred with placebo.[171,172]

Botulinum toxin

Botulinum toxin has been tried for trigeminal neuralgia[173] and has been shown to have long-lasting antinociceptive effects in carpal tunnel syndrome, with no electrophysiologic restoration.[174]

NONPHARMACOLOGIC TREATMENT OF PAINFUL DIABETIC NEUROPATHY

Because there is no entirely satisfactory pharmacotherapy for painful DN, nonpharmacologic treatment options should always be considered. A recent systematic review assessed the evidence from rigorous clinical trials and meta-analyses of complementary and alternative therapies for treating neuropathic and neuralgic pain. Data on the following complementary and alternative medicine treatments were identified: acupuncture, electrostimulation, herbal medicine, magnets, dietary supplements, imagery, and spiritual healing. The conclusion was that the evidence is not fully convincing for most complementary and alternative medicine modalities in relieving neuropathic pain. The evidence can be classified as encouraging and warrants further study for cannabis extract, magnets, carnitine, and electrostimulation (III/C).[175]

Psychological Support

A psychological component to pain should not be underestimated. Hence, an explanation to the patient that even severe pain may remit, particularly in poorly controlled patients with acute painful neuropathy or in those painful symptoms precipitated by intensive insulin treatment, is justified. Addressing the concerns and anxieties of patients with neuropathic pain is essential for their successful management.[176]

Physical Measures

The temperature of the painful neuropathic foot may be increased because of arteriovenous shunting. Cold-water immersion may reduce shunt flow and relieve pain. Allodynia may be relieved by wearing silk pajamas or the use of a bed cradle. Patients who describe painful symptoms on walking as comparable to walking on pebbles may benefit from the use of comfortable footwear.[176]

GUIDELINES FOR THE TREATMENT OF PAINFUL NEUROPATHY

Fig. 4 is an algorithm that the authors use for the management of painful neuropathy in diabetes. The identification of neuropathic pain as being focal or diffuse dictates the initial course of action. Focal neuropathic pain is best treated with diuretics to reduce edema in the canal, with splinting and surgery to release entrapment. Diffuse neuropathies are treated with medical therapy and, in a majority of cases, need multidrug therapy. Essential to the evaluation is the identification of the comorbidities and the choice of drugs that can serve dual actions: for example, pregabalin improves sleep and pain by both direct and indirect pathways, whereas duloxetine may reduce the depression and anxiety that accompany pain. Immune-mediated neuropathies are treated with intravenous immunoglobulin, steroids, or other immunomodulators. When single agents fail, combinations of drugs with different mechanisms of action are in order.

DIABETIC CARDIAC AUTONOMIC NEUROPATHY
Pathogenesis

The etiology of cardiovascular autonomic dysfunction seen early after the diagnosis of diabetes is not well understood. Hyperglycemia increases protein glycation and causes a gradual accumulation of AGEs in body tissues. These AGEs form on intracellular and extracellular proteins, lipids, and nucleic acids in complex arrangements that lead to cross-linking. The authors hypothesize that in metabolic syndrome and diabetes there is a constant increase in low-grade inflammation mediated by a large cadre of exogenous and endogenous ligands in combination with the central and autonomic nervous systems. Thus, the loss of autonomic control with reduction of parasympathetic activity, which is the hallmark of loss of autonomic balance in diabetes, initiates a cascade of inflammatory responses which, if continued unabated, will culminate in considerable morbidity and mortality.

Epidemiology of CAN

Establishing the prevalence of CAN has been hampered by heterogeneous and inadequate diagnostic criteria and population selection. A recent Consensus Panel on Diabetic Neuropathy, after extensive review of the literature, concluded that the prevalence of confirmed CAN in unselected people with type 1 and type 2 DM is approximately 20%, but can be as high as 65% with increasing age and diabetes duration. Clinical correlates or risk markers for CAN are age, diabetes duration, glycemic control, microvascular complications (peripheral polyneuropathy, retinopathy, and nephropathy), hypertension, and dyslipidemia. Established risk factors for CAN are glycemic control in type 1 DM, and a combination of hypertension, dyslipidemia, obesity, and glycemic control in type 2 DM.[177]

CAN is a significant cause of morbidity and mortality associated with a high risk of cardiac arrhythmias and sudden death, possibly related to silent myocardial ischemia. Results from the Action to Control Cardiovascular Risk in Diabetes (ACCORD) trial confirmed that individuals with baseline CAN were 1.55 to 2.14 times as likely to die as individuals without CAN.[68] Furthermore, CAN in the presence of peripheral neuropathy was the highest predictor of mortality from cardiovascular disease (ie, hazard ratio 2.95, $P<.008$). Indeed, combining indices of autonomic dysfunction have been shown to be associated with the risk of mortality.[178–180]

Clinical Manifestations

CAN has been linked to resting tachycardia, postural hypotension, exercise intolerance, enhanced intraoperative or perioperative cardiovascular liability, increased incidence of asymptomatic ischemia, MI, and decreased rate of survival after myocardial infarction.

Resting tachycardia
Whereas abnormalities in heart-rate variability (HRV) are early findings of CAN, resting tachycardia and a fixed heart rate are characteristic late findings in diabetic patients with vagal impairment. A blunted heart-rate response to adenosine receptor agonists was described in both patients with diabetes and patients with metabolic syndrome, and was attributed to earlier stages of CAN.[181] The prognostic value of resting heart

rate is a useful tool for cardiovascular risk stratification and as a therapeutic target in high-risk patients.[18,19,177]

Exercise intolerance
Diabetic patients who are likely to have CAN should be tested for cardiac stress before undertaking an exercise program. Patients with CAN need to rely on their perceived exertion, not heart rate, to avoid hazardous levels of intensity of exercise.

Intraoperative cardiovascular lability
Perioperative cardiovascular morbidity and mortality are increased 2- to 3-fold in patients with diabetes, manifested as greater declines in heart rate and blood pressure during induction of anesthesia; a greater need for vasopressor support[182]; and more severe intraoperative hypothermia with consequent impaired wound healing.[183] Preoperative cardiovascular autonomic screening of diabetic patient may help anesthesiologists identify those at greater risk of intraoperative complications.[17]

Orthostatic hypotension
Orthostatic hypotension is defined as a decrease in blood pressure (ie, >20 mm Hg for systolic or >10 mm Hg for diastolic) in response to postural change, from supine to standing.[184] In patients with diabetes, orthostatic hypotension is usually a result of damage to the efferent sympathetic vasomotor fibers, particularly in the splanchnic vasculature.[185] Patients may present with light-headedness and presyncopal symptoms, or may remain asymptomatic despite significant drops in blood pressure. Orthostatic symptoms can also be misjudged as hypoglycemia and can be aggravated by several drugs, including vasodilators, diuretics, phenothiazines, and particularly TCAs and insulin.[17]

Diagnosis and Staging of CAN

Methods of CAN assessment in clinical practice include assessment of symptoms and signs, cardiovascular autonomic reflex tests (CARTs) based on heart rate and blood pressure, and ambulatory blood pressure monitoring (ABPM).[177]

Screening for autonomic dysfunction should be performed at the diagnosis of type 2 DM and 5 years after the diagnosis of type 1 DM, particularly in patients at greater risk because of a history of poor glycemic control, cardiovascular risk factors, DPN, and macroangiopathic or microangiopathic diabetic complications.

The Toronto Consensus Panel on Diabetic Neuropathy has concluded the following regarding diagnosis of CAN (**Table 9**):

- The following CARTs are the gold standard for clinical autonomic testing: heart-rate response to deep breathing, standing, and Valsalva maneuver, and blood-pressure response to standing (class II evidence).
- These CARTs are sensitive, specific, reproducible, easy to perform, safe, and standardized (classes II and III).
- The Valsalva maneuver is not advisable in the presence of proliferative retinopathy and when there is an increased risk of retinal hemorrhage (class N).
- CARTs are subject to several confounding or interfering factors (class III).
- Age is the most relevant factor affecting heart-rate tests (class I).
- A definite diagnosis of CAN and CAN staging requires more than 1 heart-rate test and the orthostatic hypotension test (class III).

Staging of CANs is based on the number of abnormal test results:

- The presence of 1 abnormal cardiovagal test result identifies the condition of possible or early CAN, to be confirmed over time.

Table 9
Cardiovascular autonomic tests and suggested indications for their use

Test	Clinical Diagnosis	Research	End Point in Clinical Trials
Heart rate cardiovascular tests	Yes	Yes	Yes
Orthostatic hypotension test	Yes	Yes	No (low sensitivity)
QT interval	Yes (additional information and risk stratification)	Yes	No (low sensitivity)
Ambulatory blood pressure monitoring for dipping status (ABPM)	Yes (risk stratification)	Yes	No (low sensitivity)
HRV time and frequency domain indices	Yes (additional information and risk stratification)	Yes	Yes
Baroreflex sensitivity measures	No (early additional information and risk stratification but low availability)	Yes	Yes
Scintigraphic studies	No (low availability, limited standardization)	Yes	Yes
Muscle sympathetic nerve activity	No (low availability, limited data in cardiovascular autonomic neuropathy)	Yes	Possible (used in lifestyle intervention trials in obesity)
Catecholamine assessment	No (low availability)	Yes	Possible (used in lifestyle intervention trials in obesity)

Abbreviation: HRV, heart-rate variability.
Reproduced from Spallone V, Ziegler D, Freeman R, et al. Cardiovascular autonomic neuropathy in diabetes: clinical impact, assessment, diagnosis, and management. Diabetes Metab Res Rev 2011;27:639–53.

- At least 2 abnormal cardiovagal results are required for a definite or confirmed diagnosis of CAN.
- The presence of orthostatic hypotension in addition to heart-rate test abnormalities identifies severe or advanced CAN (level B).
- CARTs allow CAN staging from early to advanced involvement (level C).
- Progressive stages of CAN are associated with increasingly worse prognosis (level B).

Treatment of Autonomic Dysfunction

Intervention studies have documented the protective effects of glycemic control on autonomic function in type 1 diabetic patients (DCCT trial). In the Steno memorial trial, Gaede and colleagues[72,186] showed that a multifactorial strategy aimed at lifestyle change with pharmacologic correction of hyperglycemia, hypertension, dyslipidemia, and microalbuminuria in type 2 diabetic patients reduces abnormalities in autonomic function by 68%.

The Toronto Consensus Panel on Diabetic Neuropathy concluded the following in relation to CAN treatment:

- Intensive diabetes therapy retards the development of CAN in type 1 DM (level A).

Table 10 Diagnosis and management of autonomic dysfunction		
Symptoms	**Assessment Modalities**	**Management**
Resting tachycardia, exercise intolerance, early fatigue and weakness with exercise	HRV, respiratory HRV, MUGA thallium scan, ^{123}I MIBG scan	Graded supervised exercise, β-blockers, ACE inhibitors
Postural hypotension, dizziness, light-headedness, weakness, fatigue, syncope, tachycardia/bradycardia	HRV, blood pressure measurement lying and standing	Mechanical measures, clonidine, midodrine, octreotide, erythropoietin, pyridostigmine
Hyperhidrosis	Sympathetic/parasympathetic balance	Clonidine, amitriptyline, trihexyphenidyl, propantheline, or scopolamine, botulinum toxin, glycopyrrolate

Abbreviations: ACE, angiotensin-converting enzyme; HRV, heart-rate variability; MIBG, metaiodo-benzylguanidine; MUGA, multigated acquisition.

Reproduced from Vinik AI, Suwanwalaikorn S, Stansberry KB, et al. Quantitative measurement of cutaneous perception in diabetic neuropathy. Muscle Nerve 1995;18:574–84.

- Intensive multifactorial cardiovascular risk intervention retards the development and progression of CAN in type 2 DM (level B).
- Lifestyle intervention might improve HRV in prediabetes (level B) and diabetes (level B).
- Symptomatic orthostatic hypotension might be improved by nonpharmacologic measures (level B), and by midodrine (level A) and/or fludrocortisone (level B).

Specific assessment modalities and therapeutic interventions for CAN are detailed in **Table 10**.

Diabetic CAN is a serious complication found in one-quarter of type 1 and one-third of type 2 diabetic patients. It is associated with increased mortality and silent myocardial ischemia, and with a poor prognosis. Symptoms usually occur with advanced disease, and screening of diabetic patients for CAN is essential. The CARTs are the gold standard. Restoration of autonomic balance is possible and has been shown with therapeutic lifestyle changes, increased physical activity, and diabetes treatment (β-adrenergic blockers and potent antioxidants, such as α-lipoic acid). There are exciting new prospects for pathogenesis-oriented intervention.

SUMMARY

DN is the most common and troublesome complication of DM, leading to the greatest morbidity and mortality and resulting in a huge economic burden for diabetes care. It results in a variety of syndromes for which there is no universally accepted classification, and may even be asymptomatic for years while progressing insidiously. DPN has been recently defined as a symmetric, length-dependent sensorimotor polyneuropathy attributable to metabolic and microvascular alterations as a result of chronic hyperglycemia exposure (diabetes) and cardiovascular risk covariates. Both the clinical assessment and treatment options are multifactorial, as detailed herein. Patients with DN should be screened for autonomic neuropathy, as there is a high degree of coexistence of the 2 complications.

Painful neuropathy is an important complication of diabetes. Pathogenesis is multifactorial and requires attention to detailed management if one is to achieve success. Two drugs, pregabalin and duloxetine, have been approved for neuropathic pain in the United States, but neither of these have afforded complete relief, even when used in combination. Indeed, a sobering view is that few drugs achieve a greater than 30% reduction in pain in more than 50% of patients, dictating a need to use more than 1 drug with different mechanisms of action. There is a great need to understand pathogenic mechanisms more fully, particularly the differences in origin of peripheral and central pain. One needs to be aware of the conditions that masquerade as painful neuropathy and the treatment directed toward the underlying disorder as suggested in the algorithm provided. Treatment of peripheral neuropathic pain conditions can benefit from further understanding of the impact of pain response on QOL, activities in daily life, and sleep. As Winston Churchill said, "We need to go from failure to failure without losing our enthusiasm and ultimately we will succeed..."

REFERENCES

1. Vinik AI, Mitchell BD, Leichter SB, et al. Epidemiology of the complications of diabetes. In: Leslie RD, Robbins DC, editors. Diabetes: clinical science in practice. Cambridge (United Kingdom): Cambridge University Press; 1995. p. 221–87.
2. Holzer SE, Camerota A, Martens L, et al. Costs and duration of care for lower extremity ulcers in patients with diabetes. Clin Ther 1998;20:169–81.
3. Caputo GM, Cavanagh PR, Ulbrecht JS, et al. Assessment and management of foot disease in patients with diabetes. N Engl J Med 1994;331:854–60.
4. Herman WH, Kennedy L. Underdiagnosis of peripheral neuropathy in type 2 diabetes. Diabetes Care 2005;28:1480–1.
5. Young MJ, Boulton AJ, MacLeod AF, et al. A multicenter study of the prevalence of diabetic peripheral neuropathy in the United Kingdom hospital clinic population. Diabetologia 1993;36:150–4.
6. Dyck PJ, Kratz KM, Karnes JL, et al. The prevalence by staged severity of various types of diabetic neuropathy, retinopathy, and nephropathy in a population-based cohort: The Rochester Diabetic Neuropathy Study. Neurology 1993;43:817–24.
7. Vinik A. Diabetic neuropathy: pathogenesis and therapy. Am J Med 1999; 107(2B):17S–26S.
8. Armstrong DG, Lavery LA, Harkless LB. Validation of a diabetic wound classification system. The contribution of depth, infection, and ischemia to risk of amputation. Diabetes Care 1998;21:855–9.
9. Vinik EJ, Hayes RP, Oglesby A, et al. The development and validation of the Norfolk QOL-DN, a new measure of patients' perception of the effects of diabetes and diabetic neuropathy. Diabetes Technol Ther 2005;7:497–508.
10. Levitt NS, Stansberry KB, Wychanck S, et al. Natural progression of autonomic neuropathy and autonomic function tests in a cohort of IDDM. Diabetes Care 1996;19:751–4.
11. Rathmann W, Ziegler D, Jahnke M, et al. Mortality in diabetic patients with cardiovascular autonomic neuropathy. Diabet Med 1993;10:820–4.
12. Vinik A, Ullal J, Parson HK, et al. Diabetic neuropathies: clinical manifestations and current treatment options. Nat Clin Pract Endocrinol Metab 2006; 2:269–81.
13. Sadosky A, McDermott AM, Brandenburg NA, et al. A review of the epidemiology of painful diabetic peripheral neuropathy, postherpetic neuralgia,

and less commonly studied neuropathic pain conditions. Pain Pract 2008;8: 45–56.

14. Tesfaye S, Boulton AJ, Dyck PJ, et al. Diabetic neuropathies: update on definitions, diagnostic criteria, estimation of severity, and treatments. Diabetes Care 2010;33:2285–93.

15. Ziegler D. Painful diabetic neuropathy: treatment and future aspects. Diabetes Metab Res Rev 2008;24(Suppl 1):S52–7.

16. Boulton AJ, Malik RA, Arezzo JC, et al. Diabetic somatic neuropathies. Diabetes Care 2004;27:1458–86.

17. Vinik AI, Ziegler D. Diabetic cardiovascular autonomic neuropathy. Circulation 2007;115:387–97.

18. Vinik AI, Maser RE, Ziegler D. Neuropathy: the crystal ball for cardiovascular disease? Diabetes Care 2010;33:1688–90.

19. Vinik AI, Maser RE, Ziegler D. Autonomic imbalance: prophet of doom or scope for hope? Diabet Med 2011;28:643–51.

20. Dieleman JP, Kerklaan J, Huygen FJ, et al. Incidence rates and treatment of neuropathic pain conditions in the general population. Pain 2008;137:681–8.

21. Cornblath DR, Vinik A, Feldman E, et al. Surgical decompression for diabetic sensorimotor polyneuropathy. Diabetes Care 2007;30:421–2.

22. Ziegler D, Rathmann W, Dickhaus T, et al. Prevalence of polyneuropathy in pre-diabetes and diabetes is associated with abdominal obesity and macroangiopathy: the MONICA/KORA Augsburg Surveys S2 and S3. Diabetes Care 2008;31:464–9.

23. Smith AG, Russell J, Feldman EL, et al. Lifestyle intervention for pre-diabetic neuropathy. Diabetes Care 2006;29:1294–9.

24. Ziegler D, Rathmann W, Meisinger C, et al. Prevalence and risk factors of neuropathic pain in survivors of myocardial infarction with pre-diabetes and diabetes. The KORA Myocardial Infarction Registry. Eur J Pain 2009;13:582–7.

25. Ziegler D, Rathmann W, Dickhaus T, et al. Neuropathic pain in diabetes, prediabetes and normal glucose tolerance: the MONICA/KORA Augsburg Surveys S2 and S3. Pain Med 2009;10:393–400.

26. Vinik AI, Holland MT, LeBeau JM, et al. Diabetic neuropathies. Diabetes Care 1992;15:1926–75.

27. Vinik A, Mehrabyan A. Diabetic neuropathies. Med Clin North Am 2004;88:947–99.

28. Vinik A, Mehrabyan A, Colen L, et al. Focal entrapment neuropathies in diabetes. Diabetes Care 2004;27:1783–8.

29. Wilbourn AJ. Diabetic entrapment and compression neuropathies. In: Dyck PJ, Thomas PK, editors. Diabetic neuropathy. Toronto: WB Saunders; 1999. p. 481–508.

30. Watanabe K, Hagura R, Akanuma Y, et al. Characteristics of cranial nerve palsies in diabetic patients. Diabetes Res Clin Pract 1990;10:19–27.

31. Perkins B, Olaleye D, Bril V. Carpal tunnel syndrome in patients with diabetic polyneuropathy. Diabetes Care 2002;25:565–9.

32. Llewelyn JG, Thomas PK, King RH. Epineurial microvasculitis in proximal diabetic neuropathy. J Neurol 1998;245:159–65.

33. Vinik AI, Pittenger GL, Milicevic Z, et al. Autoimmune mechanisms in the pathogenesis of diabetic neuropathy. In: Eisenbarth RG, editor. Molecular mechanisms of endocrine and organ specific autoimmunity. 1st edition. Georgetown, Texas: Landes Company; 1998. p. 217–51.

34. Steck AJ, Kappos L. Gangliosides and autoimmune neuropathies: classification and clinical aspects of autoimmune neuropathies. J Neurol Neurosurg Psychiatry 1994;57(Suppl):26–8.

35. Ayyar DR, Sharma KR. Chronic inflammatory demyelinating polyradiculoneuropathy in diabetes mellitus. Curr Diab Rep 2004;4:409–12.
36. Krendel DA, Costigan DA, Hopkins LC. Successful treatment of neuropathies in patients with diabetes mellitus. Arch Neurol 1995;52:1053–61.
37. Barada A, Reljanovic M, Milicevic Z, et al. Proximal diabetic neuropathy—response to immunotherapy. Diabetes 1999;48(Suppl 1):A148.
38. Boulton AJ, Malik RA. Diabetic neuropathy. Med Clin North Am 1998;82:909–29.
39. Thomas PK. Classification, differential diagnosis, and staging of diabetic peripheral neuropathy. Diabetes 1997;46(Suppl 2):S54–7.
40. Oyibo SO, Prasad YD, Jackson NJ, et al. The relationship between blood glucose excursions and painful diabetic peripheral neuropathy: a pilot study. Diabet Med 2002;19:870–3.
41. Sinnreich M, Taylor BV, Dyck PJ. Diabetic neuropathies. Classification, clinical features, and pathophysiological basis. Neurologist 2005;11:63–79.
42. Vinik A. Management of the patient with neuropathic pain. In: Wartofsky L, editor. Endocrine Society; 2012. p. 177–94. J Clin Endocrinol Metab 2010;95:4802–11 [reprint].
43. Archer AG, Watkins PJ, Thomas PK, et al. The natural history of acute painful neuropathy in diabetes mellitus. J Neurol Neurosurg Psychiatry 1983;46:491–9.
44. Partanen J, Niskanen L, Lehtinen J, et al. Natural history of peripheral neuropathy in patients with non-insulin-dependent diabetes mellitus. N Engl J Med 1995;333:89–94.
45. Harris M, Eastman R, Cowie C. Symptoms of sensory neuropathy in adults with NIDDM in the U.S. population. Diabetes Care 1993;16:1446–52.
46. Singleton JR, Smith AG, Bromberg MB. Painful sensory polyneuropathy associated with impaired glucose tolerance. Muscle Nerve 2001;24:1225–8.
47. Singleton JR, Smith AG, Bromberg MB. Increased prevalence of impaired glucose tolerance in patients with painful sensory neuropathy. Diabetes Care 2001;24:1448–53.
48. Novella SP, Inzucchi SE, Goldstein JM. The frequency of undiagnosed diabetes and impaired glucose tolerance in patients with idiopathic sensory neuropathy. Muscle Nerve 2001;24:1229–31.
49. Sumner C, Sheth S, Griffin J, et al. The spectrum of neuropathy in diabetes and impaired glucose tolerance. Neurology 2003;60:108–11.
50. Pittenger GL, Ray M, Burcus NI, et al. Intraepidermal nerve fibers are indicators of small-fiber neuropathy in both diabetic and nondiabetic patients. Diabetes Care 2004;27:1974–9.
51. Dyck PJ, Lais A, Karnes JL, et al. Fiber loss is primary and multifocal in sural nerves in diabetic polyneuropathy. Ann Neurol 1986;19:425–39.
52. Cavanagh PR, Simoneau GG, Ulbrecht JS. Ulceration, unsteadiness, and uncertainty: the biomechanical consequences of diabetes mellitus. J Biomech 1993; 26(Suppl 1):23–40.
53. Katoulis EC, Ebdon-Parry M, Lanshammar H, et al. Gait abnormalities in diabetic neuropathy. Diabetes Care 1997;20:1904–7.
54. Vinik AI, Strotmeyer ES, Nakave AA, et al. Diabetic neuropathy in older adults. Clin Geriatr Med 2008;24:407–35.
55. England JD, Gronseth GS, Franklin G, et al. Distal symmetric polyneuropathy: a definition for clinical research: report of the American Academy of Neurology, the American Association of Electrodiagnostic Medicine, and the American Academy of Physical Medicine and Rehabilitation. Neurology 2005;64:199–207.

56. Ziegler D, Hidvegi T, Gurieva I, et al. Efficacy and safety of lacosamide in painful diabetic neuropathy. Diabetes Care 2010;33:839–41.
57. Young RJ, Ewing DJ, Clarke BF. Chronic and remitting painful diabetic polyneuropathy. Correlations with clinical features and subsequent changes in neurophysiology. Diabetes Care 1988;11:34–40.
58. England JD, Gronseth GS, Franklin G, et al. Practice Parameter: evaluation of distal symmetric polyneuropathy: role of autonomic testing, nerve biopsy, and skin biopsy (an evidence-based review). Report of the American Academy of Neurology, American Association of Neuromuscular and Electrodiagnostic Medicine, and American Academy of Physical Medicine and Rehabilitation. Neurology 2009;72:177–84.
59. Feldman EL, Stevens MJ, Thomas PK, et al. A practical two-step quantitative clinical and electrophysiological assessment for the diagnosis and staging of diabetic neuropathy. Diabetes Care 1994;17:1281–9.
60. Haanpaa ML, Backonja MM, Bennett MI, et al. Assessment of neuropathic pain in primary care. Am J Med 2009;122:S13–21.
61. Boulton AJ, Vinik AI, Arezzo JC, et al. Diabetic neuropathies: a statement by the American Diabetes Association. Diabetes Care 2005;28:956–62.
62. Boulton AJ, Gries FA, Jervell JA. Guidelines for the diagnosis and outpatient management diabetic peripheral neuropathy. Diabet Med 1998;15:508–14.
63. Vinik AI, Suwanwalaikorn S, Stansberry KB, et al. Quantitative measurement of cutaneous perception in diabetic neuropathy. Muscle Nerve 1995;18:574–84.
64. Abbott CA, Carrington AL, Ashe H, et al. The North-West Diabetes Foot Care Study: incidence of, and risk factors for, new diabetic foot ulceration in a community-based patient cohort. Diabet Med 2002;19:377–84.
65. Dyck PJ, Melton LJ III, O'Brien PC, et al. Approaches to improve epidemiological studies of diabetic neuropathy: insights from the Rochester Diabetic Neuropathy Study. Diabetes 1997;46(Suppl 2):S5–8.
66. Vileikyte L, Peyrot M, Bundy C, et al. The development and validation of a neuropathy- and foot ulcer-specific quality of life instrument. Diabetes Care 2003; 26:2549–55.
67. Cameron NE, Eaton SE, Cotter MA. Vascular factors and metabolic interactions in the pathogenesis of diabetic neuropathy. Diabetologia 2001;44:1973–88.
68. Albers JW, Herman WH, Pop-Busui R, et al. Effect of prior intensive insulin treatment during the Diabetes Control and Complications Trial (DCCT) on peripheral neuropathy in type 1 diabetes during the Epidemiology of Diabetes Interventions and Complications (EDIC) Study. Diabetes Care 2010;33:1090–6.
69. Pop-Busui R, Low PA, Waberski BH, et al. Effects of prior intensive insulin therapy on cardiac autonomic nervous system function in type 1 diabetes mellitus: The Diabetes Control and Complications Trial/Epidemiology of Diabetes Interventions and Complications study (DCCT/EDIC). Circulation 2009;119: 2886–93.
70. Intensive blood-glucose control with sulphonylureas or insulin compared with conventional treatment and risk of complications in patients with type 2 diabetes (UKPDS 33). UK Prospective Diabetes Study (UKPDS) Group. Lancet 1998;352: 837–53.
71. The ADVANCE Collaborative Group. Intensive blood glucose control and vascular outcomes in patients with type 2 diabetes. N Engl J Med 2008;358:2560–72.
72. Gaede P, Lund-Andersen H, Parving HH, et al. Effect of a multifactorial intervention on mortality in type 2 diabetes. N Engl J Med 2008;358:580–91.

73. Ziegler D, Sohr CG, Nourooz-Zadeh J. Oxidative stress and antioxidant defense in relation to the severity of diabetic polyneuropathy and cardiovascular autonomic neuropathy. Diabetes Care 2004;27:2178–83.

74. Pittenger G, Vinik A. Nerve growth factor and diabetic neuropathy. Exp Diabesity Res 2003;4:271–85.

75. Vinik AI. Treatment of diabetic polyneuropathy (DPN) with recombinant human nerve growth factor (rhNGF). Diabetes 1999;48(Suppl 1):A54–5.

76. Rivard A, Silver M, Chen D, et al. Rescue of diabetes-related impairment of angiogenesis by intramuscular gene therapy with adeno-VEGF. Am J Pathol 1999;154:355–63.

77. Tam J, Rosenberg L, Maysinger D. INGAP peptide improves nerve function and enhances regeneration in streptozotocin-induced diabetic C57BL/6 mice. FASEB J 2004;18:1767–9.

78. Dungan KM, Buse JB, Ratner RE. Effects of therapy in type 1 and type 2 diabetes mellitus with a peptide derived from islet neogenesis associated protein (INGAP). Diabetes Metab Res Rev 2009;25:558–65.

79. Bussolino F, Di Renzo MF, Ziche M, et al. Hepatocyte growth factor is a potent angiogenic factor which stimulates endothelial cell motility and growth. J Cell Biol 1992;119:629–41.

80. Nakagami H, Kaneda Y, Ogihara T, et al. Hepatocyte growth factor as potential cardiovascular therapy. Expert Rev Cardiovasc Ther 2005;3:513–9.

81. Matsumoto K, Nakamura T. Emerging multipotent aspects of hepatocyte growth factor. J Biochem 1996;119:591–600.

82. Jayasankar V, Woo YJ, Pirolli TJ, et al. Induction of angiogenesis and inhibition of apoptosis by hepatocyte growth factor effectively treats postischemic heart failure. J Card Surg 2005;20:93–101.

83. Hashimoto N, Yamanaka H, Fukuoka T, et al. Expression of HGF and cMet in the peripheral nervous system of adult rats following sciatic nerve injury. Neuroreport 2001;12:1403–7.

84. Ajroud-Driss S, Christiansen M, Allen JA, et al. Phase 1/2 open-label dose-escalation study of plasmid DNA expressing two isoforms of hepatocyte growth factor in patients with painful diabetic peripheral neuropathy. Mol Ther 2013;21(6):1279–86.

85. Milicevic Z, Newlon PG, Pittenger GL, et al. Anti-ganglioside GM1 antibody and distal symmetric "diabetic polyneuropathy" with dominant motor features. Diabetologia 1997;40:1364–5.

86. Sharma K, Cross J, Farronay O, et al. Demyelinating neuropathy in diabetes mellitus. Arch Neurol 2002;59:758–65.

87. Granberg V, Ejskjaer N, Peakman M, et al. Autoantibodies to autonomic nerves associated with cardiac and peripheral autonomic neuropathy. Diabetes Care 2005;28:1959–64.

88. Vinik AI, Anandacoomaraswamy D, Ullal J. Antibodies to neuronal structures: innocent bystanders or neurotoxins? Diabetes Care 2005;28:2067–72.

89. Mantyselka P, Ahonen R, Kumpusalo E, et al. Variability in prescribing for musculoskeletal pain in Finnish primary health care. Pharm World Sci 2001;23:232–6.

90. Treede RD, Jensen TS, Campbell JN, et al. Neuropathic pain: redefinition and a grading system for clinical and research purposes. Neurology 2008;70:1630–5.

91. Jensen MP, Chodroff MJ, Dworkin RH. The impact of neuropathic pain on health-related quality of life: review and implications. Neurology 2007;68:1178–82.

92. Bouhassira D, Lanteri-Minet M, Attal N, et al. Prevalence of chronic pain with neuropathic characteristics in the general population. Pain 2008;136:380–7.
93. Vinik E, Paulson J, Ford-Molvik S, et al. German-Translated Norfolk Quality of Life (QOL-DN) identifies the same factors as the English version of the tool and discriminates different levels of neuropathy severity. J Diabetes Sci Technol 2008;2:1075–86.
94. Vinik AI, Casellini CM. Guidelines in the management of diabetic nerve pain: clinical utility of pregabalin. Diabetes Metab Syndr Obes 2013;6:57–78.
95. Vinik A, Emir B, Raymond C, et al. The relationship between pain relief and improvements in patient function/quality of life in patients with painful diabetic peripheral neuropathy or post-herpetic neuralgia treated with pregabalin. Clin Ther 2013;35(5):612–23.
96. Castro MM, Daltro C. Sleep patterns and symptoms of anxiety and depression in patients with chronic pain. Arq Neuropsiquiatr 2009;67:25–8.
97. Gore M, Brandenburg NA, Dukes E, et al. Pain severity in diabetic peripheral neuropathy is associated with patient functioning, symptom levels of anxiety and depression, and sleep. J Pain Symptom Manage 2005;30:374–85.
98. Boulanger L, Zhao Y, Foster TS, et al. Impact of comorbid depression or anxiety on patterns of treatment and economic outcomes among patients with diabetic peripheral neuropathic pain. Curr Med Res Opin 2009;25:1763–73.
99. Gupta A, Silman J, Ray D, et al. The role of psychosocial factors in predicting the onset of chronic widespread pain: results from a prospective population-based study. Rheumatology 2007;46:666–71.
100. O'Connor AB. Neuropathic pain: quality-of-life impact, costs and cost effectiveness of therapy. Pharmacoeconomics 2009;27:95–112.
101. Daousi C, MacFarlane IA, Woodward A, et al. Chronic painful peripheral neuropathy in an urban community: a controlled comparison of people with and without diabetes. Diabet Med 2004;21:976–82.
102. Bennett MI, Attal N, Backonja MM, et al. Using screening tools to identify neuropathic pain. Pain 2007;127:199–203.
103. Bastyr E, Zhang D, Bril V, The MBBQ Study Group. Neuropathy Total symptom Score-6 Questionnaire (NTSS-6) is a valid instrument for assessing the positive symptoms of diabetic peripheral neuropathy (DPN). Diabetes 2002; 51:A199.
104. Scholz J, Mannion RJ, Hord DE, et al. A novel tool for the assessment of pain: validation in low back pain. PLoS Med 2009;6:e1000047.
105. Spallone V, Morganti R, D'Amato C, et al. Clinical correlates of painful diabetic neuropathy and relationship of neuropathic pain with sensorimotor and autonomic nerve function. Eur J Pain 2011;15(2):153–60.
106. Young RJ. Structural functional interactions in the natural history of diabetic polyneuropathy: a key to the understanding of neuropathic pain? Diabet Med 1993; 10(Suppl 2):89S–90S.
107. Loeser JD, Treede RD. The Kyoto protocol of IASP basic pain terminology. Pain 2008;137:473–7.
108. Bouhassira D, Attal N, Fermanian J, et al. Development and validation of the neuropathic pain symptom inventory. Pain 2004;108:248–57.
109. Bennett MI, Smith BH, Torrance N, et al. The S-LANSS score for identifying pain of predominantly neuropathic origin: validation for use in clinical and postal research. J Pain 2005;6:149–58.
110. Krause S, Backonja M. Development of a neuropathic pain questionnaire. Clin J Pain 2003;19:306–14.

111. Bouhassira D, Attal N, Alchaar H, et al. Comparison of pain syndromes associated with nervous or somatic lesions and development of a new neuropathic pain diagnostic questionnaire (DN4). Pain 2005;114:29–36.

112. Freyhagen R, Baron R, Gockel U. Pain detect: a new screening questionnaire to detect neuropathic components in patients with back pain. Curr Med Res Opin 2006;22:1911–20.

113. Portenoy R. Development and testing of a neuropathic pain screening questionnaire: ID pain. Curr Med Res Opin 2006;22:1555–65.

114. Dworkin RH, Turk DC, Revicki DA, et al. Development and initial validation of an expanded and revised version of the Short-form McGill Pain Questionnaire (SF-MPQ-2). Pain 2009;144:35–42.

115. Daut RL, Cleeland CS, Flanery RC. Development of the Wisconsin Brief Pain Questionnaire to assess pain in cancer and other diseases. Pain 1983;17:197–210.

116. Dworkin RH, Turk DC, Wyrwich KW, et al. Interpreting the clinical importance of treatment outcomes in chronic pain clinical trials: IMMPACT recommendations. J Pain 2008;9:105–21.

117. Cruccu G, Truini A. Tools for assessing neuropathic pain. PLoS Med 2009;6: e1000045.

118. Stephenson DT, Arneric SP. Neuroimaging of pain: advances and future prospects. J Pain 2008;9:567–79.

119. Chao CC, Hsieh SC, Tseng MT, et al. Patterns of contact heat evoked potentials (CHEP) in neuropathy with skin denervation: correlation of CHEP amplitude with intraepidermal nerve fiber density. Clin Neurophysiol 2008;119:653–61.

120. Atherton DD, Facer P, Roberts KM, et al. Use of the novel Contact Heat Evoked Potential Stimulator (CHEPS) for the assessment of small fibre neuropathy: correlations with skin flare responses and intra-epidermal nerve fibre counts. BMC Neurol 2007;7:21.

121. Casanova-Molla J, Grau-Junyent JM, Morales M, et al. On the relationship between nociceptive evoked potentials and intraepidermal nerve fiber density in painful sensory polyneuropathies. Pain 2011;152:410–8.

122. Chao CC, Tseng MT, Lin YJ, et al. Pathophysiology of neuropathic pain in type 2 diabetes: skin denervation and contact heat-evoked potentials. Diabetes Care 2010;33:2654–9.

123. Finnerup NB, Otto M, McQuay HJ, et al. Algorithm for neuropathic pain treatment: an evidence based proposal. Pain 2005;118:289–305.

124. Finnerup NB, Sindrup SH, Jensen TS. The evidence for pharmacological treatment of neuropathic pain. Pain 2010;150:573–81.

125. Dworkin RH, O'Connor AB, Backonja M, et al. Pharmacologic management of neuropathic pain: evidence-based recommendations. Pain 2007;132:237–51.

126. Dworkin RH, O'Connor AB, Audette J, et al. Recommendations for the pharmacological management of neuropathic pain: an overview and literature update. Mayo Clin Proc 2010;85:S3–14.

127. Edelsberg J, Oster G. Summary measures of number needed to treat: how much clinical guidance do they provide in neuropathic pain? Eur J Pain 2009; 13:11–6.

128. Said G, Bigo A, Ameri A, et al. Uncommon early-onset neuropathy in diabetic patients. J Neurol 1998;245:61–8.

129. Dogrul A, Uzbay IT. Topical clonidine antinociception. Pain 2004;111:385–91.

130. Tesfaye S, Vileikyte L, Rayman G, et al. Painful diabetic peripheral neuropathy: consensus recommendations on diagnosis, assessment and management. Diabetes Metab Res Rev 2011;27:629–38.

131. Bril V, England J, Franklin GM, et al. Evidence-based guideline: treatment of painful diabetic neuropathy: report of the American Academy of Neurology, the American Association of Neuromuscular and Electrodiagnostic Medicine, and the American Academy of Physical Medicine and Rehabilitation. Neurology 2011;76:1758–65.

132. Vinik A. The approach to the management of the patient with neuropathic pain. J Clin Endocrinol Metab 2010;95:4802–11.

133. Ziegler D, Nowak H, Kempler P, et al. Treatment of symptomatic diabetic poly-neuropathy with the antioxidant alpha-lipoic acid: a meta-analysis. Diabet Med 2004;21:114–21.

134. Ziegler D, Low PA, Boulton AJ. Antioxidant treatment with alpha-lipoic acid in diabetic polyneuropathy: a 4-year randomized double-blind trial (NATHAN 1). Diabetologia 2011;50:S63.

135. Rains C, Bryson HM. Topical capsaicin. A review of its pharmacological proper-ties and therapeutic potential in post-herpetic neuralgia, diabetic neuropathy and osteoarthritis. Drugs Aging 1995;7:317–28.

136. Mason L, Moore RA, Derry S, et al. Systematic review of topical capsaicin for the treatment of chronic pain. BMJ 2004;328:991.

137. Backonja M, Wallace MS, Blonsky ER, et al. NGX-4010, a high-concentration capsaicin patch, for the treatment of postherpetic neuralgia: a randomised, double-blind study. Lancet Neurol 2008;7:1106–12.

138. Baron R, Mayoral V, Leijon G, et al. Efficacy and safety of combination therapy with 5% lidocaine medicated plaster and pregabalin in post-herpetic neuralgia and diabetic polyneuropathy. Curr Med Res Opin 2009;25:1677–87.

139. Jarvis B, Coukell AJ. Mexiletine. A review of its therapeutic use in painful dia-betic neuropathy. Drugs 1998;56:691–707.

140. Harati Y, Gooch C, Swenson M, et al. Double-blind randomized trial of tramadol for the treatment of the pain of diabetic neuropathy. Neurology 1998;50:1842–6.

141. Harati Y, Gooch C, Swenson M, et al. Maintenance of the long-term effective-ness of tramadol in treatment of the pain of diabetic neuropathy. J Diabetes Complications 2000;14:65–70.

142. Nelson KA, Park KM, Robinovitz E, et al. High-dose oral dextromethorphan versus placebo in painful diabetic neuropathy and postherpetic neuralgia. Neurology 1997;48:1212–8.

143. Sang CN. NMDA-receptor antagonists in neuropathic pain: experimental methods to clinical trials. J Pain Symptom Manage 2000;19:S21–5.

144. Watson CP, Moulin D, Watt-Watson J, et al. Controlled-release oxycodone re-lieves neuropathic pain: a randomized controlled trial in painful diabetic neurop-athy. Pain 2003;105:71–8.

145. Gilron I, Bailey JM, Tu D, et al. Morphine, gabapentin, or their combination for neuropathic pain. N Engl J Med 2005;352:1324–34.

146. Max M, Lynch S, Muir J. Effects of desipramine, amitriptyline and fluoxetine on pain in diabetic neuropathy. N Engl J Med 1992;326:1250–6.

147. Hardy T, Sachson R, Shen S, et al. Does treatment with duloxetine for neuro-pathic pain impact glycemic control? Diabetes Care 2007;30:21–6.

148. Sansone RA, Sansone LA. Pain, pain, go away: antidepressants and pain man-agement. Psychiatry (Edgmont) 2008;5:16–9.

149. Simpson DA. Gabapentin and venlafaxine for the treatment of painful diabetic neuropathy. J Clin Neuromuscul Dis 2001;3:53–62.

150. Blom S. Trigeminal neuralgia: its treatment with a new anticonvulsant drug (g-32883). Lancet 1962;21:839–40.

151. LaRoche SM, Helmers SL. The new antiepileptic drugs: scientific review. JAMA 2004;291:605–14.
152. Dworkin RH, Backonja M, Rowbotham MC, et al. Advances in neuropathic pain: diagnosis, mechanisms, and treatment recommendations. Arch Neurol 2003;60: 1524–34.
153. Landefeld CS, Steinman MA. The Neurontin legacy—marketing through misinformation and manipulation. N Engl J Med 2009;360:103–6.
154. Backonja M, Beydoun A, Edwards KR, et al. Gabapentin for the symptomatic treatment of painful neuropathy in patients with diabetes mellitus: a randomized controlled trial. JAMA 1998;280:1831–6.
155. DeToledo JC, Toledo C, DeCerce J, et al. Changes in body weight with chronic, high-dose gabapentin therapy. Ther Drug Monit 1997;19:394–6.
156. Lesser H, Sharma U, LaMoreaux L, et al. Pregabalin relieves symptoms of painful diabetic neuropathy: a randomized controlled trial. Neurology 2004;63: 2104–10.
157. Richter RW, Portenoy R, Sharma U, et al. Relief of painful diabetic peripheral neuropathy with pregabalin: a randomized, placebo-controlled trial. J Pain 2005;6:253–60.
158. Rosenstock J, Tuchman M, LaMoreaux L, et al. Pregabalin for the treatment of painful diabetic peripheral neuropathy: a double-blind, placebo-controlled trial. Pain 2004;110:628–38.
159. Freynhagen R, Strojek K, Griesing T, et al. Efficacy of pregabalin in neuropathic pain evaluated in a 12-week, randomised, double-blind, multicentre, placebo-controlled trial of flexible- and fixed-dose regimens. Pain 2005;115:254–63.
160. Freeman R, Durso-Decruz E, Emir B. Efficacy, safety, and tolerability of pregabalin treatment for painful diabetic peripheral neuropathy: findings from seven randomized, controlled trials across a range of doses. Diabetes Care 2008; 31:1448–54.
161. Kalso E. Sodium channel blockers in neuropathic pain. Curr Pharm Des 2005; 11:3005–11.
162. Dogra S, Beydoun S, Mazzola J, et al. Oxcarbazepine in painful diabetic neuropathy: a randomized, placebo-controlled study. Eur J Pain 2005;9:543–54.
163. Vinik AI. Diabetic neuropathies: endpoints in clinical research studies. In: LeRoith D, Vinik AI, editors. Contemporary endocrinology: controversies in treating diabetes: clinical and research aspects. Totowa (NJ): Humana Press; 2008. p. 135–56.
164. Pittenger G, Mehrabyan A, Simmons K, et al. Small fiber neuropathy is associated with the metabolic syndrome. Metab Syndr Relat Disord 2005;3:113–21.
165. Raskin P, Donofrio PD, Rosenthal NR, et al. Topiramate vs placebo in painful diabetic neuropathy: analgesic and metabolic effects. Neurology 2004;63: 865–73.
166. Quilici S, Chancellor J, Lothgren M, et al. Meta-analysis of duloxetine vs. pregabalin and gabapentin in the treatment of diabetic peripheral neuropathic pain. BMC Neurol 2009;9:6–19.
167. Burke J, Sanchez R, Joshi A, et al. Health care costs in patients with painful diabetic peripheral neuropathy prescribed pregabalin or duloxetine. Pain Pract 2012;12:209–18.
168. De Salas-Cansado M, Perez C, Saldana MT, et al. An economic evaluation of pregabalin versus usual care in the management of community-treated patients with refractory painful diabetic peripheral neuropathy in primary care settings. Prim Care Diabetes 2012;6:303–12.

169. Bellows BK, Dahal A, Jiao T, et al. A cost-utility analysis of pregabalin versus duloxetine for the treatment of painful diabetic neuropathy. J Pain Palliat Care Pharmacother 2012;26:153–64.

170. Gilron I, Bailey JM, Tu D, et al. Nortriptyline and gabapentin, alone and in combination for neuropathic pain: a double-blind, randomised controlled crossover trial. Lancet 2009;374:1252–61.

171. Thethi TK, Fonseca VA, Lavery LA, et al. Metanx in Type 2 Diabetes with Peripheral Neuropathy, A Randomized Trial. Am J Med 2013;126(2):141–9.

172. Vinik AJ. A medicinal food provides food for thought in managing diabetic neuropathy. Am J Med 2013;126(2):95–6.

173. Piovesan EJ, Teive HG, Kowacs PA, et al. An open study of botulinum-A toxin treatment of trigeminal neuralgia. Neurology 2005;65:1306–8.

174. Tsai CP, Liu CY, Lin KP, et al. Efficacy of botulinum toxin type A in the relief of carpal tunnel syndrome: a preliminary experience. Clin Drug Investig 2006;26:511–5.

175. Pittler MH, Ernst E. Complementary therapies for neuropathic and neuralgic pain: systematic review. Clin J Pain 2008;24:731–3.

176. Tesfaye S. Painful diabetic neuropathy. Aetiology and nonpharmacological treatment. In: Veves A, editor. Clinical management of diabetic neuropathy. Totowa (NJ): Humana Press; 1998. p. 369–86.

177. Spallone V, Ziegler D, Freeman R, et al. Cardiovascular autonomic neuropathy in diabetes: clinical impact, assessment, diagnosis, and management. Diabetes Metab Res Rev 2011;27:639–53.

178. Maser RE, Mitchell BD, Vinik AI, et al. The association between cardiovascular autonomic neuropathy and mortality in individuals with diabetes: a meta-analysis. Diabetes Care 2003;26:1895–901.

179. Ziegler D, Zentai CP, Perz S, et al. Prediction of mortality using measures of cardiac autonomic dysfunction in the diabetic and nondiabetic population: the MONICA/KORA Augsburg Cohort Study. Diabetes Care 2008;31:556–61.

180. Lykke JA, Tarnow L, Parving HH, et al. A combined abnormality in heart rate variation and QT corrected interval is a strong predictor of cardiovascular death in type 1 diabetes. Scand J Clin Lab Invest 2008;68:654–9.

181. Hage FG, Iskandrian AE. Cardiovascular imaging in diabetes mellitus. J Nucl Cardiol 2011;18:959–65.

182. Burgos LG, Ebert TJ, Assiddao C, et al. Increased intraoperative cardiovascular morbidity in diabetics with autonomic neuropathy. Anesthesiology 1989;70:591–7.

183. Kitamura A, Hoshino T, Kon T, et al. Patients with diabetic neuropathy are at risk of a greater intraoperative reduction in core temperature. Anesthesiology 2000;92:1311–8.

184. The definition of orthostatic hypotension, pure autonomic failure, and multiple system atrophy. J Auton Nerv Syst 1996;58:123–4.

185. Low PA, Walsh JC, Huang CY, et al. The sympathetic nervous system in diabetic neuropathy. A clinical and pathological study. Brain 1975;98:341–56.

186. Gaede P, Vedel P, Parving HH, et al. Intensified multifactorial intervention in patients with type 2 diabetes mellitus and microalbuminuria: the Steno type 2 randomized study. Lancet 1999;353:617–22.

Diabetic Kidney Disease and the Cardiorenal Syndrome
Old Disease, New Perspectives

Ankur Jindal, MD[a,b], Mariana Garcia-Touza, MD[b,c],
Nidhi Jindal, MD[d], Adam Whaley-Connell, DO, MSPH[b,c,d,e],
James R. Sowers, MD[b,c,e,f],*

KEYWORDS

- Diabetes • Cardiorenal syndrome • Diabetic nephropathy • Chronic kidney disease
- Blood pressure variability • Albuminuria • Proteinuria

KEY POINTS

- Diabetic nephropathy should be studied and treated in the context of cardiorenal syndrome, with a focus on the complex intertwined metabolic changes, which increase risk for chronic kidney disease and cardiovascular disease.
- Blood pressure and glycemic control are crucial for prevention and treatment of diabetic kidney disease.
- Newer drugs for achieving glycemic control have an important role in the treatment of type 2 diabetes mellitus in patients with cardiorenal syndrome.

Funding Sources: NIH (R01 HL73101-01A1 & R01 HL107910-01), Veterans Affairs Merit System 0019 (J.R. Sowers); NIH (R-03 AG040638), Veterans Affairs System (CDA-2), ASN-ASP Junior Development Grant in Geriatric Nephrology, supported by a T. Franklin Williams Scholarship Award (A. Whaley-Connell).
Conflict of Interest: Merck Pharmaceuticals Advisory Board (J.R. Sowers).
[a] Hospital Medicine, Department of Internal Medicine, University of Missouri, One Hospital Drive, Columbia, MO 65212, USA; [b] Diabetes and Cardiovascular Research Center, University of Missouri, One Hospital Drive, Columbia, MO 65212, USA; [c] Division of Endocrinology, Diabetes & Metabolism, Department of Internal Medicine, University of Missouri Columbia School of Medicine, One Hospital Drive, Columbia, MO 65212, USA; [d] Division of Nephrology and Hypertension, Department of Internal Medicine, University of Missouri Columbia School of Medicine, One Hospital Drive, Columbia, MO 65212, USA; [e] Department of Internal Medicine, Harry S Truman Memorial Veterans Hospital, Five Hospital Drive, Columbia, MO 65201, USA; [f] Department of Medical Physiology and Pharmacology, University of Missouri, One Hospital Drive, Columbia, MO 65212, USA
* Corresponding author. University of Missouri, D109 Diabetes Center HSC, One Hospital Drive, Columbia, MO 65212.
E-mail address: sowersj@health.missouri.edu

Endocrinol Metab Clin N Am 42 (2013) 789–808
http://dx.doi.org/10.1016/j.ecl.2013.06.002
0889-8529/13/$ – see front matter © 2013 Elsevier Inc. All rights reserved.

INTRODUCTION

Prevalent chronic kidney disease (CKD) in the United States has increased over last few decades and comprises an alarming 13% of the US general population.[1] Diabetes is recognized as the leading cause of CKD and end-stage renal disease (ESRD), and accounts for about 40% of ESRD cases in the United States.[2-4] It is estimated that CKD affects more than 35% of adults with diabetes and nearly 20% of adults with hypertension.[5] The expansion of CKD can be explained, in part, by the increased prevalence of obesity and diabetes, thus raising concerns for even more pronounced trends in the future.[1] Regardless of cause, CKD is prevalent enough to be considered a critical public health concern, especially with the associated increased morbidity and mortality from cardiovascular disease (CVD).[1,6] In this context, diabetic kidney disease (DKD) is a clinical syndrome characterized by early glomerular hyperfiltration and albuminuria, followed by increasing proteinuria and a decline in glomerular filtration rate (GFR), blood pressure increase, and high risk of CVD morbidity and mortality.[7] The cause of this disease, although it is increasingly common because of the global expansion of diabetes and obesity, is poorly understood.

PATHOLOGY OF DKD

DKD has been studied extensively over the years, but our understanding of this complex disease process is far from complete. It is generally accepted that diabetes is associated with diverse structural changes in the kidney; all structural compartments are affected, leading to functional impairments at all levels of the nephron. Three basic steps have been described in progression of DKD[8]: (1) glomerular hypertrophy and hyperfiltration, (2) inflammation of the glomeruli and tubulointerstitial area, and (3) apoptosis of cells and accumulation of extracellular matrix.

The hyperglycemia observed in diabetes contributes to a microinflammatory, oxidative stress milieu and extracellular matrix expansion within the kidney.[8] There are 3 critical abnormalities including intracellular metabolism, formation of advanced glycation end products, and intraglomerular hypertension implicated in development of glomerular endothelial and mesangial cell injury. These pathologic changes are associated with cellular injury, expression of adhesion molecules, and macrophage infiltration in kidney tissue.[8]

Expansion of the mesangium, thickening of the glomerular basement membrane (GBM), and hyalinosis of afferent and efferent arterioles are the characteristic lesions of DKD.[9] It is generally believed that thickening of GBM and expansion of mesangium occur early in the course of diabetes. Diffuse global mesangial expansion is seen in diabetes, and it is primarily caused by an increase in extracellular matrix, with limited contribution from increase in mesangial cell volume.[9] Kimmelstiel-Wilson nodules (acellular to paucicellular nodular accumulations of mesangial matrix) have been described in DKD. These nodular sclerotic lesions occur in patients with advanced DKD, and their presence is considered to mark the transition from early to more advanced stages of DKD.[10] Kimmelstiel-Wilson nodules are not pathognomonic of DKD, because these lesions can be seen in other conditions like monoclonal immunoglobulin deposition disorders, membranoproliferative glomerulonephritis, postinfectious glomerulonephritis, and amyloidosis.[9,10] In parallel, hyaline deposition in the glomerular arterioles is another typical histologic feature of DKD. Hyalinosis and the resultant hyaline appearance (homogeneous and glassy) is caused by insinuation of plasma proteins into the vascular wall.

Alternatively, loss of integrity of the filtration barrier and podocyte injury with effacement of foot processes and loss of podocytes are other microscopic changes evident in DKD that play important roles in the development of progressive sclerosis and proteinuria.[9]

Recently, DKD in type 1 diabetes mellitus and type 2 diabetes mellitus (T2DM) has been classified based on severity of glomerular lesions. Classification based on glomerular lesions has been chosen over interstitial or vascular lesions, because of ease of recognition and good interobserver reproducibility. In addition, it has been suggested that severity of chronic interstitial and glomerular lesions corelate closely. The pathologic classification of DKD as proposed by the Renal Pathology Society[10] is: class 1, diabetic injury with GBM thickening (>2 standard deviations from normal); class 2, mesangial expansion; 2a, mild mesangial expansion; 2b, severe mesangial expansion; class 3, nodular sclerosis (Kimmelstiel-Wilson lesion); class 4, advanced diabetic glomerulosclerosis: global sclerosis involving more than 50% of glomeruli in addition to the changes described earlier. Ongoing basic science and clinical research is helping shape our understanding of DKD pathogenesis and correlation between histologic lesions of DKD and progression of clinical DKD.

THE CARDIORENAL SYNDROME AND DKD

Involvement of both kidneys and the cardiovascular system is common in conjunction with overweight/obesity, metabolic abnormalities, hypertension and early T2DM. Thus, it is important to understand how involvement of 1 organ system contributes to the dysfunction of the other, and these complex interactions have been captured with the emergence of the concept of cardiorenal syndrome (CRS).[7,11–13] Risk factors that influence heart and kidney disease like overweight or obesity, hypertension, insulin resistance, and metabolic dyslipidemic function are the defining components of CRS (**Fig. 1**).[11] The presence of hypertension, obesity, and hyperinsulinemia are independently associated with reductions in kidney function.[12] The interaction of these factors and their metabolic and immunologic effect should be referred to as the CRS. Obesity is associated with altered intrarenal physical forces, inappropriate activation of the renin-angiotensin system (RAS) and sympathetic nervous system, and decreased activity of endogenous natriuretic peptides, which contribute to increases in blood pressure and altered responses to handling of glucose in individuals with insulin resistance.[14] Thus, the various components of CRS interact via complex intertwined pathways and result in the loss of renal structure and function.

IMPACT OF HYPERTENSION ON DKD

There have been several seminal studies describing the importance of hypertension to cardiovascular mortality in individuals with DKD. In this context, approximately 66% of individuals with an estimated GFR (eGFR) less than 60 mL/min/1.73 m^2 have hypertension and as eGFR diminishes over time, the prevalence rates increase from 36% in stage 1 to 84% in stages 4 to 5 CKD.[15] Because increases in blood pressure dictate cardiovascular mortality to some extent, it has been noted that mortality caused by CVD is 10 to 30 times higher in individuals with kidney disease compared with the general population: a relationship that extends into earlier stages of DKD.[16] This relationship has been described as a continuous relationship: with reductions in GFR and increases in proteinuria comes a graded increase in CVD.[17] Moreover, recent studies support the notion that even early stages of CKD pose a significant risk of CVD.[18]

Control of blood pressure in diabetes has been studied extensively, and stricter blood pressure targets have been tested overtime. Many studies have shown the beneficial effects of blood pressure control on various outcomes in patients with diabetes; however, blood pressure targets have been a source of debate for several

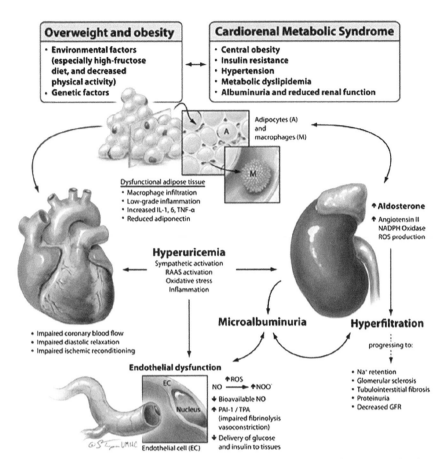

Fig. 1. The interrelationship between adiposity and maladaptive changes in the heart and kidney in CRS. IL, interleukin; PAI, plasminogen activator inhibitor; RAAS, renin-angiotensin-aldosterone system; ROS, reactive oxygen species; TNF, tumor necrosis factor; TPA, tissue plasminogen activator. (*From* Sowers JR, Whaley-Connell A, Hayden MR. The role of overweight and obesity in the cardiorenal syndrome. Cardiorenal Med 2011;1:5–12; with permission.)

years.[19] There are sufficient data to support blood pressure control in T2DM, because this control reduces proteinuria and progression of DKD.[20] The United Kingdom Prospective Diabetes Study (UKPDS) suggests the potential microvascular benefits of blood pressure control in patients with diabetes, wherein 758 patients with T2DM were randomized to tight blood pressure control (<150/85 mm Hg) and 390 to less tight control (<180/105 mm Hg). Mean blood pressures of 144/82 mm Hg and 154/87 mm Hg were achieved in the 2 groups, respectively. Fewer patients in the tight control group had urine albumin concentration greater than 50 mg/L than in the less tight control group at 6 years, although these differences were not significant at 9 years of follow-up.[21] Data from the ADVANCE (Action in Diabetes and Vascular Disease: Preterax and Diamicron Modified Release Controlled Evaluation) trial along with the AASK (African American Study of Kidney Disease and Hypertension) trial suggest that tight blood pressure control (<120/70 mm Hg) in the context of diabetes and proteinuria improves kidney-specific outcomes. In the ADVANCE trial, there were

11,140 enrolled patients with T2DM, who were randomly assigned to blood pressure treatment with fixed combination perindopril-indapamide or placebo. During the follow-up, mean systolic blood pressure (SBP) 134.7 and 140.3, and mean diastolic blood pressure (DBP) 74.8 and 77.0 mm Hg was attained in the active treatment and placebo groups, respectively. Active treatment not only decreased the risk for onset and progression of microalbuminuria, it also increased the chance of regression of microalbuminuria.[20]

Over time, evidence has accumulated to suggest renal benefits of tight blood pressure control in hypertensive patients with diabetes, and has raised questions about treatment threshold. This question was addressed in the Appropriate Blood Pressure Control in Diabetics (Normotensive ABCD) study. Normotensive ABCD is a prospective randomized trial designed to study the effects of decreasing blood pressure in normotensive (blood pressure <140/90 mm Hg) patients with diabetes. A total of 480 patients were randomly assigned to intensive DBP control (target DBP of 10 mm Hg < baseline) and moderate DBP control (target DBP 80–89 mm Hg). The intensive treatment group was treated with nisoldipine or enalapril, and the moderate-treatment group with placebo. Over a 5-year follow-up period, intensive blood pressure control (mean blood pressure 128/75 mm Hg) was associated with decreased risk for progression to incipient nephropathy and diabetic nephropathy in patients who were normotensive at baseline.[22]

The importance of blood pressure control in patients with diabetes cannot be overemphasized. Blood pressure control is paramount for preservation of kidney function in patients with diabetes, especially because risk for progression to ESRD is increased up to 7-fold in patients with concomitant T2DM and hypertension.[23]

NONDIPPING BLOOD PRESSURE/PULSE PATTERN IN DIABETES

A characteristic of diabetes includes a disproportionate increase in SBP, with a loss of nocturnal dipping of blood pressure and heart rate, commonly referred to as nondipping.[24] In normotensive patients, there is a circadian regulation of blood pressure wherein there are nocturnal drops in blood pressure of approximately 10% to 15%, commonly referred to as dipping. Alternatively, nondippers have less than the usual 10% decline at night. Nondipping is frequent among diabetic patients, as shown on ambulatory blood pressure monitoring. This nondipping pattern is caused, in part, by dysfunction of the autonomic nervous system, which is often present in individuals with T2DM and is characterized by a reduction in relative parasympathetic activity; it is believed to contribute to the 5-fold to 7-fold increase in sudden death in diabetic patients.[24,25] Studies have shown that the nondipping pattern of blood pressure is associated with microalbuminuria, overt proteinuria, and higher morbidity and mortality in patients with diabetes.[26] In this context, use of ambulatory blood pressure for measurement of dipping status is superior to office blood pressure in predicting target organ involvement, such as proteinuria and left ventricular hypertrophy.[24]

BLOOD PRESSURE VARIABILITY AS A RISK FACTOR FOR DKD

There are several modifiable risk factors that predict development of incipient and overt kidney disease in people with obesity and diabetes.[27,28] Traditional risk factors for DKD include long-term poor glycemic control, systemic and glomerular hypertension, hypercholesterolemia, urine albumin excretion (UAE) rate, intrauterine growth retardation, and smoking.[27–29] With regard to hypertension, attention has traditionally been focused on systolic, diastolic, and mean blood pressure with the assumption that conventional clinic readings depict a patient's true blood pressure and predict adverse outcomes.[30] Blood pressure variability has been considered a random phenomenon of little clinical significance, although accumulating data suggest that visit-to-visit variability in blood pressure and episodic hypertension might affect cardiovascular and other target organ outcomes.[30,31] Emerging data also suggest that different drug classes affect blood pressure variability differently. Calcium channel blockers and nonloop diuretics decrease blood pressure variability, whereas β-blockers, angiotensin-converting enzyme (ACE) inhibitors, and angiotensin receptor blockers (ARB) increase the blood pressure variability.[32]

A post hoc analysis of data from DCCT (Diabetes Control and Complications Trial) shows that a patient with SBP variability of 13.3 mm Hg has a risk 2.34 times higher for kidney disease compared with a patient with variability of 3.7 mm Hg.[33] Observational data from a retrospective cohort study involving 354 patients with T2DM suggest that individuals who have greater visit-to-visit SBP variability might be at risk for development and progression of proteinuria.[34] Recent data from multiple cohorts involving patients with previous transient ischemic attacks and treated hypertension show a strong predictive value of visit-to-visit variability in SBP and maximum SBP for stroke and coronary events, independent of mean systolic pressures. Data from this study emphasize the risks of episodic hypertension, but do not prove a causal link between stroke and blood pressure variability or maximum SBP.[35] Data from a relatively small longitudinal retrospective observational study involving 374 elderly patients with CKD showed association between visit-to-visit blood pressure variability and all-cause mortality. This study failed to show association between blood pressure variability and progression of CKD.[36] Data accumulating from other studies points that visit-to-visit SBP variability might be associated with all-cause mortality and progression of vascular disease independent of mean arterial pressures in patients with or without diabetes.[34–39]

Results of a meta-analysis[40] suggest that variability of SBP between arms could be helpful for identification of people at increased risk for vascular disease. These findings have prompted investigators to study the role of blood pressure difference between arms further and to explore its predictive value for other outcomes. Recently, investigators have studied the role of difference in SBP between arms and between lower limbs, in predicting risk for DKD. Initial data suggest that such blood pressure differences could be novel risk markers for DKD.[41]

Accumulating data challenges the notion that mean arterial pressure or usual blood pressure is a sufficient predictor of vascular events and stresses the need to analyze the available data and to explore the roles of other factors like blood pressure variability. Blood pressure variability is difficult to quantify and it is unclear how to incorporate it in to clinical practice. Further research is needed to better quantify associated risks and treatment parameters.

USE OF ACE INHIBITORS OR ARBS IN DKD

The treatment of hypertension in those with DKD includes both nonpharmacologic and pharmacologic approaches. However, in the presence of reduced blood pressure in DKD, use of pharmacologic strategies with interruption of the RAS with ACE inhibitors or ARBs is a primary risk-reduction strategy.[23,42–45] Available data suggest that ARBs might have renal benefits independent of the SBP decreasing effect in patients with T2DM.[43,44,46] Data from a study that compared the renoprotective effects of telmisartan and enalapril suggest that ARBs and ACE inhibitors are equally effective in preventing loss of kidney function in patients with T2DM and early DKD.[47] Data from another large study show that losartan has significant beneficial effects on kidney function in patients with T2DM. Small differences in blood pressure were noted between the losartan and placebo-treated groups, and it remains unclear to what extent the renal benefits in the group treated with losartan could be attributed to the lower blood pressure.[46] Data from the ROADMAP (Randomized Olmesartan and Diabetes Microalbuminuria Prevention) trial also showed that the use of olmesartan was associated with delay in onset of microalbuminuria, but again there were subtle differences in blood pressure between the 2 treatment groups.[45]

However, the benefit of dual RAS blockade has been in question. Data from ONTARGET (Ongoing Telmisartan Alone and in Combination with Ramipril Global Endpoint Trial) suggest that combined treatment with an ACE inhibitor and ARB was more effective than ACE inhibitor alone in reducing proteinuria, but the combination was associated with less desirable renal outcomes and faster decline in GFR.[48] Available data suggest that individual components of RAS blockade help preserve kidney function better than other antihypertensives, at least in people with proteinuria.[48]

EFFECTS OF CKD ON GLUCOSE HOMEOSTASIS AND ASSESSMENT OF GLYCEMIC CONTROL

Diabetes has been implicated in the development and progression of CKD, but progressive renal dysfunction also induces complex changes in insulin metabolism and clearance and affects glucose homeostasis in patients with diabetes. CKD is associated with increased insulin resistance on one hand and decreased insulin clearance on other. A decrease in GFR is associated with decrease in metabolic clearance of insulin, which becomes apparent as GFR decreases lower than 15 to 20 mL/min/1.73 m^2. Usually, as renal function declines, peritubular insulin uptake increases and maintains insulin clearance, but as GFR declines to levels lower than 15 to 20 mL/min/1.73 m^2, peritubular insulin uptake is unable to compensate for decreased renal function.[49] With progression of CKD, the degradation of insulin in the liver and muscle is also impaired because of accumulation of the uremic by-products. This decreased insulin clearance can decrease the insulin requirements in diabetes and can lead to hypoglycemic episodes. The decreased insulin clearance in CKD is counterbalanced by increased insulin resistance and decreased insulin production in patients with CKD.[50] Many other factors like loss of appetite, malnutrition and deficient renal gluconeogenesis and catecholamine release affect glucose homeostasis in renal disease.[50] Complex interactions of multiple divergent pathways make the determination of insulin requirement challenging in patients with DKD.

Lack of a standardized clinical test for monitoring glycemic control in DKD complicates management of diabetes in this patient subgroup. Glycated hemoglobin (HbA1c), which is widely used to evaluate glycemic control in diabetes, provides a retrospective assessment of glycemic control. HbA1c has been found to reliably access glycemic control in patients with diabetes, but its accuracy in patients with DKD is questionable. HbA1c levels are affected by high urea levels, uremic acidosis, reduced red blood cell survival, and frequent blood transfusions, and hence there is a potential for erroneous glycemic control estimates in patients with DKD.[51]

Other markers of glycemic control such as glycated albumin and serum fructosamine assess glycemic control over 2 weeks, but these are unreliable in conditions affecting albumin metabolism.[52] These tests have not been standardized and are not used frequently in clinical practice.[53] Further studies are required to assess their use for diagnosis of diabetes and evaluation of glycemic control.

MARKERS OF DKD AND PROGNOSTIC VALUE OF EGFR AND MICROALBUMINURIA

Traditionally, eGFR and UAE have been used to define and to follow progression of DKD. In clinical practice, eGFR is estimated using clearance of endogenous creatinine. Release of creatinine into circulation is variable and depends on factors like age, gender, muscle mass, diet, volume status, medications, and so forth. Creatinine clearance further tends to overestimate GFR, because of tubular secretion of creatinine. Several equations like Cockcroft-Gault and Modification of Diet in Renal Disease 4-variable (MDRD) have been used to improve the accuracy of GFR estimation, but these equations are less than perfect.[2] Recently, the Chronic Kidney Disease Epidemiologic Collaboration) (CKD-EPI) equation was developed in an attempt to overcome the limitations of the MDRD equation. The CKD-EPI equation estimates GFR more accurately, especially at eGFR greater than 60 mL/min/1.73 m[2].[54]

Other markers of GFR such as cystatin C have been studied, but have not received widespread acceptance in clinical practice because of associated costs. Limitations of biomarkers for acute kidney injury and CKD have prompted active interest in study of biomarkers. Many biomarkers are under investigation, including urinary podocytes, neutrophil gelatinase-associated lipocalin, kidney injury molecule 1, Smad-1, connective tissue growth factor, and transforming growth factor β.[2]

Along with eGFR, UAE is used to monitor progression and for staging of DKD. Although debatable, microalbuminuria is considered a risk predictor for progression to overt DKD and for CVD. Screening for microalbuminuria is widely recommended for risk stratification. Numerous population-based and intervention studies support microalbuminuria as a risk factor for CVD and as a strong predictor of cardiovascular morbidity and mortality in patients with diabetes.[55,56] Data from a study of 3431 diabetic patients in the United Kingdom[57] show that eGFR declined rapidly in people with macroalbuminuria and microalbuminuria, at rates of 5.7% and 1.5% per annum, respectively. The progression of DKD was slower in patients with normoalbuminuria: an eGFR decline of only 0.3% per year. Recently, a post hoc analysis of the HUNT-2 (Nord-Trøndelag Health) study[58] showed that CKD progression risk increases substantially, in presence of microalbuminuria or macroalbuminuria. Data from this analysis suggest a strong synergistic interaction between albuminuria and reduced eGFR, which together confer higher risk of progression to ESRD than is attributable to either risk factor individually.[58] This study highlights the importance of using UAE in combination with eGFR for better classification and risk stratification of patients with CKD.[58]

The risk for all-cause and cardiovascular mortality increases with increase in UAE and decrease in eGFR. Data from a large retrospective study involving 1,120,295 adult patients showed that low eGFR ($\leq$60 mL/min/1.73 m[2]) was independently associated with increased risk of death, cardiovascular events, and hospitalization. The risks were substantially increased when eGFR decreased further to levels lower than 45 mL/min/1.73 m[2]. The adjusted hazard ratios for death were 1.2 (95% confidence interval [CI], 1.1–1.2), 1.8 (95% CI, 1.7–1.9), 3.2 (95% CI, 3.1–3.4), and 5.9 (95% CI, 5.4–6.5) for eGFR 45 to 59, 30 to 44, 15 to 29, and less than 15, respectively.[17] Data from RIACE (Renal Insufficiency And Cardiovascular Events), a cross-sectional study involving 15,773 patients with T2DM,[59] led to similar conclusions. The data further showed that low eGFR and albuminuria $\geq$10.5 mg/24 h are associated with coronary artery disease in patients with T2DM. A meta-analysis of albumin-to-creatinine ratio (ACR) data from more than 1 million participants and urine protein dipstick data from 112,310 participants showed a significant increase in mortality risk at low eGFR ($\leq$60 mL/min/1.73 m[2]) compared with optimum eGFR (90–104 mL/min/1.73 m[2]).[6] Albuminuria was measured by ACR or urine dipstick in the included studies. The analyses showed that even trace protein on urine dipstick is associated with increased mortality in the general population, independent of eGFR and traditional cardiovascular risk factors.[6] The hazard ratios for all-cause mortality were 1.20 (95% CI, 1.15–1.26), 1.63 (95% CI, 1.50–1.77) and 2.22 (95% CI, 1.97–2.51) for ACR 1.1 mg/mmol, 3.4 mg/mmol, and

33.9 mg/mmol, respectively, compared with ACR of 0.6 mg/mmol.[6] These findings highlight the importance of urine dipstick, an imprecise but inexpensive measure of albuminuria, in detection of DKD.[6]

Although some data suggest that CKD is not an independent risk factor for cardio-vascular mortality,[60,61] many believe that CKD is independently associated with cardiovascular mortality and all-cause mortality.[62–67] Confounding by previous CVD and by traditional and nontraditional CVD risk in patients with established CKD makes data interpretation challenging.[17] It is unclear if the increased cardiovascular mortality in CKD is an independent effect or if it can be attributed to confounding factors. The role of other pathologic changes like hypercoagulability, endothelial dysfunction, arterial stiffness, and increased inflammatory response as cardiovascular outcome modulators in people with CKD is an area of active interest.[17]

The literature supports the simultaneous use of eGFR and UAE for better risk stratification of patients with DKD. When used simultaneously, these markers help predict CKD progression and cardiovascular risk in patients with DKD.

DKD WITHOUT ALBUMINURIA

Proteinuria has traditionally been considered a diagnostic and prognostic marker of DKD, and its presence prompts interventions such as initiation of ACE inhibitors or ARBs. Absence of proteinuria can render a false sense of reassurance for clinicians and often delays diagnosis and treatment of DKD. Development and progression of microalbuminuria in patients with DKD are not rules, and there is a distinct population who do not develop any level of proteinuria until late in disease. There is a possibility of stabilization and even regression of microalbuminuria in patients with diabetes.[68] DKD is believed to arise from microvascular damage, which leads to increased UAE.[69] Over time, data have accumulated to suggest a high prevalence of kidney disease in patients with diabetes and normal UAE, suggesting the presence of renal lesions other than classic diabetic glomerulosclerosis in this population subgroup. This finding has prompted investigators to consider other explanations like interstitial fibrosis, ischemic vascular disease, cholesterol microemboli, atherosclerotic involvement of the renal vasculature, and so forth.[69,70]

Recently, researchers studied the development of nephropathy in the Cohen diabetic rat (an experimental model of human T2DM). The Cohen diabetic sensitive rats develop CKD with reduced eGFR and histologic changes consistent with DKD, as shown by light and electron microscopy, in absence of proteinuria, when fed a diabetogenic diet. These rats develop changes suggestive of nonproliferative retinopathy as well, although these changes appeared later than development of DKD.[71]

The characteristic histologic lesions seen in classic diabetic glomerulosclerosis are often seen with other systemic manifestations of microvascular disease. These lesions include increased basement membrane thickness, diffuse mesangial sclerosis with nodular formation, hyalinosis, microaneurysm, and hyaline arteriosclerosis.[70,71]

Data from DEMAND (Developing Education on Microalbuminuria for Awareness of Renal and Cardiovascular Risk in Diabetes), a global cross-sectional study,[72] showed that kidney dysfunction is not uncommon in T2DM with normal UAE. Kramer and colleagues[70] performed a cross-sectional analysis of a nationally representative sample of adults with T2DM and found that about 30% individuals with eGFR less than 60 did not have retinopathy or microalbuminuria. Data from other cross-sectional studies like RIACE, and longitudinal studies like ARIC (Atherosclerosis Risk in Communities) and UKPDS suggest that normoalbuminuric renal impairment occurs frequently in patients with T2DM.[68,73–75] Macroangiopathy could be the underlying renal disease as opposed to microangiopathy, in diabetic patients with normoalbuminuric CKD.[73] This change in phenotype of DKD could be related to better control of risk factors like hyperglycemia, hyperlipidemia, hypertension, and early use of ACE inhibitors and ARBs.[73]

Recent findings have encouraged investigators to think of microalbuminuria and reduced eGFR as markers of different pathologic processes. Microalbuminuria could be a phenotypic expression of endothelial dysfunction, whereas reduced eGFR could be a renal manifestation of systemic atherosclerosis.[67]

DOES BETTER GLYCEMIC CONTROL REDUCE DKD?

Data from DCCT and UKPDS have shaped the understanding and management of diabetes over the years for risk reduction of cardiovascular and kidney disease. In UKPDS, patients with T2DM were randomly assigned to intensive or conventional glycemic control using insulin or oral hypoglycemic agents. Over 10 years, HbA1c levels of 7% and 7.9% were achieved in the intensive and conventional groups, respectively. The patients assigned to intensive treatment protocols had decreased risk of microvascular complications, but the intensive treatment was associated with more hypoglycemic episodes and weight gain. The data also suggested that intensive control was associated with decreased progression of albuminuria.[76] Posttrial monitoring of patients enrolled in UKPDS, without any attempt to maintain previous diabetes therapies, showed an early loss (at 1 year) of glycemic differences between the 2 cohorts. Over a 10-year follow-up, sustained benefit and continued risk reduction for microvascular complications were observed in the cohort previously subject to intensive diabetes therapy.[77]

ADVANCE is a multicenter randomized controlled trial designed to study the effects of intensive glucose control (target HbA1c <6.5%) on vascular outcomes in T2DM. Mean HbA1c levels of 6.5% and 7.3% were achieved in the intensive and standard therapy groups, respectively. Data from this trial showed significant reduction in the incidence of nephropathy with intensive glycemic control. Intensive treatment was also associated with decreased need for renal replacement therapy and death from complications related to kidney disease.[78]

Previously, data from DCCT showed beneficial effects of intensive versus conventional glycemic control on kidney function in patients with type 1 diabetes. Conventional therapy aimed at prevention of symptoms attributable to glycosuria or hyperglycemia and maintenance of normal growth and development, whereas intensive therapy aimed at achieving preprandial blood glucose levels of 70 to 120 mg/dL and postprandial blood glucose concentration less than 180 mg/dL. Over a mean follow-up period of 6.5 years, microalbuminuria and albuminuria developed in fewer patients on intensive treatment, compared with patients on conventional treatment, leading to conclusions that intensive management of blood glucose in patients with insulin-dependent diabetes can delay the onset and slow the progression of diabetic nephropathy.[79] The DCCT participants were followed in the EDIC (Epidemiology of Diabetes Interventions and Complications) study, an observational study after the DCCT closeout. The DCCT intensive treatment cohort were encouraged to continue the intensive treatment, and the conventional treatment cohort were encouraged to switch to intensive treatment. Over 8 years of further follow-up, the HbA1c difference between the 2 groups narrowed, with mean values of 8.0% and 8.2% in the 2 cohorts, respectively. The incidence of microalbuminuria and clinical albuminuria was significantly lower in the group subject to intensive treatment during the DCCT trial.[80] Further follow-up data have shown the extension of benefits of early intensive diabetes treatment in patients with insulin-dependent diabetes for up to 22 years. The patients in the intensive treatment arm of DCCT had a 50% lower risk of impaired GFR at 22 years of follow-up, compared with patients in the conventional treatment arm, suggesting a metabolic memory effect.[81] These data further suggest that intensive therapy for insulin-dependent diabetes in 29 patients for 6.5 years can prevent impaired GFR in 1 patient over 20 years.[82]

Data from these well-designed prospective trials indicate that better glycemic control has an important role in delaying the onset and slowing the progression of nephropathy in patients with diabetes.

Although good glycemic and blood pressure control remain the cornerstones of treatment strategy, to prevent or to slow progression of DKD, other treatment approaches are being explored. Recently, effects of treatment with linagliptin, either alone or in combination with telmisartan, were studied in a mouse model of diabetic nephropathy. The combination seemed to have beneficial effects on albuminuria in mice, but its role in treatment or prevention of DKD in humans needs to be explored.[83]

PHARMACOLOGIC TREATMENT OF HYPERGLYCEMIA IN DKD/USE OF OLD AND NEW DRUGS OTHER THAN INSULIN

CKD affects metabolism of oral hypoglycemic agents and leads to accumulation of their metabolites, thus limiting the therapeutic options for patients with DKD. As discussed previously, renal dysfunction alters glucose homeostasis in unpredictable ways via multiple mechanisms in patients with DKD. This finding makes management of diabetes, especially glycemic control, challenging in DKD. The alterations in glucose and insulin handling by kidneys and other body tissues in DKD lead to a state of glycemic dysregulation, which is associated with increased risk of hypoglycemia as well as hyperglycemia.[53]

Selection of an appropriate therapeutic modality is complicated by pharmacokinetic alterations caused by reduced kidney function (**Table 1**).

Sulfonylureas

Sulfonylureas are insulin secretagogues and they increase endogenous insulin secretion. There is a high risk of hypoglycemia, especially with the use of longer-acting sulfonylureas like glyburide.[84]

Second-generation sulfonylureas like glipizide and glimepiride can be used in patients with diabetes and CKD. Glyburide should be avoided because of its long half-life. Glimepiride should be initiated at a low dose in patients with CKD and should be avoided in patients on dialysis.

Glipizide is the preferred second-generation sulfonylurea for patients with diabetes and CKD, and no dosage adjustment is required for patients with CKD or for those on dialysis.[84]

Meglitinides

These are insulin secretagogues with rapid onset of action and short half-life. Repaglinide and nateglinide are the 2 meglitinides available in the United States.[85]

No dose adjustment is required while using repaglinide in patients with CKD or for those on dialysis, but it is recommended that repaglinide be initiated at a lower dose (0.5 mg before each meal) in patients with GFR less than 40.[84] Use in people with GFR less than 20 or those on dialysis has not been studied. Nateglinide should be initiated at a lower dose (60 mg before each meal) in patients with CKD and should be avoided in patients on dialysis.[84]

Table 1
Dosage of drugs used to manage hyperglycemia in patients with diabetes and CKD/DKD

Drug Class	Drug	Major Action	Dosing Recommendation in CKD	Dosing Recommendation in Dialysis
Sulfonylureas	Glipizide	Insulin secretagogue	No dose adjustment required	No dose adjustment required
	Glimepiride	Insulin secretagogue	Initiate at 1 mg/d and titrate slowly	Avoid
	Glyburide	Insulin secretagogue	Not recommended	Not recommended
α-Glucosidase inhibitors	Acarbose	Slow carbohydrate absorption	Not recommended in sCr >2 mg/dL	Not recommended
	Miglitol	Slow carbohydrate absorption	Not recommended if sCr >2 mg/dL	Not recommended
Meglitinides	Repaglinide	Insulin secretagogue	Initiate at a lower dose 0.5 mg before each meal if GFR <40	Use not studied
	Nateglinide	Insulin secretagogue	Initiate at a low dose 60 mg before each meal	Avoid
Biguanides	Metformin	Liver insulin sensitizer	Contraindicated if sCr ≥1.5 mg/dL in men, and ≥1.4 mg/dL in women	Not recommended
Thiazolidinediones	Rosiglitazone	Peripheral insulin sensitizer	No dose adjustment	No dose adjustment
	Pioglitazone	Peripheral insulin sensitizer	No dose adjustment	No dose adjustment

Class	Drug	Mechanism	Dosing	Recommendation
Incretin mimetics	Exenatide	Improved insulin secretion	GFR >50 no dose adjustment GFR 30–50 cautious use, but no dose adjustment suggested GFR <30 use not recommended	Use not recommended
	Liraglutide	Improved insulin secretion	No dose adjustment	No dose adjustment
Dipeptidylpeptidase-4 inhibitors	Sitagliptin	Improved insulin secretion	GFR >50 no dose adjustment, use 100 mg/d GFR 30–50 use 50 mg/d GFR <30 use 25 mg/d	Use 25 mg/d
	Alogliptin	Improved insulin secretion	GFR >50 no dose adjustment GFR 50–30 use 12.5 mg/d GFR <30 use 6.25 mg/d	Use 6.25 mg/d
	Linagliptin	Improved insulin secretion	No dose adjustment	No dose adjustment
	Saxagliptin	Improved insulin secretion	GFR >50 no dose adjustment GFR <50 use 2.5 mg/d	Use 2.5 mg/d
Amylin analogue	Pramlintide	Increased satiety and decreased glucagon	GFR >20 no dose adjustment	Lacks clinical data
Sodium glucose cotransporter 2 inhibitors	Canagliflozin	Glucuresis	GFR ≥60 no dose adjustment (use 100–300 mg daily) GFR 45–60 (maximum dose 100 mg/d) GFR 30–45 use not recommended GFR <30 contraindicated	Contraindicated

Abbreviation: sCr, serum creatinine level.
Adapted from Refs.[84,86–90]

α-Glucosidase Inhibitors

α-Glucosidase inhibitors prevent or decrease postprandial hyperglycemia. They work by decreasing the rate of breakdown of complex carbohydrates in the intestine, and thus decrease the amount of glucose available for absorption.[86] Acarbose has minimal systemic absorption, but the drug and its metabolite tend to accumulate in patients with severe renal dysfunction. Similarly, higher plasma levels of miglitol are present in patients with severe renal failure compared with patients with normal renal function, when on equal doses of miglitol. Acarbose and miglitol are available in the United States, but are not recommended for patients with serum creatinine greater than 2 mg/dL or on dialysis, because long-term safety of these drugs in patients with CKD has not been studied.[84]

Biguanides

Metformin suppresses gluconeogenesis by decreasing hepatic insulin resistance. It effectively decreases glucose concentration in fasting as well as postprandial states.[85]

Metformin should be avoided in patients with moderate and severe renal failure, because renal clearance of metformin is decreased in patients with renal impairment, leading to accumulation of the drug and increased risk of lactic acidosis. Its use in contraindicated in men with serum creatinine level 1.5 mg/dL or greater and women with serum creatinine level 1.4 mg/dL or greater.[84]

Thiazolidinedione

Thiazolidinediones are agonists of peroxisome proliferator-activated receptor γ. The stimulation of this receptor increases insulin-stimulated glucose uptake in muscles and adipose tissue and decreases hepatic glucose production and insulin resistance.[85]

Rosiglitazone and pioglitazone are available in the United States, and these can be used in patients with CKD without dose adjustment. However, these drugs should be used with caution in those with advanced CKD, because of concerns of volume retention. Careful attention should be given to volume status of patients, because thiazolidinediones can cause fluid retention, hemodilution, and exacerbation of heart failure.[84]

Incretin Mimetics

Glucagonlike peptide 1 (GLP-1) is an incretin that increases glucose-dependent insulin secretion. It also slows gastric emptying and increases satiety, and thus decreases food intake.[85] Exenatide and liraglutide are the GLP-1 analogues available in the United States. Use of an exenatide is not recommended in patients with creatinine clearance less than 30 mL/min, or in those on dialysis.[84] Close monitoring is required while initiating or up-titrating the dose of exenatide, especially in patients with mild to moderate renal dysfunction, because use of exenatide is associated with nausea and vomiting, and potential for volume depletion and worsening of renal function. No renal dose adjustment is required for liraglutide, and it can be used safely in patients with CKD or ESRD, although attention to volume status is warranted because of associated nausea and vomiting.[84]

Dipeptidylpeptidase-4 Inhibitors

Dipeptidylpeptidase-4 (DPP-4) inhibitors inhibit DPP-4 and thus prevent degradation of GLP-1. Sitagliptin, linagliptin, saxagliptin, and alogliptin are the DPP-4 inhibitors available in the United States. The dose of sitagliptin and alogliptin needs to be decreased by 50% and 75% for GFR 50 to 30 mL/min/1.73 m^2 and less than 30 mL/min/1.73 m^2, respectively.[84] Saxagliptin can be dosed at 2.5 to 5 mg daily if the GFR is greater than 50, but for patients with lower GFR or ESRD, a dose of 2.5 mg/d should be used.[87] No dosage adjustment is required in patients with CKD for linagliptin.[88]

Amylin Analogue

Amylin is secreted along with insulin by pancreatic β cells. Pramlintide is a synthetic analogue of amylin, and preprandial administration of pramlintide is associated with decreased plasma glucagon, slower gastric emptying, and increased satiety.[85] This medication is metabolized primarily in the kidney, but no change in dose is required if the creatinine clearance is more than 20 mL/min/1.73 m^2. Data are lacking to recommend use of pramlintide in patients on dialysis.[84]

Sodium Glucose Cotransporter 2 Inhibitors

Sodium glucose cotransporter 2 (SGLT2) inhibitors decrease renal threshold for glucose and induce glucuresis independent of insulin action. These agents induce renal excretion of glucose and have the potential to cause weight loss, by disposing excess calories/glucose.[89] Canagliflozin is an SGLT2 inhibitor that has been recently approved in the United States. Its efficacy in patients with diabetes and stage 3 CKD (eGFR $\geq$30 and <50 mL/min/1.73 m^2) has been shown in a placebo-controlled randomized, controlled trial.[90] Efficacy of canagliflozin depends on renal function and this drug is not expected to be effective in patients with eGFR less than 30 mL/min/1.73 m^2 or in those on dialysis.[90] SGLT2 inhibitors have an osmotic diuretic effect and can lead to plasma volume depletion, so kidney function should be monitored while initiating this drug in patients with DKD.

Many new therapeutic agents have been introduced for treatment of diabetes in patients with or without CKD, but special attention to renal function is warranted when choosing the appropriate agent, and dose adjustments should be made to prevent any deleterious effects.

SUMMARY

Diabetes is increasingly prevalent and is an important cause of CKD and ESRD. Recently, attention has been focused on DKD without albuminuria, and its pathogenesis is being studied. There are some indications that pathogenesis of diabetic nephropathy, in the absence of albuminuria, might differ from that of traditional diabetic nephropathy with microalbuminuria. Review of recent trial data indicates that better glycemic and blood pressure control can delay the onset and slow the progression of kidney disease in patients with diabetes. Use of several older oral hypoglycemic agents is either contraindicated or requires dosage adjustment in CKD. New medications for diabetes have been approved recently and many can be used safely in patients with CKD, thus providing treatment alternatives for better glycemic control in patients who are reluctant to use insulin. We further suggest that DKD should be considered in a broader context of cardiorenal metabolic syndrome rather than just diabetes, and close attention should be paid to other modifiable cardiorenal risk factors.

REFERENCES

1. Coresh J, Selvin E, Stevens LA, et al. Prevalence of chronic kidney disease in the United States. JAMA 2007;298:2038–47.

2. Reeves WB, Rawal BB, Abdel-Rahman EM, et al. Therapeutic modalities in diabetic nephropathy: future approaches. Open J Nephrol 2012;2:5–18.
3. Molitch ME, DeFronzo RA, Franz MJ, et al. Nephropathy in diabetes. Diabetes Care 2004;27:S79–83.
4. Whaley-Connell A, Chaudhary K, Misra M, et al. A case for early screening for diabetic kidney disease. Cardiorenal Med 2011;1:235–42.
5. Centers for Disease Control and Prevention. National chronic kidney disease fact sheet 2010. Available at: http://www.cdc.gov/diabetes/pubs/factsheets/kidney.htm. Accessed April 5, 2013.
6. Matsushita K, van der Velde M, Astor BC, et al. Association of estimated glomerular filtration rate and albuminuria with all-cause and cardiovascular mortality in general population cohorts: a collaborative meta-analysis. Lancet 2010;375:2073–81.
7. Sowers JR. Metabolic risk factors and renal disease. Kidney Int 2007;71: 719–20.
8. Wada J, Makino H. Inflammation and the pathogenesis of diabetic nephropathy. Clin Sci 2013;124:139–52.
9. Najafian B, Alpers CE, Fogo AB. Pathology of human diabetic nephropathy. Contrib Nephrol 2011;170:36–47.
10. Tervaert TW, Mooyaart AL, Amann K, et al. Pathologic classification of diabetic nephropathy. J Am Soc Nephrol 2010;21:556–63.
11. Sowers JR, Whaley-Connell A, Hayden MR. The role of overweight and obesity in the cardiorenal syndrome. Cardiorenal Med 2011;1:5–12.
12. Jindal A, Brietzke S, Sowers JR. Obesity and the cardiorenal metabolic syndrome: therapeutic modalities and their efficacy in improving cardiovascular and renal risk factors. Cardiorenal Med 2012;2:314–27.
13. Bakris G, Vassalotti J, Ritz E, et al. National Kidney Foundation consensus conference on cardiovascular and kidney diseases and diabetes risk: an integrated therapeutic approach to reduce events. Kidney Int 2010;78:726–36.
14. Whaley-Connell A, Pavey BS, Afroze A, et al. Obesity and insulin resistance as risk factors for chronic kidney disease. J Cardiometab Syndr 2006;1:209–14.
15. US Renal Data System. USRDS 2010 annual data report: atlas of chronic kidney disease and end-stage renal disease in the United States. Bethesda (MD): National Institutes of Health, National Institute of Diabetes and Digestive and Kidney Diseases; 2010.
16. Sarnak MJ, Levey AS, Schoolwerth AC, et al. Kidney disease as a risk factor for development of cardiovascular disease: a statement from the American Heart Association Councils on Kidney in Cardiovascular Disease, High Blood Pressure Research, Clinical Cardiology, and Epidemiology and Prevention. Circulation 2003;108:2154–69.
17. Go AS, Chertow GM, Fan D, et al. Chronic kidney disease and the risks of death, cardiovascular events, and hospitalization. N Engl J Med 2004;351:1296–305.
18. Anavekar NS, McMurray JJ, Velazquez EJ, et al. Relation between renal dysfunction and cardiovascular outcomes after myocardial infarction. N Engl J Med 2004;351:1285–95.
19. Jindal A, Connell AW, Sowers JR. Type 2 diabetes in older people: the importance of blood pressure control. Curr Cardiovasc Risk Rep 2013;7(3):233–7.
20. de Galan BE, Perkovic V, Ninomiya T, et al. Lowering blood pressure reduces renal events in type 2 diabetes. J Am Soc Nephrol 2009;20:883–92.
21. Tight blood pressure control and risk of macrovascular and microvascular complications in type 2 diabetes: UKPDS 38. UK Prospective Diabetes Study Group. BMJ 1998;317:703–13.

22. Schrier RW, Estacio RO, Esler A, et al. Effects of aggressive blood pressure control in normotensive type 2 diabetic patients on albuminuria, retinopathy and strokes. Kidney Int 2002;61:1086–97.
23. Ruggenenti P, Perna A, Ganeva M, et al. Impact of blood pressure control and angiotensin-converting enzyme inhibitor therapy on new-onset microalbuminuria in type 2 diabetes: a post hoc analysis of the BENEDICT trial. J Am Soc Nephrol 2006;17:3472–81.
24. Pickering TG, Kario K. Nocturnal non-dipping: what does it augur? Curr Opin Nephrol Hypertens 2001;10:611–6.
25. Nielsen FS, Hansen HP, Jacobsen P, et al. Increased sympathetic activity during sleep and nocturnal hypertension in type 2 diabetic patients with diabetic nephropathy. Diabet Med 1999;16:555–62.
26. Ohkubo T, Hozawa A, Yamaguchi J, et al. Prognostic significance of the nocturnal decline in blood pressure in individuals with and without high 24-h blood pressure: the Ohasama study. J Hypertens 2002;20:2183–9.
27. Rossing P, Hougaard P, Parving HH. Risk factors for development of incipient and overt diabetic nephropathy in type 1 diabetic patients: a 10-year prospective observational study. Diabetes Care 2002;25:859–64.
28. Gall MA, Hougaard P, Borch-Johnsen K, et al. Risk factors for development of incipient and overt diabetic nephropathy in patients with non-insulin dependent diabetes mellitus: prospective, observational study. BMJ 1997;314:783–8.
29. Parving HH. Renoprotection in diabetes: genetic and non-genetic risk factors and treatment. Diabetologia 1998;41:745–59.
30. Rothwell PM. Limitations of the usual blood-pressure hypothesis and importance of variability, instability, and episodic hypertension. Lancet 2010;375:938–48.
31. Rossignol P, Kessler M, Zannad F. Visit-to-visit blood pressure variability and risk for progression of cardiovascular and renal diseases. Curr Opin Nephrol Hypertens 2013;22:59–64.
32. Webb AJ, Fischer U, Mehta Z, et al. Effects of antihypertensive-drug class on interindividual variation in blood pressure and risk of stroke: a systematic review and meta-analysis. Lancet 2010;375:906–15.
33. Kilpatrick ES, Rigby AS, Atkin SL. The role of blood pressure variability in the development of nephropathy in type 1 diabetes. Diabetes Care 2010;33:2442–7.
34. Okada H, Fukui M, Tanaka M, et al. Visit-to-visit blood pressure variability is a novel risk factor for the development and progression of diabetic nephropathy in patients with type 2 diabetes. Diabetes Care 2013;36(7):1908–22.
35. Rothwell PM, Howard SC, Dolan E, et al. Prognostic significance of visit-to-visit variability, maximum systolic blood pressure, and episodic hypertension. Lancet 2010;375:895–905.
36. Di Iorio B, Pota A, Sirico ML, et al. Blood pressure variability and outcomes in chronic kidney disease. Nephrol Dial Transplant 2012;27:4404–10.
37. Hsieh YT, Tu ST, Cho TJ, et al. Visit-to-visit variability in blood pressure strongly predicts all-cause mortality in patients with type 2 diabetes: a 5.5-year prospective analysis. Eur J Clin Invest 2012;42:245–53.
38. Okada H, Fukui M, Tanaka M, et al. Visit-to-visit variability in systolic blood pressure is correlated with diabetic nephropathy and atherosclerosis in patients with type 2 diabetes. Atherosclerosis 2012;220:155–9.
39. Muntner P, Shimbo D, Tonelli M, et al. The relationship between visit-to-visit variability in systolic blood pressure and all-cause mortality in the general population: findings from NHANES III, 1988 to 1994. Hypertension 2011;57:160–6.

40. Clark CE, Taylor RS, Shore AC, et al. Association of a difference in systolic blood pressure between arms with vascular disease and mortality: a systematic review and meta-analysis. Lancet 2012;379:905–14.

41. Okada H, Fukui M, Tanaka M, et al. A difference in systolic blood pressure between arms and between lower limbs is a novel risk marker for diabetic nephropathy in patients with type 2 diabetes. Hypertens Res 2013;17:207.

42. Ravid M, Brosh D, Levi Z, et al. Use of enalapril to attenuate decline in renal function in normotensive, normoalbuminuric patients with type 2 diabetes mellitus. A randomized, controlled trial. Ann Intern Med 1998;128:982–8.

43. Parving HH, Lehnert H, Brochner-Mortensen J, et al. The effect of irbesartan on the development of diabetic nephropathy in patients with type 2 diabetes. N Engl J Med 2001;345:870–8.

44. Lewis EJ, Hunsicker LG, Clarke WR, et al. Renoprotective effect of the angiotensin-receptor antagonist irbesartan in patients with nephropathy due to type 2 diabetes. N Engl J Med 2001;345:851–60.

45. Haller H, Ito S, Izzo JL Jr, et al. Olmesartan for the delay or prevention of microalbuminuria in type 2 diabetes. N Engl J Med 2011;364:907–17.

46. Brenner BM, Cooper ME, de Zeeuw D, et al. Effects of losartan on renal and cardiovascular outcomes in patients with type 2 diabetes and nephropathy. N Engl J Med 2001;345:861–9.

47. Barnett AH, Bain SC, Bouter P, et al. Angiotensin-receptor blockade versus converting-enzyme inhibition in type 2 diabetes and nephropathy. N Engl J Med 2004;351:1952–61.

48. Mann JF, Schmieder RE, McQueen M, et al. Renal outcomes with telmisartan, ramipril, or both, in people at high vascular risk (the ONTARGET study): a multicentre, randomised, double-blind, controlled trial. Lancet 2008;372: 547–53.

49. Mak RH. Impact of end-stage renal disease and dialysis on glycemic control. Semin Dial 2000;13(1):4–8.

50. Kovesdy CP, Park JC, Kalantar-Zadeh K. Glycemic control and burnt-out diabetes in ESRD. Semin Dial 2010;23:148–56.

51. Ansari A, Thomas S, Goldsmith D. Assessing glycemic control in patients with diabetes and end-stage renal failure. Am J Kidney Dis 2003;41:523–31.

52. Koga M, Murai J, Saito H, et al. Glycated albumin and glycated hemoglobin are influenced differently by endogenous insulin secretion in patients with type 2 diabetes. Diabetes Care 2010;33:270–2.

53. Kovesdy CP, Sharma K, Kalantar-Zadeh K. Glycemic control in diabetic CKD patients: where do we stand? Am J Kidney Dis 2008;52:766–77.

54. Levey AS, Stevens LA, Schmid CH, et al. A new equation to estimate glomerular filtration rate. Ann Intern Med 2009;150:604–12.

55. Dinneen SF, Gerstein HC. The association of microalbuminuria and mortality in non-insulin-dependent diabetes mellitus. A systematic overview of the literature. Arch Intern Med 1997;157:1413–8.

56. Jensen T, Borch-Johnsen K, Kofoed-Enevoldsen A, et al. Coronary heart disease in young type 1 (insulin-dependent) diabetic patients with and without diabetic nephropathy: incidence and risk factors. Diabetologia 1987;30:144–8.

57. Hoefield RA, Kalra PA, Baker PG, et al. The use of eGFR and ACR to predict decline in renal function in people with diabetes. Nephrol Dial Transplant 2011;26:887–92.

58. Hallan SI, Ritz E, Lydersen S, et al. Combining GFR and albuminuria to classify CKD improves prediction of ESRD. J Am Soc Nephrol 2009;20:1069–77.

59. Solini A, Penno G, Bonora E, et al. Diverging association of reduced glomerular filtration rate and albuminuria with coronary and noncoronary events in patients with type 2 diabetes: the renal insufficiency and cardiovascular events (RIACE) Italian multicenter study. Diabetes Care 2012;35:143–9.
60. Garg AX, Clark WF, Haynes RB, et al. Moderate renal insufficiency and the risk of cardiovascular mortality: results from the NHANES I. Kidney Int 2002;61: 1486–94.
61. Culleton BF, Larson MG, Wilson PW, et al. Cardiovascular disease and mortality in a community-based cohort with mild renal insufficiency. Kidney Int 1999;56: 2214–9.
62. Drey N, Roderick P, Mullee M, et al. A population-based study of the incidence and outcomes of diagnosed chronic kidney disease. Am J Kidney Dis 2003;42: 677–84.
63. Muntner P, He J, Hamm L, et al. Renal insufficiency and subsequent death resulting from cardiovascular disease in the United States. J Am Soc Nephrol 2002;13:745–53.
64. Nakamura K, Okamura T, Hayakawa T, et al. Chronic kidney disease is a risk factor for cardiovascular death in a community-based population in Japan: NIPPON DATA90. Circ J 2006;70:954–9.
65. Manjunath G, Tighiouart H, Coresh J, et al. Level of kidney function as a risk factor for cardiovascular outcomes in the elderly. Kidney Int 2003;63:1121–9.
66. Manjunath G, Tighiouart H, Ibrahim H, et al. Level of kidney function as a risk factor for atherosclerotic cardiovascular outcomes in the community. J Am Coll Cardiol 2003;41:47–55.
67. Ninomiya T, Perkovic V, de Galan BE, et al. Albuminuria and kidney function independently predict cardiovascular and renal outcomes in diabetes. J Am Soc Nephrol 2009;20:1813–21.
68. Retnakaran R, Cull CA, Thorne KI, et al. Risk factors for renal dysfunction in type 2 diabetes: U.K. Prospective Diabetes Study 74. Diabetes 2006;55:1832–9.
69. MacIsaac RJ, Panagiotopoulos S, McNeil KJ, et al. Is nonalbuminuric renal insufficiency in type 2 diabetes related to an increase in intrarenal vascular disease? Diabetes care 2006;29:1560–6.
70. Kramer HJ, Nguyen QD, Curhan G, et al. Renal insufficiency in the absence of albuminuria and retinopathy among adults with type 2 diabetes mellitus. JAMA 2003;289:3273–7.
71. Yagil C, Barak A, Ben-Dor D, et al. Nonproteinuric diabetes-associated nephropathy in the Cohen rat model of type 2 diabetes. Diabetes 2005;54: 1487–96.
72. Dwyer JP, Parving HH, Hunsicker LG, et al. Renal dysfunction in the presence of normoalbuminuria in type 2 diabetes: results from the DEMAND study. Cardiorenal Med 2012;2:1–10.
73. Penno G, Solini A, Bonora E, et al. Clinical significance of nonalbuminuric renal impairment in type 2 diabetes. J Hypertens 2011;29:1802–9.
74. Bash LD, Selvin E, Steffes M, et al. Poor glycemic control in diabetes and the risk of incident chronic kidney disease even in the absence of albuminuria and retinopathy: Atherosclerosis Risk in Communities (ARIC) Study. Arch Intern Med 2008;168:2440–7.
75. MacIsaac RJ, Tsalamandris C, Panagiotopoulos S, et al. Nonalbuminuric renal insufficiency in type 2 diabetes. Diabetes Care 2004;27:195–200.
76. Intensive blood-glucose control with sulphonylureas or insulin compared with conventional treatment and risk of complications in patients with type 2 diabetes

(UKPDS 33). UK Prospective Diabetes Study (UKPDS) Group. Lancet 1998;352: 837–53.

77. Holman RR, Paul SK, Bethel MA, et al. 10-year follow-up of intensive glucose control in type 2 diabetes. N Engl J Med 2008;359:1577–89.

78. Patel A, MacMahon S, Chalmers J, et al. Intensive blood glucose control and vascular outcomes in patients with type 2 diabetes. N Engl J Med 2008;358: 2560–72.

79. The effect of intensive treatment of diabetes on the development and progression of long-term complications in insulin-dependent diabetes mellitus. The Diabetes Control and Complications Trial Research Group. N Engl J Med 1993;329: 977–86.

80. Writing Team for the Diabetes Control and Complications Trial/Epidemiology of Diabetes Interventions and Complications Research Group. Sustained effect of intensive treatment of type 1 diabetes mellitus on development and progression of diabetic nephropathy: the Epidemiology of Diabetes Interventions and Complications (EDIC) study. JAMA 2003;290:2159–67.

81. de Boer IH, Sun W, Cleary PA, et al. Intensive diabetes therapy and glomerular filtration rate in type 1 diabetes. N Engl J Med 2011;365:2366–76.

82. de Boer IH, Rue TC, Cleary PA, et al. Long-term renal outcomes of patients with type 1 diabetes mellitus and microalbuminuria: an analysis of the Diabetes Control and Complications Trial/Epidemiology of Diabetes Interventions and Complications cohort. Arch Intern Med 2011;171:412–20.

83. Alter ML, Ott IM, von Websky K, et al. DPP-4 inhibition on top of angiotensin receptor blockade offers a new therapeutic approach for diabetic nephropathy. Kidney Blood Press Res 2012;36:119–30.

84. Abe M, Okada K, Soma M. Antidiabetic agents in patients with chronic kidney disease and end-stage renal disease on dialysis: metabolism and clinical practice. Curr Drug Metab 2011;12:57–69.

85. Rodbard HW, Jellinger PS, Davidson JA, et al. Statement by an American Association of Clinical Endocrinologists/American College of Endocrinology consensus panel on type 2 diabetes mellitus: an algorithm for glycemic control. Endocr Pract 2009;15:540–59.

86. Hanefeld M, Schaper F. Acarbose: oral anti-diabetes drug with additional cardiovascular benefits. Expert Rev Cardiovasc Ther 2008;6:153–63.

87. Boulton DW, Li L, Frevert EU, et al. Influence of renal or hepatic impairment on the pharmacokinetics of saxagliptin. Clin Pharmacokinet 2011;50:253–65.

88. Friedrich C, Emser A, Woerle HJ, et al. Renal impairment has no clinically relevant effect on the long-term exposure of linagliptin in patients with type 2 diabetes. Am J Ther 2013;13:13.

89. Whaley JM, Tirmenstein M, Reilly TP, et al. Targeting the kidney and glucose excretion with dapagliflozin: preclinical and clinical evidence for SGLT2 inhibition as a new option for treatment of type 2 diabetes mellitus. Diabetes Metab Syndr Obes 2012;5:135–48.

90. Yale JF, Bakris G, Cariou B, et al. Efficacy and safety of canagliflozin in subjects with type 2 diabetes and chronic kidney disease. Diabetes Obes Metab 2013; 15:463–73.

Gastrointestinal Complications of Diabetes

Brigid S. Boland, MD[a],*, Steven V. Edelman, MD[b,c],
James D. Wolosin, MD[d]

KEYWORDS

- Gastrointestinal symptoms • Glycemic control • Gastroparesis • Celiac
- Nonalcoholic fatty liver disease

KEY POINTS

- Gastrointestinal symptoms are common in the general population and frequently are related to irritable bowel syndrome.
- The incidence of multiple gastrointestinal diseases is more common in diabetic patients for a variety of reasons.
- Diabetic neuropathy may lead to abnormal gastrointestinal motility that causes gastroparesis, small bacterial intestinal overgrowth, diabetic diarrhea, and fecal incontinence.

INTRODUCTION

When practitioners think about complications of diabetes, they may focus on the microvascular, macrovascular, and peripheral neuropathic complications that are known to be associated with the disease. Although gastrointestinal problems are extremely common, with upper gastrointestinal symptoms alone affecting more than 40% of the general population,[1] the incidence of certain gastrointestinal symptoms is more common in diabetes, and health care professionals should be aware of these associations. Gastrointestinal symptoms have not only a detrimental effect on quality of life but also significant medical consequences. Poor control of diabetes can affect any segment of the gut from the mouth to the rectum. However, unfamiliarity

Funding Sources: None.
Conflict of Interest: None.
[a] Division of Gastroenterology, Department of Medicine, University of California, San Diego, 9500 Gilman Drive, La Jolla, CA 92093, USA; [b] Division of Endocrinology and Metabolism, University of California, San Diego, 9350 Campus Point Drive, Suite 2G, La Jolla, CA 92093-9111G, USA; [c] Division of Endocrinology and Metabolism, Diabetes Care Clinic, Veterans Affairs Medical Center, 3350 La Jolla Village Drive (111G), San Diego, CA 92161, USA; [d] Division of Gastroenterology, Sharp Rees-Stealy Medical Group, 2929 Health Center Drive, San Diego, CA 92123, USA
* Corresponding author.
E-mail address: bboland@ucsd.edu

Endocrinol Metab Clin N Am 42 (2013) 809–832
http://dx.doi.org/10.1016/j.ecl.2013.07.006
0889-8529/13/$ – see front matter © 2013 Elsevier Inc. All rights reserved.

with these symptoms can delay treatment or referrals to appropriate specialists. The purpose of this review is to highlight the incidence, diagnosis, and treatment of some of the more common gastrointestinal complications of diabetes.

ESOPHAGEAL DISORDERS
Esophageal Motility Dysfunction in Diabetes

The term esophageal motility dysfunction is a phrase used to describe a multitude of esophageal complications that can occur in diabetic patients. Abnormalities seen include reduced lower esophageal sphincter tone, diminished amplitude of esophageal contractions, reduced coordination of esophageal contractions, prolonged esophageal transit, and increased acid reflux.[2] Esophageal motility disorders appear to be driven by neuropathy, a known complication of diabetes. Specifically, vagal nerve dysfunction is thought to drive the underlying pathophysiology. However, recent studies have also implicated motor nerve dysfunction as playing a role.[3]

Symptoms of Esophageal Motility Disorders

Symptoms of esophageal motility disorders may include heartburn after eating and/or drinking, chest pain, odynophagia, and dysphagia. More commonly, these abnormalities are asymptomatic but have been incidentally observed in clinical studies. Treatment options for esophageal hypomotility are limited but may entail lifestyle modification.

Gastroesophageal Reflux Disease in Patients with Diabetes

Just as many motility abnormalities are clinically silent in diabetic patients, the prevalence of asymptomatic gastroesophageal reflux confirmed by pH study is significantly higher in diabetic patients than in healthy controls.[4] Furthermore, the prevalence of gastroesophageal reflux disease (GERD) is higher in patients with diabetes with neuropathy as compared with the general population (41% as compared to 14%).[5] Practitioners should be mindful of this association and be aware of the incidence of GERD when a diagnosis of neuropathy is established. As GERD is a common clinical entity, it is worth familiarizing one's self with the common presentation and treatment modalities.

Risk Factors for Gastroesophageal Reflux in Diabetes
• Cardiovascular autonomic dysfunction
• Elevated body mass index
• Longer duration of disease
• Poor glycemic control

Management of GERD

In patients with reflux, initial recommendations should include lifestyle modifications, such as avoidance of trigger foods (coffee, tomato sauce, spicy foods, and alcohol being common offenders), reduction in meal size, avoidance of eating before sleeping, smoking cessation, elevation of head at night, and weight loss. Frequently, patients will require medical therapy. Management may entail antacids as needed or H2 blockers, such as rantidine, for mild disease. For more significant or persistent symptoms, proton pump inhibitors (PPIs), such as omeprazole or pantoprazole, are extremely effective in the treatment of reflux. Interestingly, a recent randomized clinical trial showed that PPIs improve glycemic control, suggesting additional benefits of

PPIs in diabetic patients with GERD.[6] In patients with classic symptoms of postprandial reflux that responds to antacids, further diagnostic testing is not necessary.

Diagnostic Testing for GERD

When the symptoms of GERD do not respond to a PPI, the underlying diagnosis should be questioned. A referral to a gastroenterologist is appropriate to guide further diagnostic evaluation, such as upper endoscopy, 24-hour esophageal pH monitoring, or manometry. Esophageal pH monitoring directly measures acid in the esophagus and quantifies acid reflux, providing a definitive diagnosis. Technological advances have significantly enhanced diagnostic capabilities with the development of a wireless pH-detection capsule that is placed during endoscopy. Manometry, a study that measures esophageal pressure and muscular contractions, may be used to evaluate for a motility disorder causing GERD-like symptoms. In patients with a long-standing history of GERD, especially middle-aged, overweight Caucasian men, upper endoscopy should be considered to evaluate for Barrett esophagus and assess for esophageal cancer risks.

Esophageal Candidiasis

Individuals with diabetes are at higher risk for oral or esophageal candidiasis that is typically caused by *Candida albicans.* Poor glycemic control allows for favorable conditions for the yeast to grow, increasing the risk of fungal infection. The incidence of esophageal candidiasis in patients with diabetes is not well defined.

Signs and Symptoms of Candidiasis
• Odynophagia
• Dysphagia with solids
• Avoidance of oral intake
• Erythematous friable lesions in oropharynx
• White patches in oropharynx

Management of Oropharyngeal and Esophageal Candidiasis

Candidiasis limited to the oropharyngeal cavity may be treated with nystatin. A typical dosage is 4 to 6 mL (400,000 to 600,000 units) 4 times per day in a swish-and-swallow fashion. Patients continue this therapy until 48 hours after symptoms have resolved. However, if the symptoms are not responding, oral fluconazole should be the treatment of choice. Similarly, the presence of odynophagia in combination with oral thrush is highly predictive of esophageal involvement and is an indication for fluconazole therapy. Therefore, the presence of thrush should always key a practitioner to inquire about pain with swallowing. A loading dose of fluconazole 200 mg is given, followed by 100 to 200 mg daily for 7 to 14 days. Symptoms should resolve in 1 week with treatment, and lack of response should prompt further evaluation with upper endoscopy.[7]

GASTRIC DISORDERS
Gastroparesis

Gastroparesis is defined as delayed gastric emptying in the absence of mechanical obstruction. The condition can result in a wide array of symptoms, ranging from none to a complete inability to tolerate oral nutrients with chronic nausea and vomiting.

Delayed gastric emptying may be seen in up to 40% of patients with diabetes but only 10% or fewer of these patients will have any symptoms. Severe symptoms can result in a significant decrease in quality of life and can further potentiate poor glycemic control, as matching mealtime insulin with slow emptying can be extremely difficult. Patients will often complain of early satiety that may be accompanied by postprandial nausea, vomiting, belching, reflux, palpitations, and/or abdominal pain. The tremendous overlap with symptoms of functional dyspepsia may obscure the diagnosis of gastroparesis.

Although gastroparesis does not independently increase mortality, it is associated with a worse prognosis as compared with age-matched and gender-matched individuals with normal gastric emptying. The 5-year survival of individuals with gastroparesis is 67% as compared with the expected 81% survival.[8]

Epidemiology

The overall incidence of gastroparesis is 4.8% in type 1 diabetes mellitus (DM1), 1% in type 2 diabetes mellitus (DM2), and 0.1% in the general population.[9] Although the incidence of gastroparesis is higher in patients with DM1 as compared with DM2, the overall higher prevalence of DM2 makes gastroparesis more commonly seen by health care providers in this patient population. The incidence and prevalence in women is nearly 4 times that in men.[8] Although onset of gastroparesis appears to occur after 10 years of disease duration, a recent population-based study found no association between diabetes duration and gastroparesis.[9–11]

Pathophysiology of Gastroparesis

Normal gastric emptying is a complex process involving synchronization of smooth muscle and autonomic nerves. This process is coordinated in the interstitial cells of Cajal (ICC), or the pacemakers of the stomach. The ICCs integrate fundic tone, antral contractions, and relaxation of the pylorus to facilitate postprandial emptying. Consequences of diabetes may lead to disruptions in different components of this process, interfering with the normal function of the stomach. Hyperglycemia, even at modest levels, disrupts gastric coordination and emptying in healthy volunteers as well as diabetic patients.[12] Reductions in ICC quantity are seen in biopsies from individuals with gastroparesis.[13]

Autonomic neuropathy, inflammation, and oxidative stress appear to be critical components driving patients with diabetic gastroparesis.[11] The effects of autonomic neuropathy have been demonstrated by gastric biopsies from diabetic patients with gastroparesis showing reduced number of nerve fibers.[14] Vagal nerve functional studies are abnormal in diabetic patients with gastroparesis, showing reduction in postprandial gastric acid section.[15] Oxidative stress has been implicated, given that loss of nitric oxide from enteric cells has been documented in mouse and human

---

Symptoms of Gastroparesis

- Nausea
- Vomiting
- Early satiety
- Bloating
- Upper abdominal discomfort

models of patients with diabetic gastroparesis and appears to occur early after diabetes onset.[16,17] Similarly, loss of a cytoprotective enzyme, heme oxidase-1, has been linked to the pathogenesis of gastroparesis in mouse models.[18] Further, oxidative stress and loss of survival signals from insulin and insulinlike growth factor (IGF)-1 contribute to ICC death.[11,18]

Diagnosis of Gastroparesis

- Symptoms of gastroparesis
- Absence of gastric outlet obstruction based on imaging or endoscopy
- Presence of retained food in the stomach on endoscopy after a fast of more than 12 hours
- Slowed gastric emptying based on scintigraphy

Overall, the symptoms lack sensitivity and specificity, but nausea, vomiting, and early satiety are the best predictors of gastroparesis.[19] The presence of food in the stomach on endoscopy after a 12-hour fast suggests delayed gastric emptying and should raise suspicion for gastroparesis. Consensus guidelines recommend diagnostic testing to confirm the diagnosis of gastroparesis, and scintigraphy is typically the test of choice.[20] For this examination, patients ingest radioisotope technetium-99m–labeled test meals of defined caloric amount. After ingestion of the solid-phase meal, images will be obtained at 60 minutes, 120 minutes, 180 minutes, and 240 minutes. The most reliable predictor of gastroparesis is percentage of retained food at 4 hours. If possible, medications that delay or accelerate gastric emptying, should be discontinued approximately 48 to 72 hours before the study. Acute hyperglycemia may delay gastric emptying, so practitioners may want to delay scintigraphy until blood sugar has been stabilized.[21] Many patients with diabetes may have abnormal emptying studies in the absence of symptoms, and others may have mildly abnormal gastric emptying along with functional dyspepsia that is not directly related to diabetes. It is important to take a good history and be certain that symptoms are suggestive of delayed gastric emptying before making a diagnosis of gastroparesis.

Management of Gastroparesis

- Evaluation and correction of nutritional status
- Improvement of gastric emptying
- Symptomatic treatment

Nutritional Optimization

Gastroparesis may interfere with oral intake and nutritional status; therefore, the first goals of management are to restore hydration, replete electrolytes, and ensure sufficient long-term oral intake. Alcohol and cigarette smoking should be avoided, as they slow gastric emptying. Dietary modifications for gastroparesis aim to optimize emptying of the stomach, while avoiding foods that may delay motility, such as those with high fat and fiber content. A gastroparesis diet entails small, frequent, low-fat, and low-residue meals. If individuals are unable to tolerate modified diets, liquid meals may be trialed, as gastric emptying of liquids is frequently maintained in gastroparesis.

Consultation with a nutritionist may be quite useful in helping patients deal with multiple dietary restrictions. In severe cases, unintentional weight loss greater than 10% of body weight over 3 to 6 months suggests refractory gastroparesis and should prompt consideration for feeding tube placement. To bypass abnormal gastric motility, feeding tubes should be placed beyond the pylorus to bypass the abnormal motility in the stomach.[20]

Management of Glycemic Control in Gastroparesis

Based on experimental models, hyperglycemia delays gastric emptying in patients with diabetes as well as healthy patients.[12,22] Management of gastroparesis should include optimization of glycemic control that may improve short-term symptoms. For patients on mealtime insulin, the timing of their mealtime bolus may have to be adjusted. Rapid-acting insulin can be dosed at the start of the meal or 15 minutes *after* starting a meal in an attempt to match peak insulin levels with glucose appearance. Similarly, switching from rapid-acting analogues to regular insulin may be appropriate for the same reason. Using the square and dual-wave bolus function that is a feature with insulin pumps can be helpful. In addition, current medical treatments, including pramlintide and GLP-1 analogs, cause delayed gastric emptying and may exacerbate symptoms of gastroparesis.[23,24] The drugs may still be used in mild cases, but their use should be discouraged in any case where prokinetic agents must be initiated.

Management of Gastroparesis in Diabetes

Metoclopramide is the first-line prokinetic drug for treatment of gastroparesis. Metoclopramide is a D2 dopamine receptor antagonist (with less potent stimulation of 5-HT4) that increases lower esophageal sphincter tone, gastric pressure, and antral contractions that aids in emptying of the stomach. Metoclopramide also provides antiemetic action by acting centrally and inhibiting the D2 dopamine and 5-HT3 receptors in the chemoreceptor trigger zone, a center in the medulla that integrates sensory input and stimulates vomiting.[25] Although this is the only prokinetic medication for gastroparesis that is approved by the Food and Drug Administration (FDA), its use is approved for only 3 months. The strongest evidence supporting use of metoclopramide comes from 4 placebo-controlled studies that showed improvement in symptoms ranging from 25% to 50%. However, these studies were of shorter duration, on the order of 3 weeks.[26–29] Prolonged use of the medication necessitates an evaluation of the benefits versus potential risks of ongoing therapy.

Metoclopramide carries a black box warning for an increased risk of tardive dyskinesia; a disorder characterized by involuntary movements of the face or extremities induced by dopamine inhibition.[25] Although the incidence of tardive dyskinesia is estimated at approximately 0.2%, the potential irreversible nature of the condition makes even a low incidence concerning. Groups at higher risk for developing tardive dyskinesia include patients on higher doses, those of younger age, and women.[30] Other side effects include QT prolongation, parkinsonian movements, akathisia, and hyperprolactinemia. Guidelines on use of metoclopramide recommend use of a minimal effective dose beginning with 5 mg before meals, monitoring for early signs of tardive dyskinesia, and drug holidays.[31]

Domperidone, a type II dopamine antagonist, has a similar mechanism of action as metoclopramide but with reduced central nervous system effects, and, thus, tardive dyskinesia. Three large randomized controlled trials with domperidone in patients with diabetic gastroparesis have been published and showed symptomatic improvement as compared with baseline or placebo.[32–34] Dosing typically starts at 10 mg with meals. Baseline electrocardiogram is recommended before initiation of therapy based on potential QT prolongation. Less common side effects also include prolactinemia, and potential drug interactions. Although the makers of domperidone have never applied for FDA approval, there are programs for obtaining this medication in the United States.[20]

Intravenous erythromycin lactobionate, a motilin agonist, has been shown to be effective in short-term treatment of hospitalized patients with diabetic gastroparesis. However, ongoing administration of intravenous or oral erythromycin over longer periods of time leads to tachyphylaxis by downregulation of receptors for motilin.[35] In addition, erythromycin itself may induce abnormal gastric motility with resultant nausea and vomiting.

Another technique that has been used in clinical practice is endoscopic intrapyloric injection of botulinum toxin. Manometry studies show that the pylorus has increased tone in patients with gastroparesis. Injection of botulinum toxin to block neurotransmission showed promise in open-label trials, but a randomized clinical trial including diabetic patients showed improvement in gastric emptying without symptomatic improvement.[36] Thus, routine use of botulinum toxin for the treatment of gastroparesis is not advised (**Table 1**).[20]

Management of the nausea and vomiting associated with gastroparesis typically relies on off-label use of medications. Therapies that are used include prochlorperazine, promethazine, ondansetron, scopolamine, and dronabinol; however, there are no evidence-based guidelines for management.

Pain remains extremely challenging, as opiates further slow gastric emptying and exacerbate symptoms. Clinical trials are lacking. Practitioners should discontinue opiates and recommend nonopiate alternatives, including tricyclic antidepressants (TCAs), tramadol, selective serotonin receptor inhibitors, or gabapentin. Low-dose tricyclic antidepressants and selective serotonin receptor inhibitors may modulate pain and improve glycemic control. TCAs have the added benefit of treating pain from coexisting peripheral neuropathy; however, this class of medications has varying anticholinergic effects that may worsen gastroparesis.[20]

Gastric Electric Stimulation for Refractory Gastroparesis

The gastric electrical stimulator (GES) is a neurostimulator that is implanted surgically into the abdomen and provides high-frequency stimulation to the stomach. GES was approved by the FDA under the humanitarian device exemption. A randomized

Table 1 Summary of prokinetic medications for gastroparesis			
Drug	**Starting Dose**	**Side Effects**	**Considerations**
Metoclopramide	5 mg with meals	Tardive dyskinesia, QT prolongation, akathisia, parkinsonian movements, hyperprolactinemia	Use minimum effective dose >4 wk of use needs to be re-evaluated
Domperidone	10 mg with meals	QT prolongation, hyperprolactinemia	Baseline electrocardiogram Not readily available in the United States Better side-effect profile
Erythromycin	3 mg/kg intravenous	Tachyphylaxis	Evidence supports short-term use in hospital

crossover trial showed a reduction in weekly vomiting frequency from 13 to 7, but in the subgroup of patients with diabetes there were no significant differences in symptoms and vomiting frequency.[37] A recent meta-analysis included 10 studies and concluded that GES improved symptoms with small mean differences in symptom scores, and diabetic gastroparesis was the most responsive to GES.[38] Although randomized trials and availability are lacking, GES may be an option for refractory cases.

Salvage and Alternative Therapies for Gastroparesis

There is little evidence to guide management of refractory cases of gastroparesis; however, salvage therapies for symptom management may include venting gastrostomy with or without jejunostomy feeding tube or gastectomy. Alternative treatments remain under investigation with acupuncture showing promise based on symptom improvement in a randomized study.[39]

Accelerated Gastric Emptying

Accelerated gastric emptying has emerged as a new entity, but few studies have been done to further understand this condition. Vagal dysfunction impairs gastric accommodation, leading to elevated pressures and rapid emptying. Symptoms are typically consistent with dumping syndrome, with the developmental of abdominal discomfort, nausea, vomiting, and diarrhea within an hour of eating. Although patients may have disproportionately more difficulty with postprandial glucose control and weight loss, the symptoms may be difficult to distinguish from gastroparesis. Gastric transit measured by scintigraphy typically establishes the diagnosis. Treatments are not well defined at this time, but amylin analogs and glucagonlike peptide-1 (GLP-1) agonists that can slow gastric emptying may improve symptoms.[11]

SMALL INTESTINAL DISORDERS
Celiac Disease Overview

Celiac disease is an immune-mediated enteropathy in which ingestion of gluten leads to atrophy of the small intestinal villi and malabsorption. Celiac disease affects approximately 1% of the US population; however, this risk is much higher in patients with DM1. Approximately 3% to 8% of patients with DM1 have celiac disease.[40–42] From 1951 to 2001, the incidence of celiac disease has increased incrementally; an increase that mirrors the increased incidence of DM1.[43,44] In the vast majority of cases, the diagnosis of DM1 precedes that of celiac disease.[45]

Pathogenesis of Celiac Disease

Gluten is a storage protein derived from wheat, rye, or barley. Gluten has high proline and glutamine content, which makes digestion difficult; α-gliadin is among the polypeptides that remain undigested in the small intestine. If there is a defect in the intestinal epithelium, then α-gliadin crosses into the lamina propria. In patients with celiac disease, α-gliadin initiates an innate and adaptive immune response that leads to an inflammatory infiltrate of the small bowel with villous destruction. The mechanism responsible for the epithelium defect is not well understood, but an infectious etiology has been proposed.[46,47] In the lamina propria, tissue transglutaminase, a celiac autoantigen, binds to gliadin and enhances its affinity for HLA DQ2 and DQ8 molecules on antigen-presenting cells that initiates humoral and cell-mediated immune responses. The immune response leads to significant inflammation in the small intestine as well as distant organs. Simultaneously, activation of intraepithelial lymphocytes initiates an innate immune response contributing to the pathology. Ultimately, destruction of small intestinal enterocytes leads to villous atrophy and impaired nutritional absorption, causing the classic symptoms associated with celiac disease.[46,47]

Genetic Predisposition to Celiac Disease

Celiac disease essentially develops only in genetically predisposed individuals who possess certain HLA genes that encode for antigen-presenting cell surface markers. HLA DQ2 and DQ8 are the susceptibility serotypes that are present in 25% to 40% of the general population. Only a small subset of individuals with DQ2 or DQ8 will develop celiac disease. If an individual carries multiple susceptibility alleles, there is an additive risk of celiac disease.[48]

Association of Celiac Disease and DM1

The mechanism underlying the increased incidence of celiac disease in patients with DM1 is not completely understood. Celiac disease and DM1 are autoimmune phenomena that share HLA and non-HLA susceptibility genes. A common environmental, microbial, or immunologic entity has been postulated, but has not been fully elucidated. Given this known association, diarrhea, weight loss, or new-onset hypoglycemic episodes in a patient with DM1 should prompt evaluation for celiac disease. The topic of whether to screen asymptomatic patients with DM1 for celiac disease remains somewhat controversial, although routinely occurs in the pediatric population. Furthermore, if an individual with DM1 undergoes upper endoscopy, obtaining duodenal biopsies is recommended to screen for celiac disease (**Table 2**).[49]

Childhood Presentation of Celiac Disease

Celiac disease may present with a wide variety of symptoms and historically was thought to be a disease of childhood. In infancy, typical presentations include development of abdominal pain and/or distension, steatorrhea, and vomiting after introduction of cereal into the diet. Falling off of the growth curve or failure to thrive should elicit concern for celiac disease. Older children may present with anemia or nutritional deficiencies, or in patients with diabetes, sudden improvement in hemoglobin A1c should prompt evaluation for celiac disease.

Table 2 Celiac disease	
Type of Celiac Disease	**Definition**
Classic	Patients with abnormal duodenal histology with typical gastrointestinal symptoms
Atypical	Lack of gastrointestinal symptoms but may present with extraintestinal findings related to celiac disease (eg, iron deficiency anemia, dermatitis herpetiformis)
Silent	Diagnosed based on serologies or during endoscopy for another indication. Lack of gastrointestinal symptoms
Latent	Individual with celiac disease on gluten-free diet with resolution of symptoms and duodenal changes based on histology or patients with normal duodenal histology with gluten-containing diet who will later develop celiac disease
Potential	Individuals with positive serologies but negative duodenal biopsies without symptoms who are at high risk for development of classic celiac disease

Adult Presentation of Celiac Disease
• Diarrhea
• Steatorrhea
• Abdominal pain
• Weight loss

Celiac symptoms are predominantly related to malabsorption. The severity of diarrhea and weight loss correlates with the degree of the intestinal inflammation. However, symptoms of celiac disease may be nonspecific and frequently overlap with symptoms of irritable bowel syndrome. It is important to consider the diagnosis of celiac disease in any patient undergoing evaluation for irritable bowel syndrome.

Extraintestinal Manifestations of Celiac Disease

Adults with celiac disease may present with extraintestinal manifestations of the systemic disease, rather than classic gastrointestinal symptoms. Iron deficiency anemia can result from decreased iron absorption in the proximal small intestine. Less frequently, celiac disease will affect the terminal ileum and interfere with vitamin B12 absorption. Nutritional deficiencies may lead to other extraintestinal signs or symptoms, such as peripheral neuropathy, ataxia, and osteoporosis. The most common dermatologic manifestation of celiac disease is dermatitis herpetiformis, a pruritic, erythematous blistering lesion located on extensor surfaces. Gluten mediates the pathogenesis of dermatitis herpetiformis, and recent studies suggest that immunoglobulin A (IgA) antiepidermal tissue transglutaminase antibody deposition in the dermis may cause the rash.[50]

Diagnosis of Celiac Disease: Utility of Serologic Testing

The first step in evaluating for celiac disease should be serologic testing; however, definitive diagnosis of celiac disease is made by duodenal biopsies in the setting of gluten exposure. Current guidelines recommend testing for tissue transglutaminase IgA (TTG IGA) as the preferred serologic test for celiac disease. Based on multiple studies, the overall specificity is greater than 95%, with sensitivity ranging from 89% to 96%.[51,52] The antiendomysial antibody (EMA) test has a similar profile but is more expensive. Antigliadin antibodies are of limited value because of decreased sensitivity and specificity. Patients with IgA deficiency will not, however, have detectable serum TTG IGA antibodies. It may be reasonable to routinely check IgA levels when evaluating individuals at high risk for celiac with the TTG IGA antibody. In individuals with low or absent IgA levels, deamidated gliadin peptide IgG antibody may be a useful screening tool. In the setting of DM1, the overlapping susceptibility genes render HLA-DQ2 and DQ8 testing less useful.

Duodenal Biopsies: Gold Standard for Diagnosis

If serologies are positive, upper endoscopy with duodenal bulb and distal duodenal biopsies should be obtained to confirm the diagnosis. Upper endoscopy should also be performed in the setting of negative serologies if there is high clinical suspicion. Endoscopic appearance of the duodenum may be abnormal with scalloping or flattening of folds. Duodenal biopsies may reveal a spectrum of changes including crypt hypertrophy, villous atrophy, and a lymphocytic inflammatory infiltrate. Dietary intake at time of endoscopy must be assessed and taken into account when interpreting the results of the endoscopy, as reductions in gluten consumption may lessen the intestinal inflammation and damage. Initiation of a 4-week gluten challenge may enable diagnosis of celiac disease in patients adhering to a gluten-free diet.[52,53]

Treatment of Celiac Disease: Gluten-Free Diet

Elimination of dietary wheat, rye, and barley is the current therapy for celiac disease. A gluten-free diet has been shown to improve symptoms, improve mortality, and possibly reduce the risk of cancer.[54,55] Nutritional consultation and support groups may offer assistance in helping patients adhere to a gluten-free diet. In a patient with concomitant diabetes, competing dietary restrictions may further complicate management of both diseases, and adequate nutrition remains a significant concern in the patients. Patients should be assessed for nutritional deficiencies in folic acid, vitamin B12, iron, calcium, and fat-soluble vitamins, as well as osteoporosis.[46]

Failure of a Gluten-Free Diet

Inadvertent exposure to gluten is the most common reason for failure to respond to a gluten-free diet. Failure should prompt reevaluation of the diagnosis of celiac disease and assessment of adherence to diet. If this evaluation is unrevealing, practitioners should consider alternative etiologies for the symptoms. Diseases that are associated with celiac disease and may cause similar symptoms include pancreatic insufficiency, small intestinal bacterial overgrowth, microscopic colitis, lactose intolerance, and irritable bowel syndrome.[56] In addition, celiac disease is associated with increased risk of small bowel adenocarcinoma and enteropathy-associated T-cell lymphoma.[46]

Small Bowel Bacterial Overgrowth Overview

Small bowel bacterial overgrowth (SIBO) is characterized by alterations in the type and quantity of bacteria within the small intestine. Significant changes in the microbiota of the small intestine may cause gastrointestinal symptoms, such as bloating, abdominal pain, diarrhea, and gas, and may lead to nutritional deficiencies.

Epidemiology

The prevalence of SIBO in the general population is difficult to estimate, although studies of healthy controls suggest a prevalence of 6% that increases with aging.[57] In one recent study, 43% of patients with diabetes with diarrhea had SIBO and improved with antibiotic therapy.[58]

Pathogenesis

The physiologic mechanisms for controlling intestinal bacterial growth include secretion of acid in the stomach and normal gastrointestinal motility. Specifically, in the small bowel, the migrating motor complex (MMC) clears any residual intestinal contents every 90 to 120 minutes. However, gastroparesis or abnormal motility of the small intestine enables bacterial stasis and subsequent overgrowth. Furthermore, any structural abnormalities from surgeries, particularly blind loops, may also create reservoirs that enable overgrowth of bacteria. The excessive growth of organisms leads to generation of ammonia, inflammatory cytokines, short-chain fatty acids, bile acid deconjugation, and toxins. Ultimately, the bacterial by-products interfere with normal absorption of fat and carbohydrates.[59]

Nutritional Complications of Untreated SIBO

If the bacterial overgrowth is severe and goes untreated, individuals may eventually develop nutritional deficiencies. Bacterial deconjugation of bile salts creates bile acids that may cause direct toxic damage to villi. This process impairs absorption and disrupts micelle formation. Disruption of fat absorption leads to deficiencies in vitamins A, D, E, and K. In addition, anaerobic intestinal bacteria metabolize vitamin B12 before absorption can occur.[60]

Symptoms of Bacterial Overgrowth

The typical symptoms associated with SIBO are abdominal pain with bloating, gas, and diarrhea. Other frequently reported symptoms include flatulence, abdominal distension, and weakness. The symptoms are frequently vague and overlap significantly with those of irritable bowel syndrome. Practitioners should consider this diagnosis when diabetic patients develop diarrhea and abdominal bloating.

Jejunal Aspirate: Gold Standard for Diagnosis of SIBO

SIBO is generally defined as greater than 100,000 colony-forming units(CFU)/mL in the small bowel as compared with the normal value of less than 10,000 CFU/mL. Historically, the gold standard for diagnosis is quantification of bacteria obtained from proximal jejunal aspirate during upper endoscopy; however, costs associated with endoscopy, rigorous specimen handling procedures, and difficulty culturing bacteria limit the widespread use of the test.[61]

Use of Breath Tests in Diagnosis of SIBO

Breath tests for diagnosis of SIBO are used to evaluate the ability of intestinal bacteria to produce analytes, such as hydrogen or radiolabeled carbon dioxide. In healthy individuals, glucose is absorbed in the small intestines; however, the excess bacteria in SIBO metabolize glucose into carbon dioxide and hydrogen that can be detected by breath test. The specificity and sensitivity of each specific test varies and fails in the setting of abnormal motility. In comparison with small bowel aspirate, the glucose hydrogen test has a sensitivity and specificity of 62% and 83%, respectively.[62] Given the low sensitivity, there is some debate over the utility of testing as compared with empiric treatment.

Treatment of Underlying Etiology

Treatment and reversal of the underlying etiology of SIBO may be difficult in certain circumstances. In the setting of gastroparesis or slow small intestinal transit as a predisposing factor, one should aim to optimize treatment of the motility disorder. Goals should include improvement of glycemic control and potential use of a prokinetic agent, such as metoclopramide or domperidone, as mentioned previously.

Nutritional Assessment

Individuals should be assessed for weight loss, malnutrition, or electrolyte imbalances. Significant weight loss should prompt discussion about nutritional supplementation. One may consider evaluating for deficiencies in fat-soluble vitamins and vitamin B12.

Antibiotic Treatment in SIBO

Antibiotic treatment for SIBO typically provides significant symptomatic relief. Although many different antibiotics are used, few randomized clinical trials have rigorously compared different regimens and durations. The most extensively studied medication in treatment of SIBO is rifaximin, a minimally absorbed antibiotic with activity against gram-negative and gram-positive bacteria. Based on a review of existing trials, rifaximin improved symptoms in 33% to 92% with eradication of SIBO in more than 80%.[63] Rifaximin, 1200 to 1600 mg daily for 7 to 10 days, is the first-line treatment; however, other antibiotics, such as doxycycline, augmentin, and flagyl, are less expensive and frequently used in clinical practice with success. Recurrence of SIBO is common and may respond to repeated courses of antibiotics. In refractory cases, patients may require continuous cycling of antibiotics to control symptoms.

Diabetic Diarrhea

Diarrhea is a frequent gastrointestinal symptom encountered in diabetic patients with a wide variety of potential etiologies. Diarrhea may be related to ingestion of artificial sweeteners, concomitant celiac disease, bacterial overgrowth, irritable bowel syndrome, or medication side effects. The biguanide derivative, metformin, frequently causes diarrhea. This effect may occur either early or late in use. The α-glucosidase inhibitors, such as acarbose, may also cause diarrhea in a significant proportion of patients. Diabetic diarrhea typically occurs in insulin-dependent patients who have had diabetes for at least 8 years. Many of these patients suffer from peripheral and autonomic neuropathy.[64,65]

Epidemiology of Diabetic Diarrhea

Significant variation in estimates of the prevalence of diabetic diarrhea may be related to referral basis in tertiary care settings. The prevalence of diabetic diarrhea is higher in patients with DM1 when compared with DM2, with rates of 5.0% and 0.4% respectively. Factors associated with diabetic diarrhea are disease duration, A1c levels, male sex, and autonomic neuropathy.[64] The lack of specific diagnostic markers for diabetic diarrhea makes differentiation from irritable bowel syndrome very difficult and undoubtedly there is some degree of overlap.

Pathogenesis of Diabetic Diarrhea

The pathogenesis of diabetic diarrhea is not well understood but appears to be closely related to autonomic neuropathy. The MMC, organized small bowel contractions while fasting, may be abnormal in patients with diabetes, slowing motility. Sympathetic denervation is found frequently in patients with autonomic neuropathy. Interruption of sympathetic nerves and adrenergic stimulation of electrolyte and fluid absorption may be the etiology of diarrhea.[66]

Symptoms of Diabetic Diarrhea

- Watery, voluminous diarrhea
- Nocturnal symptoms
- Steatorrhea
- Fecal incontinence
- Episodic symptoms with intervening normal bowel habits or constipation
- Absence of abdominal pain

Diabetic diarrhea is typically watery, voluminous, and explosive, with or without steatorrhea. Although the symptoms of diabetic diarrhea may relatively straightforward, patients may accept these symptoms and fail to disclose these symptoms.

Diagnosis

Diabetic diarrhea is a diagnosis of exclusion, and diagnostic evaluation includes obtaining a detailed history about diet and medication use for alternative etiologies. Specifically, diarrhea is a frequent side effect of metformin. Diagnostic evaluation may include stool studies for parasitic infection, serology for celiac disease, and consideration of flexible sigmoidoscopy or colonoscopy to evaluate for inflammatory bowel disease or microscopic colitis. If there is a significant history of incontinence, one may consider anorectal manometry to evaluate defecation.[64]

Treatment

Treatment may begin with optimization of glycemic control and removal of medications that may be exacerbating symptoms. Medications are almost uniformly needed to control symptoms. Initial treatment should be empiric with use of standard antidiarrheal agents, such as loperamide, diphenoxylate with atropine, and codeine sulfate, as well as fiber supplementation. Cholestyramine may be of benefit, especially if there is a component of bile salt malabsorption. A trial of fiber supplementation or probiotics may also be helpful. The $\alpha2$-adrenergic agonist, clonidine, may provide adrenergic stimuli to facilitate fluid and electrolyte absorption in the intestines that appears to be disrupted in diabetic diarrhea. Small studies demonstrated that clonidine reduced stool volume in diabetic patients with profuse diarrhea.[67] Clonidine should be started at 0.1 mg twice daily but may be increased to 0.6 mg twice daily. If the medication is discontinued, a slow taper is recommended to prevent rebound hypertension. Octreotide, a long-acting somatostatin, has also been used to treat diabetic diarrhea with symptomatic improvement in small case series; however, it may slow small bowel motility and increase risk of bacterial overgrowth.[68] Additionally, octreotide is an inhibitor of glucagon and insulin, which places patients with diabetes at risk for both hyperglycemia and hypoglycemia.

LARGE INTESTINE DISORDERS
Fecal Incontinence

Fecal incontinence, the involuntary passage of fecal matter, appears to be a consequence of autonomic neuropathy. Incidence in the general population is estimated at 1%, although increases with age.[69] Symptoms of fecal incontinence frequently start with concomitant low-volume diarrhea. Nocturnal symptoms are frequent, and a subset of patients may have steatorrhea. Fecal incontinence typically occurs in patients with long disease duration and management is frequently challenging. Most of these patients are older and may have alternative etiologies for fecal incontinence, such as prior anal sphincter injuries from childbirth or surgery.

Pathophysiology of Fecal Incontinence

Autonomic neuropathy in diabetes appears to be responsible for nerve damage that leads to fecal incontinence. Multiple mechanisms help maintain fecal continence, and numerous insults are required to disrupt the process. Diabetic patients with incontinence have abnormal resting tone of the internal anal sphincter that is responsible for maintaining continence. Sensation of rectal distension also appears to be diminished in patients with diabetes, impairing the recto-anal reflex that leads to relaxation of the internal sphincter.[70] Furthermore, studies show that hyperglycemia independently impairs internal anal sphincter tone and rectal compliance, potentiating underlying deficits.[71]

Evaluation of Fecal Incontinence

Evaluation for fecal incontinence should include an evaluation for alternative etiologies for incontinence, including fecal impaction, infection, colonic mucosal disease, or primary diarrhea. A rectal examination will indicate whether fecal impaction with overflow incontinence is responsible for the symptoms and will allow for assessment of the anal sphincter. Evaluation of diarrhea should include stool cultures and flexible sigmoidoscopy or colonoscopy to evaluate for mucosal inflammation or structural etiology for the incontinence.[72]

Diagnosis of Fecal Incontinence

Anorectal manometry is the primary method used to define the deficits in fecal incontinence and typically quantifies sphincter pressure, rectal sensation, rectal compliance, and rectal reflexes. Recent technical advances in high-resolution manometry have greatly enhanced the ability to define underlying mechanisms causing fecal incontinence and may guide potential biofeedback therapy.[72]

Treatment of Fecal Incontinence

- Optimization of glycemic control
- Supportive lifestyle modification
- Antidiarrheal medications
- Biofeedback therapy
- Sacral stimulator or surgery

Management of fecal incontinence primarily begins with optimization of glycemic control and initiation of antidiarrheal medications. Loperamide and diphenoxylate with atropine reduce incontinence episodes and may suffice in managing modest symptoms. Cholestyramine may decrease diarrhea and improve continence. Biofeedback therapy aims to train individuals to become more aware of, and increase control of, anorectal muscles. It may improve anal sphincter strength, coordination of muscles, and sensory perception. Clinical improvement appears to be variable, as a result of differing symptom severity and lack of uniformity in biofeedback therapy. Small non-randomized studies of biofeedback have shown clinical efficacy in diabetic patients with fecal incontinence.[73] In refractory fecal incontinence, sacral nerve stimulation device implantation and surgery may improve symptoms; however, studies of fecal incontinence in diabetic patients have not been performed.

HEPATOBILIARY DISORDERS
Nonalcoholic Fatty Liver Disease Overview

Nonalcoholic fatty liver disease (NAFLD) is defined by fat deposition in the liver in the absence of alcohol abuse or other known hepatotoxins. It is a spectrum that includes nonalcoholic fatty liver (NAFL; fat deposition in the liver without inflammation) and nonalcoholic steatohepatitis (NASH; fat deposition with associated inflammation or hepatitis). Fatty liver is typically defined by the accumulation of fat in the liver without associated inflammation or elevated liver enzymes. In contrast, NASH is defined by the presence of fatty infiltrate in the liver with associated inflammation. Distinguishing between these 2 entities remains a significant clinical challenge (**Table 3**).

Table 3
Spectrum of nonalcoholic fatty liver disease

Term	Definition
Nonalcoholic fatty liver disease (NAFLD)	Encompasses spectrum of liver disease from fatty infiltrate without inflammation to cirrhosis
Nonalcoholic fatty liver (NAFL)	Liver fat accumulation in the liver without inflammation
Nonalcoholic steatohepatitis (NASH)	Liver fat accumulation *with* inflammation
NASH cirrhosis	End stage of NASH

Epidemiology

Incidence of NAFLD in the general population is not well defined. The incidence reported by different studies varies dramatically depending on the population, definition of NAFLD, and diagnostic modalities. Based on 2 histology-based studies of potential living liver donors, the prevalence of NAFLD is estimated to be between 20% and 51%.[74,75] The prevalence of NAFLD in DM2 may be as high as 69%, with diabetes as an independent predictor for progression of liver disease.[76] Risk factors include obesity, diabetes, hyperlipidemia, and age. The highest incidence appears to be in Hispanic individuals, and the lowest incidence occurs in African American individuals.[76]

Natural History of NAFLD

Based on limited studies, individuals with NAFLD have increased mortality as compared with matched control populations. Although liver-associated mortality is higher in NAFLD, the most common cause of death in this population is cardiovascular disease.[77] The survival of patients with NASH with associated inflammation as compared with those with benign hepatic fat is significantly worse.[78] Individuals with NASH, but probably not NAFL, have a significant risk of progression to cirrhosis, which will occur in up to 30%.[23]

Pathogenesis of NAFLD

The pathogenesis of NAFLD is poorly understood, and the lack of adequate animal models has limited research. The accumulation of fat in the liver appears to be related to an imbalance where lipogenesis exceeds lipolysis, and the amount of hepatic free-fatty acids exceeds requirements for mitochondrial oxidation, cholesterol synthesis, and phospholipid synthesis. This process appears to be driven by insulin levels and insulin resistance that drives free-fatty acid synthesis, inhibits synthesis of very low-density lipoproteins (VLDL), and enhances susceptibility to hepatic injury.[79] Free-fatty acids are toxic to hepatocytes through multiple mechanisms and play a role in induction of inflammation, but the precise mechanism underlying the progression from fatty liver to steatohepatitis is not completely understood, although it may be related to oxidative stress and mitochondrial dysfunction.[66,80]

Signs and Symptoms of NAFLD

NAFLD is typically asymptomatic and is frequently incidentally detected during an evaluation for an unrelated condition. Some individuals may report right upper quadrant abdominal pain, fatigue, or malaise. Although patients may have an enlarged liver on physical examination, concomitant obesity makes this physical finding difficult to appreciate. Serum alanine aminotransferase (ALT) and aspartate aminotransferase (AST) are frequently elevated, with ALT usually higher than AST. In the absence of advanced liver disease, total bilirubin, prothrombin time, and albumin levels remain normal. Imaging studies may show fat infiltrating the liver with the appearance varying by imaging modality.

Definition of NAFLD

- Presence of hepatic steatosis based on imaging or histology
- Absence of significant alcohol use
- Absence of secondary etiologies for liver disease
- Absence of coexisting chronic liver disease

Diagnosis of NAFLD or NASH is a clinical and pathologic diagnosis. Clinically, practitioners must exclude other etiologies for liver disease, including significant alcohol use, medications causing hepatic injury, viral hepatitis, Wilson's disease, autoimmune hepatitis, hemochromatosis, or alternative etiologies. The definition of significant alcohol use varies by gender and ultimately becomes a clinical assessment. Without histology, one cannot distinguish between benign fatty liver deposition and NASH, the latter being associated with a worse prognosis.

New Diagnostic Tools for NAFLD

Although practitioners typically begin with abdominal ultrasound when evaluating those suspected for NAFLD, this modality is not sensitive, nor specific. Computed tomography and magnetic resonance imaging (MRI) are more sensitive and specific in detecting steatosis. Newer forms of MRI are being developed to detect individuals with NASH or advanced fibrosis. Specifically, MR transient elastography measures liver stiffness noninvasively and successfully detects the presence of fibrosis in NAFLD, although is less accurate in the setting of obesity.[24] Other composite scores of simple laboratory parameters are being validated for detecting advanced fibrosis.[69]

The Role of Liver Biopsy

The role of liver biopsy in diagnosis remains somewhat debated. In some cases, biopsy is clearly needed to rule out concomitant liver disease. Although liver biopsy is an expensive and morbid procedure, it remains the gold standard for diagnosis and staging of disease. Fat deposition in the form of steatosis may be present on histology in fatty liver and NASH, but cellular damage with hepatocyte ballooning and/or fibrosis occurs only in NASH and distinguishes the progressive disease from benign fat infiltration. An active area of investigation is the development of noninvasive testing to identify NASH or advanced fibrosis.[81]

Management of NAFLD

Current management involves addressing any modifiable risk factors for NAFLD, including insulin resistance, diabetes, obesity, and hyperlipidemia, as well as the liver disease. Medications aimed at reversing the liver disease are reserved for individuals with NASH.

Lifestyle Modification

First-line treatment for NAFLD is initiation of diet and exercise. Based on current studies, weight loss of 3% to 5% of body weight may improve steatosis, but greater weight loss may be required to improve fibrosis. Exercise even without weight loss improves steatosis but may not reverse fibrosis.[77]

Medical Therapies for NASH and Diabetes

The medical therapies for NASH evaluated to date focus on enhancing insulin sensitivity but have had limited success. Metformin initially showed promise; however, a meta-analysis shows that metformin does not decrease liver enzymes or improve histology.[76] Conversely, a meta-analysis of 4 randomized clinical trials concluded that pioglitazone, a thiazolidinedione (TZD), significantly reduced steatosis and inflammation in NASH. However, the trials enrolled patients without diabetes, limiting the generalizability to diabetic patients, and long-term cardiovascular safety data are lacking.[77] Furthermore, recent associations of TZDs with bladder cancer have limited their overall use.[82] Similarly, vitamin E (800 IU per day) may improve histology in NASH; however, few data support use of vitamin E in diabetic patients with NASH, particularly given the potential association with prostate cancer.[83] Bariatric surgery appears to improve liver histology and will likely be a future treatment; however, randomized clinical trials are needed to support its use and determine which surgeries are most efficacious.[84] Overall, studies of NASH in diabetic patients are lacking and will be essential going forward to guide management; however, there are no approved treatments currently for liver disease associated with NASH.

Statin Use in NAFLD

Central to management of NAFLD is risk factor modification. Statins are extremely effective for dyslipidemia but may cause elevations in AST and ALT. As a result of this potential side effect, practitioners may be reluctant to use statins in the setting of NAFLD. The use of statins in the setting of NAFLD appears safe without increased risk of hepatotoxicity, and post hoc analyses suggest that statins improve cardiovascular outcomes and liver enzymes in NAFLD.[77] Although there are no guidelines to guide practitioners, a twofold increase in liver enzymes should be tolerated without cessation of therapy.

Cholelithiasis and Association with Diabetes

Gallstone disease and its complications, such as cholangitis, cholecystitis, and gallstone pancreatitis, occur more frequently in diabetic patients based on epidemiologic studies. However, these 2 diseases are both quite common and share risk factors, making it difficult to tease out the relationship between these entities. Mouse and human studies have shown relative bile stasis within the gallbladder and reduced cholecystokinin levels that may drive gallbladder stone formation.[85] Prophylactic cholecystectomy should not be performed for asymptomatic gallstones in diabetic patients.

PANCREATIC DISEASE
Pancreatic Insufficiency

Pancreatic exocrine insufficiency occurs in patients with DM1 and DM2. Historical studies demonstrated biochemical insufficiency in nearly 50% and 30% to 50% of patients with insulin-dependent diabetes and noninsulin-dependent diabetes, respectively.[86] Most of these patients have minor pancreatic exocrine insufficiency that is not clinically significant. If exocrine insufficiency is clinically significant and leads to fat malabsorption, individuals may benefit from mealtime pancreatic enzyme supplementation containing amylase, lipase, and protease. Clinically, pancreatic insufficiency may be a difficult entity to diagnose, and at times a clinical trial of pancreatic enzyme supplementation may be appropriate.

Acute Pancreatitis in Diabetes

Diabetic patients have an elevated risk of pancreatitis that appears to be intrinsic to the diseases as well as related to medications. Patients with DM1 have a twofold increased risk of pancreatitis, and patients with DM2 have a nearly threefold increased risk of pancreatitis as compared with the general population. The highest risk was in patients with DM2 who were younger than 30 years old.[66,87] The precise mechanism is not completely understood but may be related to ongoing inflammation. DM2 and pancreatitis share obesity and hypertriglyceridemia as common risk factors. Based on a review of the FDA adverse event reporting, GLP-1 agonists and dipeptidyl peptidase 4 inhibitors are associated with a sixfold increased risk of pancreatitis with a possible increased risk of pancreatic cancer.[88]

Pancreatic Cancer

Diabetes is a risk factor for pancreatic cancer but may also be a presenting sign. The etiologic role of diabetes in development of pancreatic cancer is poorly understood, although may be related to low-grade chronic inflammation of the pancreas. The relative risk of pancreatic cancer appears to be nearly 2 in patients with diabetes. The highest risk was in newly diagnosed diabetic patients, underscoring that new-onset diabetes may be an early sign of pancreatic malignancy.[89]

SUMMARY

The gastrointestinal complications of diabetes can affect essentially any organ in the gastrointestinal tract, are associated with significant morbidity and mortality, and can directly impair quality of life. With this in mind, the health care professional should be aware of these associated conditions, as well as the high prevalence of overlapping gastrointestinal symptoms unrelated to diabetes. Although screening for heart disease, retinopathy, neuropathy, and nephropathy typically make their way into preformed electronic records for a clinic visit, gastrointestinal symptoms are frequently not screened for and may be underreported. Abnormalities uncovered should be investigated with consideration of referral to a gastroenterology specialist when appropriate. In this way, screening and treating gastrointestinal-related complications may enhance comprehensive care of diabetic patients.

REFERENCES

1. Camilleri M, Dubois D, Coulie B, et al. Prevalence and socioeconomic impact of upper gastrointestinal disorders in the United States: results of the US Upper Gastrointestinal Study. Clin Gastroenterol Hepatol 2005;3:543–52.
2. Gatopoulou A, Papanas N, Maltezos E. Diabetic gastrointestinal autonomic neuropathy: current status and new achievements for everyday clinical practice. Eur J Intern Med 2012;23:499–505.
3. Kinekawa F, Kubo F, Matsuda K, et al. Relationship between esophageal dysfunction and neuropathy in diabetic patients. Am J Gastroenterol 2001;96: 2026–32.
4. Lluch I, Ascaso JF, Mora F, et al. Gastroesophageal reflux in diabetes mellitus. Am J Gastroenterol 1999;94:919–24.

5. Wang X, Pitchumoni CS, Chandrarana K, et al. Increased prevalence of symptoms of gastroesophageal reflux diseases in type 2 diabetics with neuropathy. World J Gastroenterol 2008;14:709–12.

6. Singh PK, Hota D, Dutta P, et al. Pantoprazole improves glycemic control in type 2 diabetes: a randomized, double-blind, placebo-controlled trial. J Clin Endocrinol Metab 2012;97:E2105–8.

7. Wilcox CM, Karowe MW. Esophageal infections: etiology, diagnosis, and management. Gastroenterologist 1994;2:188–206.

8. Jung HK, Choung RS, Locke GR 3rd, et al. The incidence, prevalence, and outcomes of patients with gastroparesis in Olmsted County, Minnesota, from 1996 to 2006. Gastroenterology 2009;136:1225–33.

9. Choung RS, Locke GR 3rd, Schleck CD, et al. Risk of gastroparesis in subjects with type 1 and 2 diabetes in the general population. Am J Gastroenterol 2012; 107:82–8.

10. Keshavarzian A, Iber FL, Vaeth J. Gastric emptying in patients with insulin-requiring diabetes mellitus. Am J Gastroenterol 1987;82:29–35.

11. Camilleri M, Bharucha AE, Farrugia G. Epidemiology, mechanisms, and management of diabetic gastroparesis. Clin Gastroenterol Hepatol 2011;9:5–12 [quiz: e17].

12. Schvarcz E, Palmer M, Aman J, et al. Physiological hyperglycemia slows gastric emptying in normal subjects and patients with insulin-dependent diabetes mellitus. Gastroenterology 1997;113:60–6.

13. Farrugia G. Interstitial cells of Cajal in health and disease. Neurogastroenterol Motil 2008;20(Suppl 1):54–63.

14. Harberson J, Thomas RM, Harbison SP, et al. Gastric neuromuscular pathology in gastroparesis: analysis of full-thickness antral biopsies. Dig Dis Sci 2010;55: 359–70.

15. Schwartz TW. Pancreatic polypeptide: a hormone under vagal control. Gastroenterology 1983;85:1411–25.

16. Tomita R, Tanjoh K, Fujisaki S, et al. The role of nitric oxide (NO) in the human pyloric sphincter. Hepatogastroenterology 1999;46:2999–3003.

17. Watkins CC, Sawa A, Jaffrey S, et al. Insulin restores neuronal nitric oxide synthase expression and function that is lost in diabetic gastropathy. J Clin Invest 2000;106:803.

18. Choi KM, Gibbons SJ, Nguyen TV, et al. Heme oxygenase-1 protects interstitial cells of Cajal from oxidative stress and reverses diabetic gastroparesis. Gastroenterology 2008;135:2055–64, 2064.e1–2.

19. Sarnelli G, Caenepeel P, Geypens B, et al. Symptoms associated with impaired gastric emptying of solids and liquids in functional dyspepsia. Am J Gastroenterol 2003;98:783–8.

20. Camilleri M, Parkman HP, Shafi MA, et al, American College of Gastroenterology. Clinical guideline: management of gastroparesis. Am J Gastroenterol 2013;108: 18–37 [quiz: 38].

21. Abell TL, Camilleri M, Donohoe K, et al, American Neurogastroenterology and Motility Society and the Society of Nuclear Medicine. Consensus recommendations for gastric emptying scintigraphy: a joint report of the American Neurogastroenterology and Motility Society and the Society of Nuclear Medicine. J Nucl Med Technol 2008;36:44–54.

22. Fraser RJ, Horowitz M, Maddox AF, et al. Hyperglycaemia slows gastric emptying in type 1 (insulin-dependent) diabetes mellitus. Diabetologia 1990; 33:675–80.

23. Fassio E, Alvarez E, Dominguez N, et al. Natural history of nonalcoholic steato-hepatitis: a longitudinal study of repeat liver biopsies. Hepatology 2004;40: 820–6.
24. Musso G, Gambino R, Cassader M, et al. Meta-analysis: natural history of non-alcoholic fatty liver disease (NAFLD) and diagnostic accuracy of non-invasive tests for liver disease severity. Ann Med 2011;43:617–49.
25. Lee A, Kuo B. Metoclopramide in the treatment of diabetic gastroparesis. Expert Rev Endocrinol Metab 2010;5:653–62.
26. McCallum RW, Ricci DA, Rakatansky H, et al. A multicenter placebo-controlled clinical trial of oral metoclopramide in diabetic gastroparesis. Diabetes Care 1983;6:463–7.
27. Perkel MS, Moore C, Hersh T, et al. Metoclopramide therapy in patients with de-layed gastric emptying: a randomized, double-blind study. Dig Dis Sci 1979;24: 662–6.
28. Snape WJ Jr, Battle WM, Schwartz SS, et al. Metoclopramide to treat gastropa-resis due to diabetes mellitus: a double-blind, controlled trial. Ann Intern Med 1982;96:444–6.
29. Miller LG, Jankovic J. Metoclopramide-induced movement disorders. Clinical findings with a review of the literature. Arch Intern Med 1989;149:2486–92.
30. Bateman DN, Rawlins MD, Simpson JM. Extrapyramidal reactions with metoclo-pramide. Br Med J (Clin Res Ed) 1985;291:930–2.
31. Parkman HP, Mishra A, Jacobs M, et al. Clinical response and side effects of metoclopramide: associations with clinical, demographic, and pharmacoge-netic parameters. J Clin Gastroenterol 2012;46:494–503.
32. Silvers D, Kipnes M, Broadstone V, et al. Domperidone in the management of symptoms of diabetic gastroparesis: efficacy, tolerability, and quality-of-life out-comes in a multicenter controlled trial. DOM-USA-5 Study Group. Clin Ther 1998;20:438–53.
33. Patterson D, Abell T, Rothstein R, et al. A double-blind multicenter comparison of domperidone and metoclopramide in the treatment of diabetic patients with symptoms of gastroparesis. Am J Gastroenterol 1999;94:1230–4.
34. Franzese A, Borrelli O, Corrado G, et al. Domperidone is more effective than cis-apride in children with diabetic gastroparesis. Aliment Pharmacol Ther 2002;16: 951–7.
35. Janssens J, Peeters TL, Vantrappen G, et al. Improvement of gastric emptying in diabetic gastroparesis by erythromycin. Preliminary studies. N Engl J Med 1990;322:1028–31.
36. Adams LA, Angulo P. Role of liver biopsy and serum markers of liver fibrosis in non-alcoholic fatty liver disease. Clin Liver Dis 2007;11:25–35, viii.
37. Abell T, McCallum R, Hocking M, et al. Gastric electrical stimulation for medi-cally refractory gastroparesis. Gastroenterology 2003;125:421–8.
38. Chu H, Lin Z, Zhong L, et al. Treatment of high-frequency gastric electrical stim-ulation for gastroparesis. J Gastroenterol Hepatol 2012;27:1017–26.
39. Wang CP, Kao CH, Chen WK, et al. A single-blinded, randomized pilot study evaluating effects of electroacupuncture in diabetic patients with symptoms suggestive of gastroparesis. J Altern Complement Med 2008;14:833–9.
40. Sjoberg K, Eriksson KF, Bredberg A, et al. Screening for coeliac disease in adult insulin-dependent diabetes mellitus. J Intern Med 1998;243:133–40.
41. Talal AH, Murray JA, Goeken JA, et al. Celiac disease in an adult population with insulin-dependent diabetes mellitus: use of endomysial antibody testing. Am J Gastroenterol 1997;92:1280–4.

42. Cronin CC, Feighery A, Ferriss JB, et al. High prevalence of celiac disease among patients with insulin-dependent (type I) diabetes mellitus. Am J Gastroenterol 1997;92:2210–2.

43. Fasano A, Berti I, Gerarduzzi T, et al. Prevalence of celiac disease in at-risk and not-at-risk groups in the United States: a large multicenter study. Arch Intern Med 2003;163:286–92.

44. Ludvigsson JF, Rubio-Tapia A, van Dyke CT, et al. Increasing incidence of celiac disease in a North American population. Am J Gastroenterol 2013;108(5):818–24.

45. Cronin CC, Shanahan F. Insulin-dependent diabetes mellitus and coeliac disease. Lancet 1997;349:1096–7.

46. Green PH, Cellier C. Celiac disease. N Engl J Med 2007;357:1731–43.

47. Kagnoff MF. Celiac disease: pathogenesis of a model immunogenetic disease. J Clin Invest 2007;117:41–9.

48. Rostom A, Dube C, Cranney A, et al. Celiac disease. Evid Rep Technol Assess (Summ) 2004;(104):1–6.

49. Sud S, Marcon M, Assor E, et al. 2010 Celiac disease and pediatric type 1 diabetes: diagnostic and treatment dilemmas. Int J Pediatr Endocrinol 2010;2010:161285.

50. Nakajima K. 2012 Recent advances in dermatitis herpetiformis. Clin Dev Immunol 2012;2012:914162.

51. van der Windt DA, Jellema P, Mulder CJ, et al. Diagnostic testing for celiac disease among patients with abdominal symptoms: a systematic review. JAMA 2010;303:1738–46.

52. Rostom A, Murray JA, Kagnoff MF. American Gastroenterological Association (AGA) Institute technical review on the diagnosis and management of celiac disease. Gastroenterology 2006;131:1981–2002.

53. Rostom A, Dube C, Cranney A, et al. The diagnostic accuracy of serologic tests for celiac disease: a systematic review. Gastroenterology 2005;128:S38–46.

54. Corrao G, Corazza GR, Bagnardi V, et al. Mortality in patients with coeliac disease and their relatives: a cohort study. Lancet 2001;358:356–61.

55. Loftus CG, Loftus EV Jr. Cancer risk in celiac disease. Gastroenterology 2002;123:1726–9.

56. Leffler DA, Dennis M, Hyett B, et al. Etiologies and predictors of diagnosis in nonresponsive celiac disease. Clin Gastroenterol Hepatol 2007;5:445–50.

57. Parlesak A, Klein B, Schecher K, et al. Prevalence of small bowel bacterial overgrowth and its association with nutrition intake in nonhospitalized older adults. J Am Geriatr Soc 2003;51:768–73.

58. Virally-Monod M, Tielmans D, Kevorkian JP, et al. Chronic diarrhoea and diabetes mellitus: prevalence of small intestinal bacterial overgrowth. Diabete Metab 1998;24:530–6.

59. Dukowicz AC, Lacy BE, Levine GM. Small intestinal bacterial overgrowth: a comprehensive review. Gastroenterol Hepatol 2007;3:112–22.

60. Saltzman JR, Russell RM. Nutritional consequences of intestinal bacterial overgrowth. Compr Ther 1994;20:523–30.

61. Bures J, Cyrany J, Kohoutova D, et al. Small intestinal bacterial overgrowth syndrome. World J Gastroenterol 2010;16:2978–90.

62. Corazza GR, Menozzi MG, Strocchi A, et al. The diagnosis of small bowel bacterial overgrowth. Reliability of jejunal culture and inadequacy of breath hydrogen testing. Gastroenterology 1990;98:302–9.

63. Pimentel M. Review of rifaximin as treatment for SIBO and IBS. Expert Opin Investig Drugs 2009;18:349–58.

64. Lysy J, Israeli E, Goldin E. The prevalence of chronic diarrhea among diabetic patients. Am J Gastroenterol 1999;94:2165–70.
65. Miller LJ. Small intestinal manifestations of diabetes mellitus. Yale J Biol Med 1983;56:189–93.
66. Feldman M, Friedman LS, Brandt LJ, editors. Sleisenger and Fordtran's gastrointesitnal and liver disease: pathophysiology/diagnosis/management. 9th edition. Philadelphia: Elsevier; 2010.
67. Fedorak RN, Field M, Chang EB. Treatment of diabetic diarrhea with clonidine. Ann Intern Med 1985;102:197–9.
68. Meyer C, O'Neal DN, Connell W, et al. Octreotide treatment of severe diabetic diarrhoea. Intern Med J 2003;33:617–8.
69. Angulo P, Hui JM, Marchesini G, et al. The NAFLD fibrosis score: a noninvasive system that identifies liver fibrosis in patients with NAFLD. Hepatology 2007;45: 846–54.
70. Schiller LR, Santa Ana CA, Schmulen AC, et al. Pathogenesis of fecal incontinence in diabetes mellitus: evidence for internal-anal-sphincter dysfunction. N Engl J Med 1982;307:1666–71.
71. Russo A, Botten R, Kong MF, et al. Effects of acute hyperglycaemia on anorectal motor and sensory function in diabetes mellitus. Diabet Med 2004;21:176–82.
72. Rao SS. Diagnosis and management of fecal incontinence. American College of Gastroenterology Practice Parameters Committee. Am J Gastroenterol 2004;99: 1585–604.
73. Wald A, Tunuguntla AK. Anorectal sensorimotor dysfunction in fecal incontinence and diabetes mellitus. Modification with biofeedback therapy. N Engl J Med 1984;310:1282–7.
74. Lee JY, Kim KM, Lee SG, et al. Prevalence and risk factors of non-alcoholic fatty liver disease in potential living liver donors in Korea: a review of 589 consecutive liver biopsies in a single center. J Hepatol 2007;47:239–44.
75. Marcos A, Fisher RA, Ham JM, et al. Selection and outcome of living donors for adult to adult right lobe transplantation. Transplantation 2000;69:2410–5.
76. Vernon G, Baranova A, Younossi ZM. Systematic review: the epidemiology and natural history of non-alcoholic fatty liver disease and non-alcoholic steatohepatitis in adults. Aliment Pharmacol Ther 2011;34:274–85.
77. Chalasani N, Younossi Z, Lavine JE, et al, American Gastroenterological Association, American Association for the Study of Liver Diseases, American College of Gastroenterologyh. The diagnosis and management of non-alcoholic fatty liver disease: practice guideline by the American Gastroenterological Association, American Association for the Study of Liver Diseases, and American College of Gastroenterology. Gastroenterology 2012;142:1592–609.
78. Soderberg C, Stal P, Askling J. Decreased survival of subjects with elevated liver function tests during a 28-year follow-up. Hepatology 2010;51:595–602.
79. Chitturi S, Abeygunasekera S, Farrell GC, et al. NASH and insulin resistance: insulin hypersecretion and specific association with the insulin resistance syndrome. Hepatology 2002;35:373–9.
80. Browning JD, Horton JD. Molecular mediators of hepatic steatosis and liver injury. J Clin Invest 2004;114:147–52.
81. Farrell GC, Larter CZ. Nonalcoholic fatty liver disease: from steatosis to cirrhosis. Hepatology 2006;43:S99–112.
82. Lewis JD, Ferrara A, Peng T, et al. Risk of bladder cancer among diabetic patients treated with pioglitazone: interim report of a longitudinal cohort study. Diabetes Care 2011;34:916–22.

83. Sanyal AJ, Chalasani N, Kowdley KV, et al. Pioglitazone, vitamin E, or placebo for nonalcoholic steatohepatitis. N Engl J Med 2010;362:1675–85.

84. Chavez-Tapia NC, Tellez-Avila FI, Barrientos-Gutierrez T, et al. Bariatric surgery for non-alcoholic steatohepatitis in obese patients. Cochrane Database Syst Rev 2010;(1):CD007340.

85. Pazzi P, Scagliarini R, Gamberini S, et al. Review article: gall-bladder motor function in diabetes mellitus. Aliment Pharmacol Ther 2000;14(Suppl 2):62–5.

86. Hardt PD, Ewald N. 2011 Exocrine pancreatic insufficiency in diabetes mellitus: a complication of diabetic neuropathy or a different type of diabetes? Exp Diabetes Res 2011;2011:761950.

87. Shen HN, Chang YH, Chen HF, et al. Increased risk of severe acute pancreatitis in patients with diabetes. Diabet Med 2012;29:1419–24.

88. Elashoff M, Matveyenko AV, Gier B, et al. Pancreatitis, pancreatic, and thyroid cancer with glucagon-like peptide-1-based therapies. Gastroenterology 2011; 141:150–6.

89. Ben Q, Xu M, Ning X, et al. Diabetes mellitus and risk of pancreatic cancer: a meta-analysis of cohort studies. Eur J Cancer 2011;47:1928–37.

Complications of the Diabetic Foot

Paul J. Kim, DPM, MS, John S. Steinberg, DPM*

KEYWORDS

- Diabetes • Ulcer • Wound • Amputation • Infection • Multidisciplinary

KEY POINTS

- A discussion should be had between the physician and the patient regarding the relationship between glucose control and complications encountered in the foot and ankle.
- Peripheral neuropathy and peripheral vascular disease create an environment that will lead to ulceration and possible amputation.
- Calluses are a sign of impending ulceration and should be debrided; the underlying cause should be addressed surgically or through offloading in a brace or shoe.
- Infection should be treated aggressively with culture-sensitive oral or parenteral antibiotic therapy, topical antimicrobials, and/or surgical intervention.
- Residual foot function should be considered when amputation is considered to prevent new ulcer formation or ulcer recurrence.
- A multidisciplinary team approach is vital to the prevention and treatment of the diabetic foot.

INTRODUCTION

The foot is a complex structure that requires delicate and deliberate orchestration for normal weight bearing and ambulation. The foot and ankle serve the dual role of being able to adapt to the ground to absorb shock as well as becoming a rigid lever necessary for forward propulsion. The result of altered biomechanics is disability and deformity. The diabetic foot is particularly at risk for complications because of its inability to tolerate stress. Prolonged uncontrolled blood glucose imparts deleterious effects on all structures related to the foot and ankle, including the skin and subcutaneous tissue, nerve, blood vessels, fascia, ligaments, tendons, muscle, and bone. The diabetic foot follows a common pathway that begins with a small ulcer or surgical wound and

Disclosures: None.
Department of Plastic Surgery, Georgetown School of Medicine, Center for Wound Healing & Hyperbaric Medicine, MedStar Georgetown University Hospital, 3800 Reservoir Road Northwest, Washington, DC 20007, USA
* Corresponding author.
E-mail address: JSS5@gunet.georgetown.edu

Endocrinol Metab Clin N Am 42 (2013) 833–847
http://dx.doi.org/10.1016/j.ecl.2013.08.002
0889-8529/13/$ – see front matter © 2013 Elsevier Inc. All rights reserved.

terminates in limb loss. This article discusses key complications in the diabetic foot and ankle caused by peripheral neuropathy, peripheral vascular disease, and soft-tissue and bone deformity that contribute to ulceration, infection, and amputation (**Fig. 1**). Treatment options are mentioned but are not discussed in great detail, the principal focus being the recognition and understanding of the complications unique to the diabetic foot.

RISK FACTORS
Peripheral Neuropathy

A spectrum of peripheral neuropathy encountered in the lower extremity affects up to 66% of patients with diabetes.[1–3] The type of peripheral neuropathy experienced in the diabetic patient encompasses both large and small nerve fibers, with size describing the relative degree of myelination. Small nerve fiber disease is classically related to the sensation of pain experienced in the diabetic patient. Furthermore, small nerve fiber disease disrupts temperature discrimination and autonomic function. In the early stages of peripheral neuropathy, patients may present with burning, tingling, radiating pain beginning at the toes and progressing proximally on the foot and leg. The pain may increase during periods of elevated blood glucose and decrease with better control of blood glucose.[4,5] Although anticonvulsant medications (gabapentin, pregabalin), vitamin supplementation (B, folic acid, thiamine), and surgical decompression have been used for the treatment of peripheral neuropathy, none have consistently shown an ability to restore sensory loss. As peripheral neuropathy advances, the patient will become insensate with a noted loss of protective sensation distally in the extremities. This problem is irreversible, and can significantly elevate the risk for limb loss in the patient with diabetes. The patient is unable to detect trauma

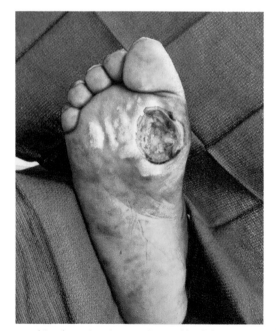

Fig. 1. Plantar neuropathic ulceration in a patient with diabetes. Note the fibrotic white base with lack of granulation tissue.

to the foot and thus does not respond by protecting or treating the area.[2] Hence, even a smaller blister can progress to a chronic ulcer because of the delay in care. The peripheral neuropathy experienced by the diabetic patient encompasses other types of nerve dysfunction, including the loss of proprioception (position sense) and motor control.[6] The decrease in proprioception can lead to falls and difficulties in ambulation.[7] Peripheral motor neuropathy can also lead to ambulation difficulties via muscle atrophy and lack of muscle coordination needed for steady ambulation. All of these challenges can contribute to increased and uneven weight-bearing pressure on the foot, which results in a heightened risk for nonhealing wounds and infections (**Fig. 2**).

Peripheral Vascular Disease

Adequate perfusion is fundamental to tissue repair and regeneration. Diabetes-induced peripheral vascular disease affects both small and large vessels in the lower extremities.[8–10] The 3 large vessels that deliver arterial blood to the foot are the posterior tibial artery, anterior tibial artery, and the peroneal artery. Specific areas of the foot (angiosomes) correspond to 1 of these 3 arteries.[10] With advancing diabetic disease, 1 or all of the arteries may be compromised. In the person with diabetes and peripheral vascular disease there is often focal or long-segment stenosis or occlusion, as seen on angiography of the lower extremity. There are redundant arterial pathways through perforator vessels that connect arteries to arteries. Furthermore, collateral vessels are formed to bypass areas of significant disease. However, even partial compromise of 1 of the major vessels can lead to chronic ulcerations with poor healing potential and tissue loss. A hand-held Doppler examination is the first means of detecting perfusion problems. If signals are any less than triphasic, assessment of segmental pressures (ankle brachial index [ABI]) should be conducted, followed by a vascular consultation. An ABI of less than 0.50 in a chronic ulcer environment has

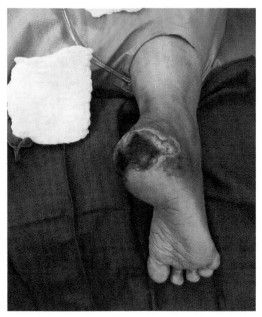

Fig. 2. Posterior neuropathic heel ulceration with ischemia caused by pressure and poor shoe gear.

a high likelihood of amputation.[11] An angiogram may reveal significant macrovascular disease requiring intervention, including angioplasty or open bypass. Microvascular disease may also develop in diabetic patients with altered local blood flow and dysregulation of vascular tone.[12–14] Hence, successful macrovascular intervention does not necessarily correlate with adequate perfusion to the tissue.

It is important to identify early signs of a vascular compromised limb before ulcer formation. The foot may appear atrophic, evidenced by the lack of hair growth, cool temperature of the limb, and thin atrophic and shiny skin. Patients may also complain of pain in the limb as the ischemia progresses, caused by oxygen and nutrient deprivation of the tissue. This environment places the foot and ankle at risk for ulceration. Once an ulcer forms it is important to determine the degree of perfusion loss to that area of the foot or ankle. Indirect blood flow to the area of ulceration may be sufficient to heal the ulcer but may take a long time to do so, placing it at risk for infection or increasing depth. Rapid recognition of compromised blood flow and optimization of perfusion to the affected limb will support ulcer healing (**Fig. 3**).

Soft-Tissue and Bone Deformity

Inherent changes in the quality of soft tissue predispose the diabetic foot to a destructive pathway. It is important to consider 2 important forces experienced by the foot

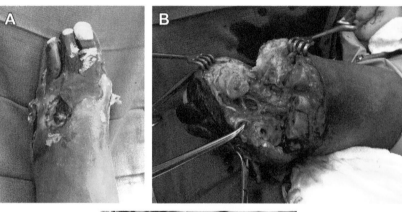

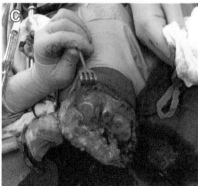

Fig. 3. (A) Forefoot gangrene with osteomyelitis and abscess in patient with diabetes and prior partial forefoot amputation. (B) Intraoperative view showing deep tissue necrosis and abscess extending to plantar tissues. (C) Status post open midfoot amputation.

during ambulation. The first is direct sagittal plane force experienced on the plantar aspect of the foot during heel strike and forefoot push-off. The force experienced is in a relatively confined surface area of the plantar foot. There is a direct correlation between peak sagittal plantar forces and ulcer location.[15,16] The second is a lesser understood force called shear, which is either a transverse force (eg, side to side or front to back) or frontal-plane force (rotational).[17,18] These shear forces are experienced between the foot and the ground or foot and the inside of the shoe. This type of force produces blister formation whereby the epidermis separates from the dermis. In the healthy foot both the peak plantar pressure and shear forces are quickly dissipated, which the soft tissue is able to tolerate. The environment of the diabetic foot is profoundly different. The epidermis is often dry, making it susceptible to tears and fissuring. Furthermore, there is atrophy of subcutaneous tissue, which negatively affects its ability to absorb shock during ambulation.[19,20]

The tendons and ligaments become stiff and lose their elasticity.[21,22] Tendon contracture produces deformities such as hammertoe, which increase the likelihood of distal toe ulcers.[23] Equinus deformity caused by Achilles tendon contracture can increase plantar forefoot pressures, creating wounds on the plantar forefoot.[16] Biomechanical surgical correction of tendon contractures can alleviate many of these weight-bearing pressures. Flexor tenotomies of the toes and tendo-Achilles lengthenings can correct these abnormalities.[24,25] Thus the combination of compromised skin-related structures and tendon contractures places the foot at high risk for ulceration (**Fig. 4**).

Bony deformity is also encountered in the diabetic foot. Standard weight-bearing radiographs are sufficient to appreciate many of these changes. Any bony prominences

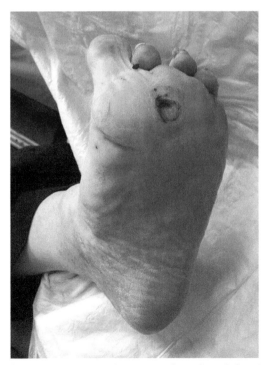

Fig. 4. Severe forefoot contracture with joint and tendon deformity causing plantar pressure and ulceration in a patient with diabetes and neuropathy.

cause increased pressure against the shoe or ground, which may result in ulcer formation or chronicity.[26,27] These bony prominences can be the result of instability of joints in the foot or frank subluxations/dislocations. Repetitive minor trauma or a discrete traumatic event may be the cause. Patients with later-stage peripheral neuropathy may not notice the change in foot structure and continue to ambulate, causing further subluxation/dislocation. These deformities require conservative offloading or surgical reconstruction. Conservative offloading involves the use of offloading camwalkers, total-contact casts, or CROW (Charcot Restraint Orthotic Walker) devices during the early stages of the deformity. Once the deformity has stabilized and no longer progresses, multidensity inserts in customized shoes or braces that offload and realign the foot and ankle are necessary. Surgical reconstruction involves exostectomies (removal of prominences) or realignment and arthrodesis of joints using screws, plates, rods, or external fixation. If the joint deformity is not manageable using shoes or braces, the surgical option should be considered.

A limb-threatening example of joint deformity is Charcot neuroarthropathy. Overt or subtle trauma may trigger a cascade of events that culminates in fractures, subluxations, and dislocations of the bones in the foot or ankle. Charcot foot is characterized by edema, erythema, and calor. During the acute stages of Charcot neuroarthropathy there is gross instability of the affected joints. Immediate non–weight bearing is critical to prevent further collapse. If left untreated, these fracture dislocations will proceed rapidly to ulceration and bone infection. After the Charcot neuroarthropathy deformity has consolidated, bony prominences develop, causing areas of high pressure resulting in ulcerations. Surgical reconstruction is not necessary if the deformity is shoeable or braceable (**Fig. 5**).

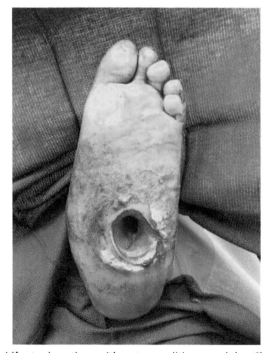

Fig. 5. Plantar midfoot ulceration with osteomyelitis caused by Charcot neuropathic osteoarthropathy.

CLINICAL FEATURES AND MANAGEMENT
Ulceration

Peripheral neuropathy, peripheral vascular disease, and bony deformity set the stage for ulceration. Approximately 15% of diabetic patients will develop ulceration over their lifetime.[28] The diabetic foot ulcer is typically located on the plantar aspect of the foot. Other common areas include the medial first metatarsal phalangeal joint, lateral aspect of the fifth metatarsal phalangeal joint, and the posterior calcaneus. All these locations are areas of higher pressure. Other chronic ulcerations related to diabetes may result from elective or nonelective surgical incisions. The diabetic foot ulcer typically evolves over time. Hyperkeratosis (callus) is the precursor to ulceration, increasing the relative risk 11-fold.[29,30] The skin reinforces areas of pressure or shear with layers of dense stratum corneum. Hyperkeratosis is counterproductive because these areas experience even greater pressure. Hence, frequent debridement is needed to remove this tissue and to uncover underlying hidden ulcers or infection. Multidensity inserts with extra-depth, wide-toebox shoes are necessary to more evenly distribute pressure and reduce shear forces.

The classic definition of a diabetic foot ulcer implies some level of peripheral neuropathy.[26] Patients continue to ambulate on the ulcer site because they lack the ability to perceive pain. Thus the ulcer continues to enlarge and begins to penetrate to deeper layers of tissue. However, diabetic foot ulcers can also be classified as ischemic, neuropathic, or decubitus wounds. For example, a diabetic patient may develop a posterior heel ulcer from prolonged pressure while being confined to bed. This patient may also have peripheral neuropathy and peripheral vascular disease. In this case the ulcer is most appropriately described as a decubitus ulcer. However, it can also be described as a diabetic foot ulcer, ischemic ulcer, or a neuropathic ulcer. Furthermore, there are wound-classification schemes that help describe the wound in relationship to depth of the ulcer, presence of infection, and ischemia.[31–33]

The duration and size of the ulcer relates directly to healing potential. Full-thickness or deeper wounds of longer than 2 months' duration are 79% less likely to heal.[34] A chronic ulcer is defined as a wound that does not decrease in size by 50% in 1 month.[35] Measurements (length × width × depth) of the wound should be taken every 1 to 2 weeks to track changes in wound size. Photographs should also be taken at every visit to remind the clinician of the appearance of the wound on prior visits. The wound should be fully explored, including all areas of undermining, and tunneling should be explored for any pus pockets or communication to bone or hardware (eg, internal screws or plates). The wound edges may have a rolled appearance indicating a chronic ulcer state. Senescent cells are found in the base and perimeter of the wound, preventing active wound healing and repair. Nonviable tissue (necrotic and fibrotic) may be evident in the wound bed, delaying wound healing. The wound with healing potential contains predominantly granulation tissue (bed of capillaries). The quality of the surrounding tissue should also be evaluated. Typically all diabetic foot ulcers have some level of serous drainage unless there is an active infection, in which case purulence may be present. Maceration about the surrounding tissue indicates drainage causing the tissue to be friable, which impedes wound healing.

Treatment of a diabetic foot ulcer involves a multimodal approach that includes conservative and surgical interventions. Paramount to ulcer healing is glucose control, which includes medical management, dietary/nutritional control, and exercise. Regarding the direct care of the diabetic ulcer, there are 4 fundamental treatment principles: optimization of perfusion (see previous discussion), biofilm/infection control, debridement, and offloading. Biofilm/infection control is discussed in detail in the next section. This section focuses on debridement and offloading.

Numerous purported effective therapies for diabetic foot ulcers exist. There are numerous claims that dressings, ointments, solutions, cellular and/or tissue-based products, and other topical therapies heal diabetic foot wounds. However, there is a paucity of evidence to support that any of these therapies is superior to another.[36] There is a role for some of these therapies, but none assist in healing wounds without addressing the 4 aforementioned treatment principles. For example, dressings can be an effective adjunctive treatment by facilitating the removal of drainage from the wound site. Furthermore, wound-healing ointments (antimicrobial, growth-factor impregnated) and solutions (cleansers, antiseptics) can promote a healthy wound environment. Bioengineered alternative tissues can include either xenografts or allografts that are impregnated with living cells or are acellular matrices.[37] Cell-impregnated allografts potentiate wound healing by introducing cells that secrete growth factors that activate native cells. Acellular matrices serve as scaffolds for organized migration of native cells. Although bioengineered alternative tissues promote wound healing, they should not be viewed as the sole agent for wound healing.

Debridement serves multiple functions that promote wound healing.[38,39] First, debridement removes detritus, foreign material, and nonviable tissue, and activates senescent cells by creating acute trauma to the wound bed and perimeter. Second, it removes infectious material associated with planktonic bacteria or biofilm. Debridement includes enzymatic debridement using collagenases, mechanical debridement using wet-to-dry dressing changes or whirlpool therapy, and biological debridement via maggot therapy. These techniques require a long duration of treatment and are not efficient in isolation. The preferred method is sharp debridement, which includes clinic-based debridement and surgery-based excisional debridement. Clinic-based debridement involves the use of scalpels, scissors, and curettes. Clinic-based debridement is constrained by the inability to aggressively debride tissue, owing to pain and the inability to control excessive bleeding. Furthermore, the clinic is not a sterile environment, with cross-contamination a real possibility. Surgery-based excisional debridement is performed in the sterile environment of an operating room, where more aggressive removal of infectious material and nonviable tissue can be conducted. However, there is expense related to surgery as well as the risks inherent with anesthesia. A combination of debridement strategies that includes all of the modalities described here should be used. Wounds should generally be debrided in the clinic with every visit. Enzymatic and mechanical debridement can be performed between clinic visits. Once the wound is sufficiently prepared in the clinic, the patient can be taken to the operating room for excisional debridement, after which the wound can be closed or covered with a split-thickness skin graft. Large soft-tissue defects require local or free tissue flaps for closure and/or coverage of deep structures and bone.

Offloading is of critical importance to successful ulcer healing, and is also perhaps the most difficult aspect of wound healing. As discussed earlier, diabetic foot ulcers are typically located on the plantar aspect of the foot. Hence, the patient with an insensate foot is likely to continue to bear weight on the affected limb. Wheelchairs, crutches, and wheeled single-limb offloading platforms are some options that may be used to completely offload a limb. Although the ideal situation is that the patient remains completely non–weight bearing, this is an unrealistic expectation. Patients will continue to bear weight on the ulcer area. Therefore, devices are needed to allow the patient to bear weight on the affected extremity while still offloading the ulcer. The use of "donut-shaped" cutouts from felt or foam is discouraged. These offloading pads can create an "edge" effect, causing increased pressure to the wound margins and resulting in the wound becoming larger.[40,41] Surgical shoes and removable cast walkers with multidensity inserts assist in offloading the ulcer by more evenly distributing pressure to varying degrees.[42,43] The multidensity aspect of these inserts allows for a gradual decline in durometry (hardness) from the most outer layer of the insert to the layer that is in contact with the dressing on the foot.[44] Some of these devices contain hexagonal plugs that can be removed. The removal of these plugs is not encouraged because this will again produce an edge effect. The advantage of the plugs is that they function to independently contour to the plantar aspect of the foot. Compliance with many of these removable offloading devices may be an issue, with patients removing the device once they are at home.

Total-contact casts are plaster or fiberglass constructs that cannot be removed and evenly distribute pressure on the plantar aspect of the foot. Total-contact casts need to be replaced every 1 or 2 weeks. There is good evidence to suggest that total-contact casts are the most effective modality of offloading, with healing rates of almost 90%.[45–47] However, there is an ulcer recurrence rate of 59% 7 months after the total-contact cast has been removed.[47] Although compliance can be maintained, the wound cannot be monitored on a daily basis. Furthermore, heavily draining wounds are not amenable to this type of offloading because the plaster or fiberglass will be become saturated with fluid. Moreover, the patient may refuse a total-contact cast because of its restrictive nature.

Surgical intervention may be the most effective way to offload an ulcer. As briefly described earlier, tendon lengthening/rebalancing, exostectomies, and bone/joint reconstruction can reduce the deforming forces that create a diabetic foot ulcer and contribute to its chronicity. The key in deciding between soft-tissue tendon lengthening/rebalancing and bone/joint reconstruction is the reducibility of the deformity. If the deformity is reducible, tendon lengthening and rebalancing may be effective. If the deformity is rigid, bone/joint reconstruction is necessary. A combined tendon and bone reconstruction may also be necessary.

Infection

The diabetic foot ulcer can have an active and/or passive (biofilm) infection. Active infection includes the classic signs of ascending erythema, edema, purulence, increased drainage, and malodor. However, the diabetic patient is not able to mount a robust immune response and can present without these signs; this is particularly the case when end-stage renal disease is superimposed with diabetes. Therefore, there may not be obvious signs of infection. Furthermore, nonelevated laboratory values (eg, white blood cell count) may not reflect an active infection, although elevated blood glucose levels may. The degree of soft-tissue infection and depth of infection (eg, to the level of muscle or bone) will dictate the course of treatment. Superficial soft-tissue infection can be managed with oral or parenteral (via peripherally inserted central catheter) antibiotics, debridement, and topical antimicrobials. Deeper soft-tissue or bone infections may require hospital admission with parenteral antibiotics and serial surgical debridement/decompression. Soft-tissue infections of the diabetic foot are often polymicrobial with gram-positive species as well as gram-negative bacteria, whereas bone infections are typically monomicrobial[48]; this includes staphylococcal and streptococcal species as well as *Pseudomonas* and *Escherichia coli*. Antibiotic therapy requires broad-spectrum coverage, based on sensitivities from deep cultures, for an extended duration until resolution of the infection (**Fig. 6**).[49]

Biofilm consists of bacterial colonies that form on the surface of chronic wounds, and certainly plays a detrimental role in ulcer healing. Biofilm is present in 60% of

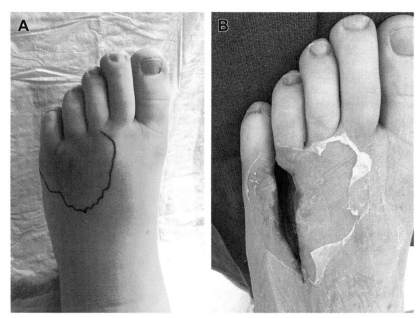

Fig. 6. (A) Dorsal forefoot abscess resulting from web-space tinea pedis in a patient with diabetes. (B) Resolved abscess and cellulitis status post incision, drainage, and intravenous antibiotics.

chronic wounds but in only 6% of acute wounds.[50] These bacterial colonies are often multispecies and differ from planktonic bacteria.[51,52] These bacteria have low metabolic activity and are encased with a glycocalyx matrix, making them resistant to oral, parenteral, and topical antibiotics.[53,54] Biofilm will reform within 10 hours of debridement.[55] A comprehensive multimodal strategy is needed that includes sharp excision of the wound to disrupt the biofilm, with immediate antimicrobial therapy to prevent its rapid reformation.[56]

Amputation

The unfortunate sequela of peripheral neuropathy, peripheral vascular disease, soft tissue/bony deformity, ulceration, and infection is often amputation. An amputation may be the result of a diabetic foot ulceration that progresses in depth, causing bone infection that is not readily amenable to antibiotic therapy and requires bone resection. Amputation may also be the result of an ischemic process whereby there is tissue necrosis and no revascularization option. The diabetic patient has a 20 to 30 times higher risk of amputation than a nondiabetic patient, with high probability of an amputation after developing a diabetic foot ulcer.[28,57–59] Amputations at any level of the foot affects the ambulatory capability of the patient, with higher-level amputations having a greater cardiovascular impact.[60] Furthermore, the survival rate diminishes with ascending amputation level. For example, in particularly high-risk type 2 diabetes populations the 5-year mortality rate for a forefoot amputation is 39%, compared with 67% for above-knee amputations.[61] Others report cumulative mortality rates after the first proximal amputation has been reported to be high as 45.8% at 5 years and 70.4% at 10 years for patients with diabetes.[62] Hence, every attempt should be made to preserve as much length as possible.

Amputations are generally performed at the level of the joints in the foot or along the rays of the foot (eg, hallux and first metatarsal). However, a commonly performed amputation is across the diaphysis of the metatarsals (ie, transmetatarsal amputation [TMA]). Multiple factors need to be assessed when amputation is considered. After serial operative debridements are performed to clear the infected tissue, the level of viable tissue needs to be assessed. The patient may require vascular intervention to maximize perfusion to the tissue before a decision is made regarding the amputation level. If the patient does not have triphasic Doppler signals, angiography should be performed to evaluate where the flow terminates. Furthermore, a qualitative assessment of tissue viability should be made, evaluating for necrosis and bleeding wound edges. Attention should then be turned to biomechanical concerns. Soft-tissue coverage is certainly important; however, the preservation of function should also play an important role in the selection of amputation level. For example, the TMA preserves the weight-bearing parabola that allows for postamputation function. This consideration is important, because an unbalanced amputation of any part of the foot can lead to ulceration in a new area as a result of changes in pressure distribution.[63–65] TMA should be selected if more than 1 ray has been wholly or partially amputated (**Fig. 7**).

It is vitally important to properly shoe or brace all feet that have had an amputation to prevent new ulcer formation. Furthermore, it is important to recognize that there is a significant alteration in gait after ulceration, even with the use of a prosthesis.[66] The use of toe and forefoot fillers is important as part of the custom insert, to prevent excessive motion of the residual foot in the shoe for amputations distal to the tarsometatarsal joint. For more proximal amputations, a brace that spans across the ankle may be necessary to facilitate ambulation. Rocker-bottom configuration of the shoe also allows for fluid transfer from heel to forefoot loading.

An amputation should not necessarily be viewed as a complication. An elective amputation may be the best option for some patients. For example, if a patient presents with gangrene of the toes and minimal perfusion to the foot that is not amenable to vascular intervention, a below-knee amputation may be considered at the first visit. Such a decision may save the patient countless operations attempting to salvage the foot as well as prolonged hospital stays and clinic visits. However, the challenge lies in trying to identify which patients would be better served by having a proximal leg amputation rather than aggressive limb salvage.

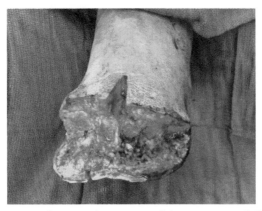

Fig. 7. Open transmetatarsal amputation as part of the treatment of diabetic foot ulceration with infection.

FUTURE CONSIDERATIONS AND SUMMARY

The diabetic foot is a complex structure that is at risk for multiple complications. The weight-bearing demands required for ambulation place the diabetic foot at particular risk. Uncontrolled glucose levels lead to peripheral neuropathy and peripheral vascular disease, which can potentiate the breakdown of soft tissue and lead to ulceration, infection, and possible amputation. Although glucose control and ulcer prevention are the key to stopping this progression, diligent monitoring and aggressive treatment are necessary after a diabetic ulcer has occurred. New devices, biologics, drugs, and therapies will assist in healing wounds. However, fundamental principles of frequent debridement, microbial control, and offloading are still crucial. Most importantly, a multidisciplinary approach is needed to prevent and treat the diabetic foot.[67] A multidisciplinary team approach can reduce amputation rates and wound-related complications by greater than 50%.[68–71] Such an approach involves both medical and surgical fields lending their expertise through intensive communication and interaction.

REFERENCES

1. Young MJ, Boulton AJ, MacLeod AF, et al. A multicentre study of the prevalence of diabetic peripheral neuropathy in the United Kingdom hospital clinic population. Diabetologia 1993;36:150–4.
2. Kumar S, Ashe HA, Parnell LN, et al. The prevalence of foot ulceration and its correlates in type 2 diabetic patients: a population-based study. Diabet Med 1994;11:480–4.
3. Cabezas-Cerrato J. The prevalence of clinical diabetic polyneuropathy in Spain: a study in primary care and hospital clinic groups. Neuropathy Spanish Study Group of the Spanish Diabetes Society (SDS). Diabetologia 1998;41:1263–9.
4. Sumner CJ, Sheth S, Griffin JW, et al. The spectrum of neuropathy in diabetes and impaired glucose tolerance. Neurology 2003;60:108–11.
5. The effect of intensive treatment of diabetes on the development and progression of long-term complications in insulin-dependent diabetes mellitus. The Diabetes Control and Complications Trial Research Group. N Engl J Med 1993;329:977–86.
6. Courtemanche R, Teasdale N, Boucher P, et al. Gait problems in diabetic neuropathic patients. Arch Phys Med Rehabil 1996;77:849–55.
7. Oliveira PP, Fachin SM, Tozatti J, et al. Comparative analysis of risk for falls in patients with and without type 2 diabetes mellitus. Rev Assoc Med Bras 2012;58:234–9.
8. Donahue RP, Orchard TJ. Diabetes mellitus and macrovascular complications. An epidemiological perspective. Diabetes Care 1992;15:1141–55.
9. Jude EB, Oyibo SO, Chalmers N, et al. Peripheral arterial disease in diabetic and nondiabetic patients: a comparison of severity and outcome. Diabetes Care 2001;24:1433–7.
10. Attinger CE, Evans KK, Bulan E, et al. Angiosomes of the foot and ankle and clinical implications for limb salvage: reconstruction, incisions, and revascularization. Plast Reconstr Surg 2006;117:261S–93S.
11. Marston WA, Davies SW, Armstrong B, et al. Natural history of limbs with arterial insufficiency and chronic ulceration treated without revascularization. J Vasc Surg 2006;44:108–14.
12. Jorneskog G, Brismar K, Fagrell B. Skin capillary circulation is more impaired in the toes of diabetic than non-diabetic patients with peripheral vascular disease. Diabet Med 1995;12:36–41.

13. Schramm JC, Dinh T, Veves A. Microvascular changes in the diabetic foot. Int J Low Extrem Wounds 2006;5:149–59.

14. Jaap AJ, Shore AC, Stockman AJ, et al. Skin capillary density in subjects with impaired glucose tolerance and patients with type 2 diabetes. Diabet Med 1996;13:160–4.

15. Boulton AJ, Hardisty CA, Betts RP, et al. Dynamic foot pressure and other studies as diagnostic and management aids in diabetic neuropathy. Diabetes Care 1983;6:26–33.

16. Lavery LA, Armstrong DG, Boulton AJ. Ankle equinus deformity and its relationship to high plantar pressure in a large population with diabetes mellitus. J Am Podiatr Med Assoc 2002;92:479–82.

17. Pollard JP, Le Quesne LP, Tappin JW. Forces under the foot. J Biomed Eng 1983; 5:37–40.

18. Delbridge L, Ctercteko G, Fowler C, et al. The aetiology of diabetic neuropathic ulceration of the foot. Br J Surg 1985;72:1–6.

19. Brash PD, Foster J, Vennart W, et al. Magnetic resonance imaging techniques demonstrate soft tissue damage in the diabetic foot. Diabet Med 1999;16: 55–61.

20. Robertson DD, Mueller MJ, Smith KE, et al. Structural changes in the forefoot of individuals with diabetes and a prior plantar ulcer. J Bone Joint Surg Am 2002; 84:1395–404.

21. Grant WP, Sullivan R, Sonenshine DE, et al. Electron microscopic investigation of the effects of diabetes mellitus on the Achilles tendon. J Foot Ankle Surg 1997; 36:272–8 [discussion: 330].

22. Reddy GK. Cross-linking in collagen by nonenzymatic glycation increases the matrix stiffness in rabbit Achilles tendon. Exp Diabesity Res 2004;5:143–53.

23. Ledoux WR, Shofer JB, Smith DG, et al. Relationship between foot type, foot deformity, and ulcer occurrence in the high-risk diabetic foot. J Rehabil Res Dev 2005;42:665–72.

24. Lavery LA. Effectiveness and safety of elective surgical procedures to improve wound healing and reduce re-ulceration in diabetic patients with foot ulcers. Diabetes Metab Res Rev 2012;28(Suppl 1):60–3.

25. Armstrong DG, Lavery LA, Stern S, et al. Is prophylactic diabetic foot surgery dangerous? J Foot Ankle Surg 1996;35:585–9.

26. Reiber GE, Vileikyte L, Boyko EJ, et al. Causal pathways for incident lower-extremity ulcers in patients with diabetes from two settings. Diabetes Care 1999;22:157–62.

27. Boyko EJ, Ahroni JH, Stensel V, et al. A prospective study of risk factors for diabetic foot ulcer. The Seattle Diabetic Foot Study. Diabetes Care 1999;22: 1036–42.

28. Reiber GE. The epidemiology of diabetic foot problems. Diabet Med 1996; 13(Suppl 1):S6–11.

29. Hazenberg CE, van Baal JG, Manning E, et al. The validity and reliability of diagnosing foot ulcers and pre-ulcerative lesions in diabetes using advanced digital photography. Diabetes Technol Ther 2010;12:1011–7.

30. Murray HJ, Young MJ, Hollis S, et al. The association between callus formation, high pressures and neuropathy in diabetic foot ulceration. Diabet Med 1996;13: 979–82.

31. Wagner FW Jr. The dysvascular foot: a system for diagnosis and treatment. Foot Ankle 1981;2:64–122.

32. Wagner FW Jr. The diabetic foot. Orthopedics 1987;10:163–72.

33. Lavery LA, Armstrong DG, Harkless LB. Classification of diabetic foot wounds. J Foot Ankle Surg 1996;35:528–31.

34. Margolis DJ, Allen-Taylor L, Hoffstad O, et al. Diabetic neuropathic foot ulcers: predicting which ones will not heal. Am J Med 2003;115:627–31.

35. Sheehan P, Jones P, Giurini JM, et al. Percent change in wound area of diabetic foot ulcers over a 4-week period is a robust predictor of complete healing in a 12-week prospective trial. Plast Reconstr Surg 2006;117:239S–44S.

36. Hinchliffe RJ, Valk GD, Apelqvist J, et al. A systematic review of the effectiveness of interventions to enhance the healing of chronic ulcers of the foot in diabetes. Diabetes Metab Res Rev 2008;24(Suppl 1):S119–44.

37. Felder JM 3rd, Goyal SS, Attinger CE. A systematic review of skin substitutes for foot ulcers. Plast Reconstr Surg 2012;130:145–64.

38. Steed DL, Donohoe D, Webster MW, et al. Effect of extensive debridement and treatment on the healing of diabetic foot ulcers. Diabetic Ulcer Study Group. J Am Coll Surg 1996;183:61–4.

39. Attinger CE, Bulan EJ. Debridement. The key initial first step in wound healing. Foot Ankle Clin 2001;6:627–60.

40. Armstrong DG, Liswood PJ, Todd WF. Potential risks of accommodative padding in the treatment of neuropathic ulcerations. Ostomy Wound Manage 1995;41: 44–6, 48–9.

41. Armstrong DG, Athanasiou KA. The edge effect: how and why wounds grow in size and depth. Clin Podiatr Med Surg 1998;15:105–8.

42. Lavery LA, Vela SA, Lavery DC, et al. Reducing dynamic foot pressures in high-risk diabetic subjects with foot ulcerations. A comparison of treatments. Diabetes Care 1996;19:818–21.

43. Lavery LA, Vela SA, Fleischli JG, et al. Reducing plantar pressure in the neuropathic foot. A comparison of footwear. Diabetes Care 1997;20:1706–10.

44. Fleischli JG, Lavery LA, Vela SA, et al. 1997 William J. Stickel Bronze Award. Comparison of strategies for reducing pressure at the site of neuropathic ulcers. J Am Podiatr Med Assoc 1997;87:466–72.

45. Mueller MJ, Diamond JE, Sinacore DR, et al. Total contact casting in treatment of diabetic plantar ulcers. Controlled clinical trial. Diabetes Care 1989;12:384–8.

46. Armstrong DG, Nguyen HC, Lavery LA, et al. Off-loading the diabetic foot wound: a randomized clinical trial. Diabetes Care 2001;24:1019–22.

47. Mueller MJ, Sinacore DR, Hastings MK, et al. Effect of Achilles tendon lengthening on neuropathic plantar ulcers. A randomized clinical trial. J Bone Joint Surg Am 2003;85:1436–45.

48. Parvez N, Dutta P, Ray P, et al. Microbial profile and utility of soft tissue, pus, and bone cultures in diagnosing diabetic foot infections. Diabetes Technol Ther 2012;14:669–74.

49. Lipsky BA, Berendt AR, Cornia PB, et al, Infectious Diseases Society of America. 2012 Infectious Diseases Society of America clinical practice guideline for the diagnosis and treatment of diabetic foot infections. Clin Infect Dis 2012;54:e132–73.

50. James GA, Swogger E, Wolcott R, et al. Biofilms in chronic wounds. Wound Repair Regen 2008;16:37–44.

51. Frank DN, Wysocki A, Specht-Glick DD, et al. Microbial diversity in chronic open wounds. Wound Repair Regen 2009;17:163–72.

52. Dowd SE, Sun Y, Secor PR, et al. Survey of bacterial diversity in chronic wounds using pyrosequencing, DGGE, and full ribosome shotgun sequencing. BMC Microbiol 2008;8:43.

53. Stewart PS, Costerton JW. Antibiotic resistance of bacteria in biofilms. Lancet 2001;358:135–8.
54. Hoiby N, Bjarnsholt T, Givskov M, et al. Antibiotic resistance of bacterial biofilms. Int J Antimicrob Agents 2010;35:322–32.
55. Harrison-Balestra C, Cazzaniga AL, Davis SC, et al. A wound-isolated pseudomonas aeruginosa grows a biofilm in vitro within 10 hours and is visualized by light microscopy. Dermatol Surg 2003;29:631–5.
56. Kim PJ, Steinberg JS. Wound care: biofilm and its impact on the latest treatment modalities for ulcerations of the diabetic foot. Semin Vasc Surg 2012;25:70–4.
57. Trautner C, Haastert B, Giani G, et al. Incidence of lower limb amputations and diabetes. Diabetes Care 1996;19:1006–9.
58. Pecoraro RE, Reiber GE, Burgess EM. Pathways to diabetic limb amputation. Basis for prevention. Diabetes Care 1990;13:513–21.
59. Armstrong DG, Lavery LA, Quebedeaux TL, et al. Surgical morbidity and the risk of amputation due to infected puncture wounds in diabetic versus nondiabetic adults. J Am Podiatr Med Assoc 1997;87:321–6.
60. Pinzur MS, Gold J, Schwartz D, et al. Energy demands for walking in dysvascular amputees as related to the level of amputation. Orthopedics 1992;15:1033–6 [discussion: 1036–7].
61. Lee ET, Russell D, Jorge N, et al. A follow-up study of diabetic Oklahoma Indians. Mortality and causes of death. Diabetes Care 1993;16:300–5.
62. Morbach S, Furchert H, Groblinghoff U, et al. Long-term prognosis of diabetic foot patients and their limbs: amputation and death over the course of a decade. Diabetes Care 2012;35:2021–7.
63. Lavery LA, Lavery DC, Quebedeax-Farnham TL. Increased foot pressures after great toe amputation in diabetes. Diabetes Care 1995;18:1460–2.
64. Armstrong DG, Lavery LA. Plantar pressures are higher in diabetic patients following partial foot amputation. Ostomy Wound Manage 1998;44:30–2, 34, 36 passim.
65. Garbalosa JC, Cavanagh PR, Wu G, et al. Foot function in diabetic patients after partial amputation. Foot Ankle Int 1996;17:43–8.
66. Dillon MP, Barker TM. Comparison of gait of persons with partial foot amputation wearing prosthesis to matched control group: observational study. J Rehabil Res Dev 2008;45:1317–34.
67. Kim PJ, Evans KK, Steinberg JS, et al. Critical elements to building an effective wound care center. J Vasc Surg 2013;57:1703–9.
68. Hellingman AA, Smeets HJ. Efficacy and efficiency of a streamlined multidisciplinary foot ulcer service. J Wound Care 2008;17:541–4.
69. Yesil S, Akinci B, Bayraktar F, et al. Reduction of major amputations after starting a multidisciplinary diabetic foot care team: single centre experience from Turkey. Exp Clin Endocrinol Diabetes 2009;117:345–9.
70. Faglia E, Favales F, Aldeghi A, et al. Change in major amputation rate in a center dedicated to diabetic foot care during the 1980s: prognostic determinants for major amputation. J Diabet Complications 1998;12:96–102.
71. Chiu CC, Huang CL, Weng SF, et al. A multidisciplinary diabetic foot ulcer treatment programme significantly improved the outcome in patients with infected diabetic foot ulcers. J Plast Reconstr Aesthet Surg 2011;64:867–72.

Periodontitis
Oral Complication of Diabetes

Philip M. Preshaw, BDS, FDSRCSEd, FDS(RestDent)RCSEd, PhD*,
Susan M. Bissett, MClinRes

KEYWORDS

- Periodontal diseases • Periodontitis • Gingivitis • Diabetes
- Diabetes complications • Inflammation • Glycated hemoglobin • HbA1c

KEY POINTS

- Periodontitis is a common, chronic inflammatory disease of the supporting structures of the teeth. It is highly prevalent (approximately 10% of adults have advanced periodontitis), and can lead to mobile teeth and premature tooth loss.
- Diabetes is a major risk factor for periodontitis, and increases the susceptibility to periodontitis approximately 3-fold.
- Similar to other diabetes complications, susceptibility to periodontitis is increased with poor glycemic control.
- Inflammation is at the heart of the mechanistic links between the 2 conditions. Key mediators include cytokines such as interleukin (IL)-1β, IL-6, tumor necrosis factor alpha, receptor activator of nuclear factor kappa B ligand, and osteoprotegerin. The advanced glycation end product (AGE) receptor for AGE (RAGE) axis also plays an important role in mediating breakdown events in the periodontal tissues in people with diabetes.
- There is evidence to support a 2-way relationship between diabetes and periodontitis; not only does diabetes increase susceptibility to periodontitis, but periodontitis has been associated with compromised glycemic control.
- Treatment of periodontitis is associated with modest, but potentially clinically relevant, hemoglobin A1c reductions of approximately 0.4%.

INTRODUCTION

Periodontitis is a common chronic inflammatory disease that affects the tissues that support and invest the teeth. These tissues include the gingiva (or gum, the visible part of pink tissue that surrounds the teeth), the periodontal ligament (the suspensory ligament that secures the teeth to the underlying bone), and the alveolar bone (that

The author has no relationship to declare with any commercial interest or any conflicts of interest associated with this article.

School of Dental Sciences, Institute of Cellular Medicine, Newcastle University, Framlington Place, Newcastle upon Tyne NE2 4BW, UK

* Corresponding author.

E-mail address: philip.preshaw@ncl.ac.uk

Endocrinol Metab Clin N Am 42 (2013) 849–867

http://dx.doi.org/10.1016/j.ecl.2013.05.012

part of the jaw bone that supports the teeth). Periodontal diseases include a spectrum of disorders ranging from gingivitis (mild inflammation that affects the gingival tissues only) to chronic periodontitis (the subject of this article, usually referred to simply as periodontitis).

Healthy gingival tissues are pink in color, with a firm texture, and are attached to the cervical margin of the tooth (that part of the tooth where the crown enamel meets the root) (**Fig. 1**). As a result of plaque accumulation at the gingival margin, the characteristic clinical signs of gingivitis develop, including erythema, edema, and an increased tendency to bleed (for example, on brushing the teeth, or when a probe is used to assess the tissues). Gingivitis is highly prevalent, and affects most of the population to a greater or lesser degree. The tissue changes that characterize gingivitis are confined to the gingiva and are reversible with professional plaque removal and improvements in oral hygiene.

In periodontitis, the inflammation extends deeper into the underlying connective tissues, resulting in breakdown of fibers of the periodontal ligament and resorption of alveolar bone (**Fig. 2**). Breakdown of the periodontal ligament results in the formation of a pocket between the gingiva and the tooth, which is measurable with a periodontal probe. Pocket formation is not apparent on simple visual inspection alone,

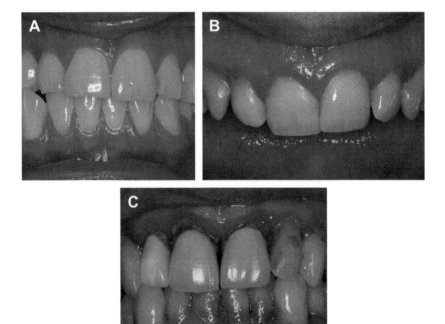

Fig. 1. Clinical appearance of health, gingivitis, and periodontitis. (*A*) Gingival health. The gingival tissues are pink and noninflamed. There is no evidence of gingival swelling or bleeding. (*B*) Gingivitis. There is generalized gingival erythema (particularly affecting the gingival margins) together with gingival edema, particularly of the interdental gingival tissues. (*C*) Periodontitis. The gingival tissues are edematous and erythematous. There is generalized gingival recession, as a result of loss of attachment between the tooth and the supporting bone, so that the roots of the teeth are partially visible. Abundant plaque deposits are also evident.

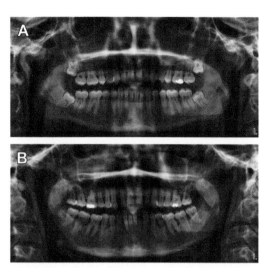

Fig. 2. Radiographic appearance of periodontitis. (*A*) Patient with minimal/no evidence of periodontitis. Alveolar bone levels are generally normal, with the alveolar bone encasing the roots of the teeth (contrast with part *B*). (*B*) Advanced periodontitis. There is generalized alveolar bone loss affecting the dentition, being particularly advanced at the maxillary molars (both right and left sides) and the upper and lower incisor teeth. The lower left lateral incisor tooth has already been lost.

and assessment of pocket depth (or probing depth) with a periodontal probe is essential for detecting the presence of disease. Disease progression is slow (characterized by progressive breakdown of the tooth supporting structures and resorption of alveolar bone), but the tissue destruction that occurs is largely irreversible. Long-term sequelae include tooth mobility, drifting and spacing of teeth (as a result of loss of attachment), sensitivity (as a result of gingival recession), compromised aesthetics, and ultimately tooth loss. Periodontitis can have significant impacts on aspects of daily living and quality of life, such as reduced confidence and self-esteem, and negative impacts on social interactions and food choices.[1]

Classification of periodontal diseases is complex and takes into account the clinical presentation, rate of disease progression, age at time of diagnosis, and also systemic and local risk factors. Chronic periodontitis (periodontitis) is prevalent, and advanced disease is typically found to affect about 10% of adults.[2,3] Mild forms of periodontitis affect approximately 40% to 60% of adults. Patients with chronic periodontitis tend to present in their 40s and 50s. Other than gingival bleeding, the condition tends to be asymptomatic (and generally does not cause pain), with the result that it can remain undetected for many years until teeth start to become mobile, by which time significant tissue damage may have already occurred. Periodontitis is therefore a highly prevalent, but largely hidden, chronic inflammatory disease.

The 2 major risk factors for periodontitis are smoking and diabetes.[4] Smoking significantly increases the risk for developing the condition, as well as increasing the severity of the disease.[5,6] Smoking also impairs treatment outcomes, and smoking cessation counseling forms a central component of therapy.[7] Treatment outcomes are significantly better in smokers who manage to quit compared with those who continue to smoke.[8] Besides smoking and diabetes, other risk factors for periodontitis include medications that can cause gingival overgrowth (eg, some calcium channel blockers, cyclosporin, phenytoin), conditions that result in compromised immune responses (eg, human immunodeficiency virus), nutritional defects, possibly osteoporosis, and local factors (eg, anatomic defects in the alveolar bone, or other plaque-retentive features).[4]

ASSOCIATIONS BETWEEN DIABETES AND PERIODONTITIS

The risk of periodontitis is increased approximately 3 times in people with diabetes compared with those who do not have diabetes.[9] The level of glycemic control is directly linked to the increased risk. In the US National Health and Nutrition Examination Survey (NHANES) III, adults with hemoglobin A1c (HbA1c) greater than 9% had a significantly higher prevalence of severe periodontitis compared with those who did not have diabetes (odds ratio [OR] 2.90; 95% confidence interval [CI] 1.40, 6.03), after controlling for smoking, age, ethnicity, and gender.[10] Evidence linking periodontitis and diabetes began to emerge in the 1990s from several studies conducted in the Pima India population in the United States. Cross-sectional and longitudinal studies identified that both the prevalence and incidence of periodontitis were significantly greater in subjects who had type 2 diabetes,[11,12] with a 3-fold increased risk for periodontitis compared with those subjects who did not have diabetes.[13] Most studies of the associations between periodontitis and diabetes have focused on type 2 diabetes, probably because both conditions have typically tended to present in individuals in their 40s and 50s. However, the risk for periodontitis is also increased in type 1 diabetes.[14–16] Therefore, all people with diabetes (including children and young adults) should be considered to be at increased risk of periodontitis, particularly if glycemic control is poor.

In the past, although dental clinicians have been aware of the associations between diabetes and periodontitis, diabetes care teams have tended to be less well informed, probably resulting from several factors including lack of knowledge, lack of integrated patient care that can result from fragmented health care delivery, and perceived divisions that exist between the medical and dental professions.[17] However, in the early 1990s, periodontitis was sometimes referred to as the sixth complication of diabetes,[18] which marked the beginning of an extensive period of research into the pathogenic links between the two conditions.

THE 2-WAY RELATIONSHIP BETWEEN PERIODONTITIS AND DIABETES

The 2-way relationship between periodontitis and diabetes holds that (1) diabetes is a risk factor for periodontitis (resulting in increased prevalence and severity of periodontitis) and (2) that periodontitis negatively affects glycemic control (rendering control of diabetes more difficult). This concept was first postulated following longitudinal studies of residents of the Gila River Indian Community, which identified that severe periodontitis was associated with an increased risk of poorer glycemic control (HbA1c$\geq$9%) when patients were followed up 2 years later.[19] The effect of periodontitis on development of nephropathy (macroalbuminuria and end-stage renal disease [ESRD]) was also assessed in 529 diabetic individuals from the Gila River Indian population who were followed for up to 22 years.[20] At baseline, individuals had glomerular filtration rate greater than or equal to 60 mL/min/1.73 m^2 and no macroalbuminuria (urinary albumin/creatine ratio $\geq$300 mg/g). Over the course of the study, 193 individuals developed macroalbuminuria (after a median follow-up of 9.4 years) and 68 developed ESRD (after a median follow-up of 14.9 years). The incidences (after adjustment for age, sex, diabetes duration, body mass index [BMI] and smoking) of macroalbuminuria and ESRD increased with the severity of periodontitis; incidence of macroalbuminuria was 2.0 and 2.1 times as high, and incidence of ESRD was

2.3 and 3.5 times as high, in those with moderate and severe periodontitis, respectively, compared with those with no/mild periodontitis ($P<.05$).

The impact of periodontitis on cardiovascular disease mortality was also studied in a population of Pima Indians with type 2 diabetes.[21] Six-hundred and twenty-eight individuals underwent periodontal assessment, all were aged 35 years or older, all had type 2 diabetes, and the median follow-up period was 11 years. Age-adjusted and sex-adjusted death rates per 1000 person-years were 3.7 (95% CI 0.7, 6.6) for those with no/mild periodontitis, 19.6 (95% CI 10.7, 28.5) for those with moderate periodontitis, and 28.4 (95% CI 22.3, 34.6) for those with severe periodontitis. Periodontitis was a statistically significant predictor of deaths from ischemic heart disease ($P = .04$) and diabetic nephropathy ($P<.01$), and, after adjusting for known risk factors (age, sex, duration of diabetes, HbA1c, BMI, macroalbuminuria, cholesterol, hypertension, smoking), subjects with severe periodontitis had a 3.2 times increased risk (95% CI 1.1, 9.3) of cardiorenal mortality (ischemic heart disease and diabetic nephropathy combined).

The impact of periodontitis on incident diabetes has also been investigated. In a 7-year prospective study of 5848 nondiabetic individuals, a tendency for increased risk of developing diabetes was reported in individuals with moderate/severe periodontitis (the association was significant in unadjusted analyses, although significance was lost after accounting for variables such as smoking, sex, BMI, hypertension, and lipid profiles).[22] The impact of periodontitis on increases in HbA1c in individuals who do not have diabetes has also been investigated. After adjusting for confounders such as age, sex, smoking, obesity and family history, those individuals who had the most advanced periodontitis at baseline showed a 5-fold greater increase in HbA1c (0.11% $\pm$ 0.03%) compared with those who had no periodontitis at baseline (0.02% $\pm$ 0.02%) over a 5-year period.[23] These findings suggest that advanced periodontitis is associated with a gradual increase in HbA1c levels in nondiabetic individuals, with the implication that periodontitis possibly increases the risk for incident diabetes.

TREATMENT OF PERIODONTITIS IS ASSOCIATED WITH IMPROVEMENTS IN GLYCEMIC CONTROL

Perhaps the most intriguing evidence to support a direct link between diabetes and periodontitis comes from studies that have identified improvements in glycemic control (reductions in HbA1c) following periodontal therapy in people with diabetes. These studies have tended to be underpowered and of short duration, but, despite variations in the methodologies that have been used, it has been possible to conduct meta-analyses to investigate the impact of periodontal treatment on glycemic control. The first of these was published in 2005, and included 10 intervention studies (involving a total of 456 patients).[24] A nonsignificant weighted mean reduction in HbA1c of 0.38% was identified following periodontal treatment in the patients with diabetes. A further meta-analysis of 9 studies (485 patients) was published in 2008, which reported a standardized mean reduction in HbA1c following periodontal treatment of 0.46% (95% CI 0.11%, 0.82%; $P<.05$).[25] In 2010, a meta-analysis of 5 studies (371 patients with type 2 diabetes) showed a weighted mean reduction in HbA1c of 0.40% (95% CI 0.04%, 0.77%; $P = .03$) over a follow-up period of 3 to 9 months following periodontal therapy, although there was heterogeneity among the studies.[26]

A further meta-analysis was provided by the Cochrane Collaboration in 2010.[27] Three studies were pooled into the meta-analysis, which identified a mean reduction in HbA1c following nonsurgical (ie, standard) periodontal therapy of 0.40% (95% CI 0.01%, 0.78%; $P = .04$). The investigators reported that there is evidence of improvements in metabolic control in people with diabetes after treating periodontal disease, but there are currently few studies available, and individual studies lack power and are at risk of bias. Further evidence in support of a beneficial impact of periodontal treatment on glycemic control was provided by a population-based cross-sectional study that evaluated the association between periodontal treatment (as a proxy for periodontitis) and HbA1c values based on medical/dental insurance data collected from more than 5000 individuals over a period of 5 years.[28] Patients who underwent at least one episode of periodontal surgery (an intense form of treatment usually reserved for late stages of advanced periodontitis) had HbA1c levels that were 0.25% lower than those who did not undergo periodontal surgery ($P = .04$).

Taken together, these studies support the contention that periodontal therapy is associated with improvements in glycemic control in people with diabetes. Most studies have focused on type 2 diabetes and mean HbA1c reductions have typically been of the order of 0.4%. Further carefully controlled randomized studies are now required to test this hypothesis further. The precise mechanisms that could account for such a reduction also require further investigation, but could result from reduced systemic inflammation (eg, reduced levels of circulating tumor necrosis factor alpha [TNF-α], and interleukin [IL]-6) as a result of resolution of periodontal inflammation. Both IL-6 and TNF-α induce the production of acute phase proteins including C-reactive protein (CRP), and evidence from animal studies[29] and cell culture studies of human adipocytes[30] has suggested that these cytokines can impair insulin signaling. Therefore, there is the possibility that periodontal treatment leading to reduced inflammation in the periodontal tissues could yield reductions in systemic inflammation (eg, reductions in the levels of cytokines such as IL-6 and TNF-α) with the potential for a beneficial impact on glycemic control. However, although increased CRP levels are a consistent finding in patients with periodontitis compared with healthy controls,[31] there is a lack of consistent evidence for increased systemic cytokine levels (eg, IL-6, TNF-α) in patients with coexisting periodontitis and diabetes, and the precise mechanisms that lead to reductions in HbA1c following periodontal treatment remain, as yet, unclear.[32]

Although the magnitude of reductions in HbA1c that has been reported following periodontal therapy is small (approximately 0.4%), it is similar to the improvements achieved by some second-line therapies for diabetes. Furthermore, it is known that each percentage point reduction in HbA1c is associated with a quantifiable reduction in complications and deaths related to diabetes.[33] Therefore, periodontal therapy is potentially an important component of the overall management strategy for patients with diabetes.

WHAT ARE THE MECHANISMS THAT LINK PERIODONTITIS AND DIABETES?

Periodontal tissue breakdown results from a prolonged, chronic, dysregulated inflammatory response to the bacteria present in the subgingival environment. Key mediators include cytokines such as IL-1β and IL-6, prostanoids such as prostaglandin E_2 (PGE$_2$), TNF-α, receptor activator of nuclear factor kappa B ligand (RANKL), and the matrix metalloproteinases (MMPs; especially MMP-8, MMP-9 and MMP-13). T-cell regulatory cytokines (eg, IL-12, IL-18) and chemokines are also likely to play a role.[34] Cytokine networks interact functionally with components of the innate and adaptive immune response to the bacteria, involving both resident cells in the periodontium and infiltrating inflammatory cells. There is significant heterogeneity in the nature of the inflammatory response between individuals, and also within individuals over time, which influences susceptibility to the disease.[35]

Dysregulated immune responses also play a role in the pathogenesis of both type 1 and type 2 diabetes, and are associated with metabolic, nutritional, and physiologic changes such as the formation of advanced glycation end products (AGEs), hyperglycemia, and hyperlipidemia. Increased levels of cytokines systemically (notably IL-6 and TNF-α) are a consistent finding in diabetes and obesity, and chronic overnutrition constitutes a proinflammatory state.[36] Increased serum levels of IL-6 and CRP have been linked to future occurrence of type 2 diabetes,[37] and hyperglycemia can result in inflammation and increased oxidative stress.[38] Inflammation is therefore of central importance to the pathogenesis of both periodontitis and diabetes, and it is important to consider those aspects of the inflammatory response that are likely to link the two conditions. This subject has recently been extensively reviewed,[32] and some of the key mechanisms that are likely to play a role in the pathogenesis of periodontitis in diabetes are shown in **Fig. 3**.

The Role of Cytokines

A large number of studies have investigated the production of various cytokines in the periodontal tissues of patients with diabetes.[32] Most studies have focused on type 2 diabetes and, despite heterogeneity among the studies, the most consistent finding has been that patients with type 2 diabetes have increased levels of IL-1β and IL-6 in the periodontal tissues compared with those with matched periodontal status but who do not have diabetes.[39–43] A possible role for TNF-α in exacerbating and prolonging the inflammatory response to periodontal bacteria has been suggested in animal models of diabetes.[44–47] However, these findings have not been consistently replicated in human studies, with no strong evidence for increased local production of TNF-α in the periodontal tissues of people with diabetes.[48–51] In one study that investigated the impact of hyperglycemia on cytokine production in the periodontal tissues, gingival crevicular fluid (GCF; a fluid exudate that flows continuously from the gingival margins, the composition of which reflects the inflammatory status of the periodontal tissues) was collected from patients with type 2 diabetes and untreated periodontitis.[52] Patients with HbA1c greater than 8% had significantly increased GCF IL-1β concentrations compared with patients with HbA1c less than 8%. Multivariate analyses identified that HbA1c and random blood glucose were independent predictors of GCF IL-1β levels, suggesting that hyperglycemia contributes to an upregulated inflammatory response in the periodontal tissues.

In a study of 39 patients with type 1 diabetes, GCF levels of IL-1β and PGE_2 were significantly higher in patients with diabetes compared with controls with similar periodontal disease status but who did not have diabetes.[53] Monocytes from the patients with type 1 diabetes also showed significantly higher secretion of PGE_2 and IL-1β in response to challenge with lipopolysaccharide (LPS) from *Escherichia coli* and *Porphyromonas gingivalis* (a key periodontal pathogen). In an experimental gingivitis study (in which volunteers abstain from oral hygiene for 3–4 weeks to permit plaque accumulation and development of gingival inflammation), those with type 1 diabetes showed a greater increase in GCF IL-1β and MMP-8 levels compared with nondiabetic controls, even though plaque accumulation was similar between the two groups.[54]

Diabetes may also result in alterations in alveolar bone homeostasis, with evidence of increased levels of RANKL in the periodontal tissues.[48,55,56] Increased RANKL/osteoprotegerin (OPG) ratios have been reported in GCF from patients with poorly controlled diabetes compared with those with either well-controlled diabetes or no diabetes.[57,58] Increased RANKL/OPG ratios, as well as increased IL-17 and IL-23 levels, have also been reported in the gingival tissues of diabetic mice compared with controls.[59,60] These studies suggest that diabetes can result in increased

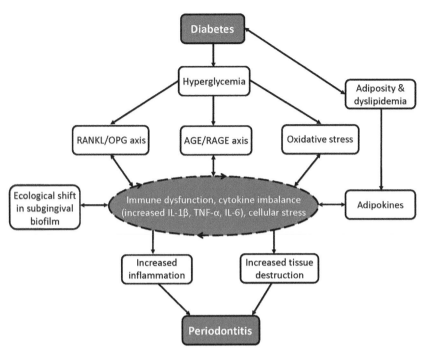

Fig. 3. Proposed mechanisms involved in the pathogenesis of periodontitis in diabetes. Hyperglycemia has multiple impacts on aspects of immune functioning, with exacerbated and dysregulated inflammatory responses being at the heart of the interactions between diabetes and periodontitis. Hyperglycemia results in the deposition of AGEs in the periodontal tissues (as well as elsewhere in the body) and binding of the receptor for AGE (RAGE) results in altered inflammatory responses and upregulated secretion of proinflammatory cytokines. Hyperglycemia also results in increased generation of ROS and a state of cellular stress resulting in further immune dysfunction. Disrupted alveolar bone homeostasis characterized by altered RANKL/OPG ratios further contributes to local tissue damage, and adipokines such as leptin also contribute to upregulated inflammatory responses. Periodontal inflammation results in alterations in the subgingival environment and an ecological shift in the subgingival microbiota, favoring more pathogenic species. A state of chronic inflammation develops, perpetuated by the subgingival microbiota and characterized by immune dysfunction and proinflammatory responses that are exacerbated by the hyperglycemic state. The net result is enhanced tissue destruction and increased progression and severity of periodontitis. Note that there is marked interindividual variation in susceptibility to periodontitis, and other risk factors such as smoking, stress, and genetic factors are highly likely to modify the mechanisms shown in the figure. OPG, osteoprotegerin; RAGE, receptor for AGEs. (*From* Taylor JJ, Preshaw PM, Lalla E. A review of the evidence for pathogenic mechanisms that may link periodontitis and diabetes. J Clin Periodontol 2013;40(Suppl 14):S129, Figure 1; with permission.)

RANKL/OPG ratios, which contribute to the exacerbated periodontal tissue breakdown observed in diabetes.

AGEs

AGEs form as a result of nonenzymatic glycosylation of structural proteins throughout the body, and their production is increased as a result of hyperglycemia in diabetes. AGEs can result in proinflammatory effects either directly or via interaction with cell-surface receptors, such as the receptor for AGE (RAGE). AGEs can be found in the periodontal tissues and may be associated with a state of enhanced oxidant stress locally,[61] and serum levels of AGE have also been shown to be associated with more advanced periodontitis in patients with type 2 diabetes.[62]

AGEs interact with RAGE to signal multiple transduction cascades and activation of proinflammatory genes, leading to chronic tissue injury and suppression of tissue repair.[63] AGEs also enhance the respiratory burst in neutrophils,[64] which potentially increases tissue damage in periodontitis. In a mouse model of diabetes and periodontitis, alveolar bone loss that resulted from inoculation with *P gingivalis* was enhanced in animals with diabetes, together with increased expression of RAGE, increased AGE deposition, and increased collagenolytic activity.[65] Using the same model, the investigators identified that blockade of RAGE using soluble RAGE resulted in a dose-dependent reduction in alveolar bone destruction, together with decreased gingival concentrations of TNF-α, IL-6, and MMPs.[44] Increased RAGE expression has also been shown in the periodontal tissues of rats with periodontitis following induction of diabetes.[66] Diabetes inducement resulted in increased expression of RAGE, TNF-α, IL-6, and RANKL, and spontaneous development of periodontitis without major changes being evident in the composition of the oral microbiota. These findings suggest that the development of spontaneous periodontitis was independent of the bacterial composition, but resulted from altered homeostasis induced by the diabetic state. Human studies have reported similar findings, with increased RAGE expression in the gingival tissues of individuals with diabetes and periodontitis.[67–69]

AGE-RAGE interactions are therefore important in the pathogenesis of periodontal disease in diabetes. AGE formation is enhanced in the periodontal tissues (as well as elsewhere in the body) as a result of hyperglycemia, and AGEs have multiple proinflammatory and prooxidant effects.[70] The proinflammatory transduction cascades that result from RAGE activation seem to contribute to the exaggerated inflammatory response and enhanced tissue breakdown that is observed in the periodontal tissues in diabetes.

Immune Functioning and Oxidative Stress

Altered immune functioning contributes to the pathogenesis of periodontitis in diabetes. Monocytic secretion of IL-1β, TNF-α, and PGE$_2$ in response to LPS has been shown to be increased in patients with type 1 diabetes.[53,71] Altered neutrophil function has also been implicated in the links between diabetes and periodontitis. For example, in patients with type 2 diabetes and periodontitis, levels of β-glucuronidase (a glycosidase enzyme that catalyzes breakdown of complex carbohydrates, and which is produced by neutrophils), and the chemokine IL-8 (a chemotactic factor for neutrophils) were reduced compared with nondiabetic controls after adjusting for periodontal status, suggesting that an inadequate local neutrophil response, possibly mediated by an altered chemokine gradient, could contribute to periodontal disease in people with diabetes.[72] Further evidence for altered gingival neutrophil function in diabetes has been provided by studies of diabetic mice in which hyperglycemia resulted in exaggerated inflammatory responses and priming of leukocytes for marginalization and superoxide production, but not for transmigration.[73,74] These findings suggest that the diabetic state could result in leukocyte defects that contribute to periodontal tissue damage by enhancing accumulation of neutrophils in the gingival tissues and tissue damage resulting from superoxide release. This suggestion is supported by studies that showed that neutrophils from patients with poorly controlled diabetes (HbA1c>7%), who also had more advanced periodontitis, released significantly more superoxide on stimulation with phorbol myristate acetate than neutrophils from patients with better controlled diabetes, or from patients who did not have diabetes.[75] Neutrophils from the patients with poorly controlled diabetes also showed increased protein kinase C (PKC) activity, suggesting that hyperglycemia can lead to priming of neutrophils characterized by increased PKC activity and superoxide release.

Production of reactive oxygen species (ROS) such as superoxide results in upregulated production of proinflammatory cytokines, for example by inducing activation of transcription factors such as nuclear factor kappa B (NF-κB) or activation of the mitogen-activated protein kinase pathway.[76] The precise role of such mechanisms in the context of diabetes and periodontitis is yet to be determined, but interactions between ROS and transcription factors that regulate osteoblast activity may result in increased bone resorption.[77] Oxidative stress has also been suggested as a common link between components of metabolic syndrome and periodontitis, with a possible role for adipokines such as leptin in modulating oxidant/antioxidant balance.[78] A potential role for leptin in modifying immune responses in diabetes is supported by evidence that leptin upregulates Toll-like receptor (TLR)-2 expression by human monocytes.[79] Expression of TLRs, particularly TLR-2, TLR-4, and TLR-9, has been reported to be higher in gingival tissue biopsies from patients with type 2 diabetes and periodontitis compared with patients with periodontitis but not diabetes.[80] Serum leptin concentrations are increased in obesity and type 2 diabetes, and therefore increased expression of TLR-2 stimulated by leptin may exacerbate inflammatory responses in these conditions.

Microbial Factors

Many investigators have attempted to determine whether the subgingival microbiota differs in people with diabetes compared with those who do not have diabetes, and whether this may explain the increased susceptibility to periodontitis associated with diabetes.[32] However, many investigations have used restricted microbiological techniques (eg, culture analyses), or have not properly controlled for periodontal status, so it is difficult to determine whether reported altered microbial profiles resulted from the diabetic state, or simply from more advanced periodontitis in the cohorts with diabetes. Studies that did account for periodontal status have not identified any meaningful differences in the periodontal microbiota between patients with or without diabetes (both type 1 diabetes and type 2 diabetes) using a variety of analytical methods including culture techniques, polymerase chain reaction, and DNA-DNA hybridization.[81–88] These findings indicate that, based on current knowledge, the presence of diabetes has no significant impact on the composition of the periodontal microbiota.

However, periodontal inflammation does influence the composition of the periodontal microbiota. In health, the subgingival biofilm is stable, in a state of homeostasis with a steady-state, low-level inflammatory response in the gingival tissues. As inflammation develops, alterations in the redox potential of the local environment and increased GCF flow favor the growth of the predominantly anaerobic pathogenic species that are associated with advanced periodontitis.[89] Thus, an ecological shift occurs in the subgingival biofilm as a result of increased periodontal inflammation, and the increased pathogenicity of the microbiota serves to perpetuate the chronic inflammatory response in the periodontal tissues. Therefore, although diabetes does not seem to directly influence the composition of the subgingival microbiota, the exacerbated periodontal inflammation associated with diabetes almost certainly does, contributing further to the chronicity of the periodontal condition.

INFLUENCE ON CLINICAL PRACTICE

Diabetes results in several complications that have significant impacts on morbidity and mortality. The cause of each complication is clearly multifactorial, but epidemiologic studies show an approximately 3-fold increased risk for periodontitis in people with diabetes. Good oral health is integral to good general health and life quality,[90] but has tended to be overlooked as a priority by health care policy makers and clinicians.[91] Management of diabetes involves aspects of patient education, self-management, and self-monitoring. Lifestyle changes are similarly important in the management of periodontitis, including patient education, smoking cessation, and optimized oral hygiene to reduce plaque levels. Improved oral hygiene by the patient together with disruption and reduction of the plaque biofilm by the clinician are the major components of periodontal therapy, with the aim being to reduce inflammation in the periodontal tissues. Structured education programs have been implemented for diabetes management,[92–94] and similar programs are also being developed for periodontitis treatment.[95,96] These programs all promote self-efficacy of patients for managing their disease, supported by the clinical team, with patient education being the key strategy for achieving lifelong behavior change.

There are therefore intriguing parallels between the therapeutic strategies that are routinely used for diabetes management and those that are used in the treatment of periodontitis. Patient education and self-efficacy are fundamental to the management of both conditions. Furthermore, given the evidence for a positive impact of periodontal treatment on glycemic control, dental screening to assess periodontal status is an important part of the management of patients with diabetes. Dental hygienists in particular are adept at instituting behavior change in their patients, and could represent an untapped source of support for diabetes health care teams in promoting healthy lifestyle messages as part of diabetes management. Closer collaboration between medical and dental health care teams would be of benefit for the management of patients with diabetes.[97]

OTHER ORAL COMPLICATIONS OF DIABETES

Several other potential oral complications of diabetes may be identified, including xerostomia, dental caries, and oral candidiasis. Furthermore, diabetes has a negative impact on the success rates for certain dental procedures such as implant placement.

Xerostomia

Dry mouth is a common complaint for patients with diabetes, and may be an early indication of the onset of diabetes. Dry mouth can result from dehydration associated with polyuria, or in long-standing cases may result from microvascular damage and/or neuropathy affecting the major salivary glands. Many commonly used medications also contribute to reduced salivary flow, such as diuretics, antidepressants, anxiolytics, and antihypertensives. Signs and symptoms of dry mouth include difficulty speaking, swallowing, and chewing, as well as dry, cracked, atrophic mucosa.[98]

Although many patients with diabetes may complain of a dry mouth, severe xerostomia is not usually a common finding. Management of dry mouth includes simple remedies (being well hydrated, taking frequent sips of water, ice chips, sugar-free gum, avoiding alcohol), that usually are sufficient to alleviate symptoms. In more advanced cases, artificial salivas may be prescribed, and liaison with the dental team is necessary to ensure that the appropriate product is used.

Dental Caries

Dental caries is not a specific complication of diabetes, but dry mouth greatly increases the risk for caries as a result of loss of the buffering and remineralizing properties of saliva and increased plaque accumulation.[98] In older patients who may have generalized gingival recession (for example, as a result of previous periodontitis), the exposed roots of the teeth are particularly susceptible to caries. Prevention is key, with a focus on oral hygiene instruction, plaque control, and fluoride therapy.

Oral Candidiasis

Candida albicans is a commensal resident of the oral cavity that may overgrow in situations of reduced salivary flow, increased salivary glucose levels, and compromised immune responses. Candidiasis is commonly found in patients with poorly controlled diabetes, particularly if dentures are worn. There are several clinical presentations of oral candidiasis. Acute pseudomembranous candidiasis is characterized by diffuse white patches that can be easily wiped off, leaving a red, raw surface, and this condition usually affects the tongue, buccal mucosa, and soft palate. Denture stomatitis (chronic erythematous candidiasis) is the most common form, associated with poorly fitting dentures and/or dentures being worn at night. Presentation varies from pinpoint erythema in the hard palate at the openings of the minor salivary glands, to generalized erythema of the denture-bearing area. Denture stomatitis is often found together with angular cheilitis, a painful condition that affects the commissures of the lips, which appear red, fissured, and sometimes ulcerated, and this is typically associated with overclosure of the mouth as a result of worn-down denture teeth.[99] Chronic hyperplastic candidiasis is another variant of candidal infections, and is linked to poor oral hygiene, trauma, smoking, denture wearing, and xerostomia. Lesions cannot be peeled off, and present with a white, rough surface with a raised red border. Biopsy is required for diagnosis, and patients require careful monitoring because this condition is considered potentially malignant.

Treatment of candidiasis involves alleviating the local factors; for example, improving oral hygiene, leaving dentures out at night, and replacing worn or ill-fitting dentures. Beyond these measures, topical antifungals such as nystatin are usually sufficient to achieve resolution. In severe cases, systemic antifungals may be indicated, such as fluconazole.

Impact of Diabetes on Implant Therapy

Titanium implants are routinely used for the replacement of missing teeth, and rely on osseointegration between the implant and the surrounding bone for long-term stability. Early studies reported high success rates for dental implants, typically greater than 95%.[100] However, more recent studies have reported less favorable outcomes, with lower implant survival rates (approximately 80% at 10–16 years), as well as a high frequency of technical (eg, implant fracture) and biologic complications (eg, periimplantitis).[101] Periimplantitis is an inflammatory condition that affects the tissues surrounding the implant, and is similar to periodontitis. Prevalence of periimplantitis is increasing rapidly; many implants have now been in situ for 10 to 20 years, and a patient's inflammatory response to plaque accumulation around an implant is likely to be similar to the inflammatory response to plaque accumulation around their natural teeth. The current estimates of prevalence of periimplantitis range from 9% to 47% according to different studies.[102–104] Several risk factors for periimplantitis have been identified, including poor oral hygiene, history of periodontitis, smoking, and diabetes.[105] Although there is less literature on the association between diabetes and periimplantitis compared with the literature linking diabetes and periodontitis, it seems from the available studies that diabetes (particularly if metabolic control is poor) does increase the risk for periimplantitis and, therefore, potentially implant failure.

Relevance of Bisphosphonate Therapy

Bisphosphonates are widely used for preventing and reducing the bone resorption that occurs in diseases such as osteoporosis and metastatic bone disorders. Diabetes is a risk factor for osteoporosis, and many patients with diabetes may be receiving bisphosphonate therapy. However, bisphosphonate-induced osteonecrosis of the jaw is a serious unwanted effect of treatment with this class of agents.[106] The condition is characterized by exposure of bone in the mandible or maxilla, which may develop spontaneously or after dental procedures such as extractions. The sites are usually painful and susceptible to infection, and surgical coverage of the exposed bone is difficult to achieve. The risk of osteonecrosis of the jaw is greater with higher doses, with intravenous administration (as opposed to oral), and after prolonged duration of therapy.[107] There is no clear evidence that patients with diabetes who are also taking bisphosphonates are at any greater risk for osteonecrosis compared with nondiabetic patients. However, given the increased risk for periodontitis and infections in general in people with diabetes, then close liaison between medical and dental teams is warranted, with an emphasis on careful monitoring and prevention of dental disease to reduce the risk of developing the condition.

SUMMARY

A large number of epidemiologic studies confirm that the risk for periodontitis is increased approximately 3-fold in people with diabetes, particularly if glycemic control is poor. Furthermore, periodontitis is associated with increased risk of macroalbuminuria, ESRD, and cardiorenal mortality (ischemic heart disease and diabetic nephropathy combined) in diabetic individuals who also have severe periodontitis, compared with diabetic individuals without severe periodontitis. The pathogenic links between the two conditions remain to be fully elucidated, but specific mediators such as IL-1β, TNF-α, and IL-6 are likely to play a key role in shared susceptibility, with emerging data supporting a role for RANKL, OPG, and the AGE-RAGE axis. Treatment of periodontitis in people with diabetes is associated with modest, but potentially clinically relevant, reductions in HbA1c, of the order of 0.4% at 3 months after treatment. Closer integration of medical and dental health care teams is warranted to improve the management of patients with diabetes and periodontitis.

REFERENCES

1. O'Dowd LK, Durham J, McCracken GI, et al. Patients' experiences of the impact of periodontal disease. J Clin Periodontol 2010;37:334–9.
2. Fox CH. New considerations in the prevalence of periodontal disease. Curr Opin Dent 1992;2:5–11.
3. White D, Pitts N, Steele JG, et al. Diseases and related disorders - a report from the Adult Dental Health Survey 2009. London: NHS Information Centre for Health and Social Care; 2011.
4. Pihlstrom BL, Michalowicz BS, Johnson NW. Periodontal diseases. Lancet 2005; 366:1809–20.
5. Grossi SG, Genco RJ, Machtei EE, et al. Assessment of risk for periodontal disease. II. Risk indicators for alveolar bone loss. J Periodontol 1995;66:23–9.

6. Kinane DF, Chestnutt IG. Smoking and periodontal disease. Crit Rev Oral Biol Med 2000;11:356–65.
7. Warnakulasuriya S, Dietrich T, Bornstein MM, et al. Oral health risks of tobacco use and effects of cessation. Int Dent J 2010;60:7–30.
8. Preshaw PM, Heasman L, Stacey F, et al. The effect of quitting smoking on chronic periodontitis. J Clin Periodontol 2005;32:869–79.
9. Mealey BL, Ocampo GL. Diabetes mellitus and periodontal disease. Periodontol 2000 2007;44:127–53.
10. Tsai C, Hayes C, Taylor GW. Glycemic control of type 2 diabetes and severe periodontal disease in the US adult population. Community Dent Oral Epidemiol 2002;30:182–92.
11. Nelson RG, Shlossman M, Budding LM, et al. Periodontal disease and NIDDM in Pima Indians. Diabetes Care 1990;13:836–40.
12. Taylor GW, Burt BA, Becker MP, et al. Glycemic control and alveolar bone loss progression in type 2 diabetes. Ann Periodontol 1998;3:30–9.
13. Emrich LJ, Shlossman M, Genco RJ. Periodontal disease in non-insulin dependent diabetes mellitus. J Periodontol 1991;62:123–31.
14. Cianciola LJ, Park PH, Bruck E, et al. Prevalence of periodontal disease in insulin-dependent mellitus (juvenile diabetes). J Am Dent Assoc 1982;104:653–60.
15. Lalla E, Cheng B, Lal S, et al. Periodontal changes in children and adolescents with diabetes: a case-control study. Diabetes Care 2006;29:295–9.
16. Lalla E, Cheng B, Lal S, et al. Diabetes mellitus promotes periodontal destruction in children. J Clin Periodontol 2007;34:294–8.
17. Bissett SM, Stone KM, Rapley T, et al. An exploratory qualitative interview study about collaboration between medicine and dentistry in relation to diabetes management. BMJ Open 2013;3. pii:e002192.
18. Loe H. Periodontal disease. The sixth complication of diabetes mellitus. Diabetes Care 1993;16:329–34.
19. Taylor GW, Burt BA, Becker MP, et al. Severe periodontitis and risk for poor glycemic control in patients with non-insulin-dependent diabetes mellitus. J Periodontol 1996;67:1085–93.
20. Shultis WA, Weil EJ, Looker HC, et al. Effect of periodontitis on overt nephropathy and end-stage renal disease in type 2 diabetes. Diabetes Care 2007;30:306–11.
21. Saremi A, Nelson RG, Tulloch-Reid M, et al. Periodontal disease and mortality in type 2 diabetes. Diabetes Care 2005;28:27–32.
22. Ide R, Hoshuyama T, Wilson D, et al. Periodontal disease and incident diabetes: a seven-year study. J Dent Res 2011;90:41–6.
23. Demmer RT, Desvarieux M, Holtfreter B, et al. Periodontal status and A1C change: longitudinal results from the Study of Health in Pomerania (SHIP). Diabetes Care 2010;33:1037–43.
24. Janket SJ, Wightman A, Baird AE, et al. Does periodontal treatment improve glycemic control in diabetic patients? A meta-analysis of intervention studies. J Dent Res 2005;84:1154–9.
25. Darre L, Vergnes JN, Gourdy P, et al. Efficacy of periodontal treatment on glycaemic control in diabetic patients: a meta-analysis of interventional studies. Diabetes Metab 2008;34:497–506.
26. Teeuw WJ, Gerdes VE, Loos BG. Effect of periodontal treatment on glycemic control of diabetic patients: a systematic review and meta-analysis. Diabetes Care 2010;33:421–7.

27. Simpson TC, Needleman I, Wild SH, et al. Treatment of periodontal disease for glycaemic control in people with diabetes. Cochrane Database Syst Rev 2010;(5):CD004714. http://dx.doi.org/10.1002/14651858.CD004714.pub2.
28. Spangler L, Reid RJ, Inge R, et al. Cross-sectional study of periodontal care and glycosylated hemoglobin in an insured population. Diabetes Care 2010;33: 1753–8.
29. Hotamisligil GS. Molecular mechanisms of insulin resistance and the role of the adipocyte. Int J Obes Relat Metab Disord 2000;24(Suppl 4):S23–7.
30. Rotter V, Nagaev I, Smith U. Interleukin-6 (IL-6) induces insulin resistance in 3T3-L1 adipocytes and is, like IL-8 and tumor necrosis factor-alpha, overexpressed in human fat cells from insulin-resistant subjects. J Biol Chem 2003; 278:45777–84.
31. Loos BG. Systemic markers of inflammation in periodontitis. J Periodontol 2005; 76:2106–15.
32. Taylor JJ, Preshaw PM, Lalla E. A review of the evidence for pathogenic mechanisms that may link periodontitis and diabetes. J Clin Periodontol 2013; 40(Suppl 14):S113–34.
33. Stratton IM, Adler AI, Neil HA, et al. Association of glycaemia with macrovascular and microvascular complications of type 2 diabetes (UKPDS 35): prospective observational study. BMJ 2000;321:405–12.
34. Preshaw PM, Taylor JJ. How has research into cytokine interactions and their role in driving immune responses impacted our understanding of periodontitis? J Clin Periodontol 2011;38(Suppl 11):60–84.
35. Kinane DF, Preshaw PM, Loos BG. Host-response: understanding the cellular and molecular mechanisms of host-microbial interactions-consensus of the Seventh European Workshop on Periodontology. J Clin Periodontol 2011; 38(Suppl 11):44–8.
36. Dandona P, Aljada A, Bandyopadhyay A. Inflammation: the link between insulin resistance, obesity and diabetes. Trends Immunol 2004;25:4–7.
37. Schmidt MI, Duncan BB, Sharrett AR, et al. Markers of inflammation and prediction of diabetes mellitus in adults (Atherosclerosis Risk in Communities study): a cohort study. Lancet 1999;353:1649–52.
38. Brownlee M. The pathobiology of diabetic complications: a unifying mechanism. Diabetes 2005;54:1615–25.
39. Duarte PM, de Oliveira MC, Tambeli CH, et al. Overexpression of interleukin-1beta and interleukin-6 may play an important role in periodontal breakdown in type 2 diabetic patients. J Periodontal Res 2007;42:377–81.
40. Kardesler L, Buduneli N, Biyikoglu B, et al. Gingival crevicular fluid PGE2, IL-1beta, t-PA, PAI-2 levels in type 2 diabetes and relationship with periodontal disease. Clin Biochem 2008;41:863–8.
41. Andriankaja OM, Barros SP, Moss K, et al. Levels of serum interleukin (IL)-6 and gingival crevicular fluid of IL-1beta and prostaglandin E(2) among non-smoking subjects with gingivitis and type 2 diabetes. J Periodontol 2009;80: 307–16.
42. Ross JH, Hardy DC, Schuyler CA, et al. Expression of periodontal interleukin-6 protein is increased across patients with neither periodontal disease nor diabetes, patients with periodontal disease alone and patients with both diseases. J Periodontal Res 2010;45:688–94.
43. Kardesler L, Buduneli N, Cetinkalp S, et al. Gingival crevicular fluid IL-6, tPA, PAI-2, albumin levels following initial periodontal treatment in chronic periodontitis patients with or without type 2 diabetes. Inflamm Res 2011;60:143–51.

44. Lalla E, Lamster IB, Feit M, et al. Blockade of RAGE suppresses periodontitis-associated bone loss in diabetic mice. J Clin Invest 2000;105:1117–24.

45. Naguib G, Al-Mashat H, Desta T, et al. Diabetes prolongs the inflammatory response to a bacterial stimulus through cytokine dysregulation. J Invest Dermatol 2004;123:87–92.

46. Graves DT, Naguib G, Lu H, et al. Inflammation is more persistent in type 1 diabetic mice. J Dent Res 2005;84:324–8.

47. Watanabe K, Petro BJ, Shlimon AE, et al. Effect of periodontitis on insulin resistance and the onset of type 2 diabetes mellitus in Zucker diabetic fatty rats. J Periodontol 2008;79:1208–16.

48. Duarte PM, Neto JB, Casati MZ, et al. Diabetes modulates gene expression in the gingival tissues of patients with chronic periodontitis. Oral Dis 2007;13: 594–9.

49. Navarro-Sanchez AB, Faria-Almeida R, Bascones-Martinez A. Effect of non-surgical periodontal therapy on clinical and immunological response and glycaemic control in type 2 diabetic patients with moderate periodontitis. J Clin Periodontol 2007;34:835–43.

50. Santos VR, Ribeiro FV, Lima JA, et al. Cytokine levels in sites of chronic periodontitis of poorly controlled and well-controlled type 2 diabetic subjects. J Clin Periodontol 2010;37:1049–58.

51. Santos VR, Ribeiro FV, Lima JA, et al. Partial- and full-mouth scaling and root planing in type 2 diabetic subjects: a 12-mo follow-up of clinical parameters and levels of cytokines and osteoclastogenesis-related factors. J Periodontal Res 2012;47:45–54.

52. Engebretson SP, Hey-Hadavi J, Ehrhardt FJ, et al. Gingival crevicular fluid levels of interleukin-1b and glycemic control in patients with chronic periodontitis and type 2 diabetes. J Periodontol 2004;75:1203–8.

53. Salvi GE, Yalda B, Collins JG, et al. Inflammatory mediator response as a potential risk marker for periodontal diseases in insulin-dependent diabetes mellitus patients. J Periodontol 1997;68:127–35.

54. Salvi GE, Franco LM, Braun TM, et al. Pro-inflammatory biomarkers during experimental gingivitis in patients with type 1 diabetes mellitus: a proof-of-concept study. J Clin Periodontol 2010;37:9–16.

55. Mahamed DA, Marleau A, Alnaeeli M, et al. G(-) anaerobes-reactive CD4+ T-cells trigger RANKL-mediated enhanced alveolar bone loss in diabetic NOD mice. Diabetes 2005;54:1477–86.

56. Lappin DF, Eapen B, Robertson D, et al. Markers of bone destruction and formation and periodontitis in type 1 diabetes mellitus. J Clin Periodontol 2009;36: 634–41.

57. Santos VR, Lima JA, Goncalves TE, et al. Receptor activator of nuclear factor-kappa B ligand/osteoprotegerin ratio in sites of chronic periodontitis of subjects with poorly and well-controlled type 2 diabetes. J Periodontol 2010;81: 1455–65.

58. Vieira Ribeiro F, de Mendonca AC, Santos VR, et al. Cytokines and bone-related factors in systemically healthy patients with chronic periodontitis and patients with type 2 diabetes and chronic periodontitis. J Periodontol 2011; 82:1187–96.

59. Silva JA, Ferrucci DL, Peroni LA, et al. Sequential IL-23 and IL-17 and increased Mmp8 and Mmp14 expression characterize the progression of an experimental model of periodontal disease in type 1 diabetes. J Cell Physiol 2012;227:2441–50.

60. Silva JA, Lopes Ferrucci D, Peroni LA, et al. Periodontal disease-associated compensatory expression of osteoprotegerin is lost in type 1 diabetes mellitus and correlates with alveolar bone destruction by regulating osteoclastogenesis. Cells Tissues Organs 2012;196:137–50.

61. Schmidt AM, Weidman E, Lalla E, et al. Advanced glycation endproducts (AGEs) induce oxidant stress in the gingiva: a potential mechanism underlying accelerated periodontal disease associated with diabetes. J Periodontal Res 1996;31:508–15.

62. Takeda M, Ojima M, Yoshioka H, et al. Relationship of serum advanced glycation end products with deterioration of periodontitis in type 2 diabetes patients. J Periodontol 2006;77:15–20.

63. Yan SF, Ramasamy R, Schmidt AM. Receptor for AGE (RAGE) and its ligands-cast into leading roles in diabetes and the inflammatory response. J Mol Med 2009;87:235–47.

64. Wong RK, Pettit AI, Quinn PA, et al. Advanced glycation end products stimulate an enhanced neutrophil respiratory burst mediated through the activation of cytosolic phospholipase A2 and generation of arachidonic acid. Circulation 2003;108:1858–64.

65. Lalla E, Lamster IB, Feit M, et al. A murine model of accelerated periodontal disease in diabetes. J Periodontal Res 1998;33:387–99.

66. Claudino M, Gennaro G, Cestari TM, et al. Spontaneous periodontitis development in diabetic rats involves an unrestricted expression of inflammatory cytokines and tissue destructive factors in the absence of major changes in commensal oral microbiota. Exp Diabetes Res 2012;2012:356841.

67. Katz J, Bhattacharyya I, Farkhondeh-Kish F, et al. Expression of the receptor of advanced glycation end products in gingival tissues of type 2 diabetes patients with chronic periodontal disease: a study utilizing immunohistochemistry and RT-PCR. J Clin Periodontol 2005;32:40–4.

68. Abbass MM, Korany NS, Salama AH, et al. The relationship between receptor for advanced glycation end products expression and the severity of periodontal disease in the gingiva of diabetic and non diabetic periodontitis patients. Arch Oral Biol 2012;57:1342–54.

69. Yu S, Li H, Ma Y, et al. Matrix metalloproteinase-1 of gingival fibroblasts influenced by advanced glycation end products (AGEs) and their association with receptor for AGEs and nuclear factor-kB in gingival connective tissue. J Periodontol 2012;83:119–26.

70. Giacco F, Brownlee M. Oxidative stress and diabetic complications. Circ Res 2010;107:1058–70.

71. Salvi GE, Collins JG, Yalda B, et al. Monocytic TNF-a secretion patterns in IDDM patients with periodontal diseases. J Clin Periodontol 1997;24:8–16.

72. Engebretson SP, Vossughi F, Hey-Hadavi J, et al. The influence of diabetes on gingival crevicular fluid beta-glucuronidase and interleukin-8. J Clin Periodontol 2006;33:784–90.

73. Gyurko R, Siqueira CC, Caldon N, et al. Chronic hyperglycemia predisposes to exaggerated inflammatory response and leukocyte dysfunction in Akita mice. J Immunol 2006;177:7250–6.

74. Sima C, Rhourida K, Van Dyke TE, et al. Type 1 diabetes predisposes to enhanced gingival leukocyte margination and macromolecule extravasation in vivo. J Periodontal Res 2010;45:748–56.

75. Karima M, Kantarci A, Ohira T, et al. Enhanced superoxide release and elevated protein kinase C activity in neutrophils from diabetic patients: association with periodontitis. J Leukoc Biol 2005;78:862–70.

76. Graves DT, Kayal RA. Diabetic complications and dysregulated innate immunity. Front Biosci 2008;13:1227–39.

77. Galli C, Passeri G, Macaluso GM. FoxOs, Wnts and oxidative stress-induced bone loss: new players in the periodontitis arena? J Periodontal Res 2011;46: 397–406.

78. Bullon P, Morillo JM, Ramirez-Tortosa MC, et al. Metabolic syndrome and periodontitis: is oxidative stress a common link? J Dent Res 2009;88:503–18.

79. Jaedicke KM, Roythorne A, Padget K, et al. Leptin up-regulates TLR2 in human monocytes. J Leukoc Biol 2013;93:561–71.

80. Rojo-Botello NR, Garcia-Hernandez AL, Moreno-Fierros L. Expression of toll-like receptors 2, 4 and 9 is increased in gingival tissue from patients with type 2 diabetes and chronic periodontitis. J Periodontal Res 2012;47:62–73.

81. Sastrowijoto SH, Hillemans P, van Steenbergen TJ, et al. Periodontal condition and microbiology of healthy and diseased periodontal pockets in type 1 diabetes mellitus patients. J Clin Periodontol 1989;16:316–22.

82. Tervonen T, Oliver RC, Wolff LF, et al. Prevalence of periodontal pathogens with varying metabolic control of diabetes mellitus. J Clin Periodontol 1994;21:375–9.

83. Pinducciu G, Micheletti L, Piras V, et al. Periodontal disease, oral microbial flora and salivary antibacterial factors in diabetes mellitus type 1 patients. Eur J Epidemiol 1996;12:631–6.

84. Sbordone L, Ramaglia L, Barone A, et al. Periodontal status and subgingival microbiota of insulin-dependent juvenile diabetics: a 3-year longitudinal study. J Periodontol 1998;69:120–8.

85. Yuan K, Chang CJ, Hsu PC, et al. Detection of putative periodontal pathogens in non-insulin-dependent diabetes mellitus and non-diabetes mellitus by polymerase chain reaction. J Periodontal Res 2001;36:18–24.

86. Lalla E, Kaplan S, Chang SM, et al. Periodontal infection profiles in type 1 diabetes. J Clin Periodontol 2006;33:855–62.

87. da Cruz GA, de Toledo S, Sallum EA, et al. Clinical and laboratory evaluations of non-surgical periodontal treatment in subjects with diabetes mellitus. J Periodontol 2008;79:1150–7.

88. Ebersole JL, Holt SC, Hansard R, et al. Microbiologic and immunologic characteristics of periodontal disease in Hispanic Americans with type 2 diabetes. J Periodontol 2008;79:637–46.

89. Marsh PD. Microbial ecology of dental plaque and its significance in health and disease. Adv Dent Res 1994;8:263–71.

90. US Department of Health and Human Services. Oral health in America: a report of the Surgeon General. Rockville (MD): US Department of Health and Human Services, National Institute of Dental and Craniofacial Research, National Institutes of Health; 2000.

91. Oral health: prevention is key. Lancet 2009;373:1.

92. Deakin TA, Cade JE, Williams R, et al. Structured patient education: the diabetes X-PERT programme makes a difference. Diabet Med 2006;23:944–54.

93. Davies MJ, Heller S, Khunti K, et al. The DESMOND educational intervention. Chronic Illn 2008;4:38–40.

94. Gillett M, Dallosso HM, Dixon S, et al. Delivering the Diabetes Education and Self Management for Ongoing and Newly Diagnosed (DESMOND) programme

for people with newly diagnosed type 2 diabetes: cost effectiveness analysis. BMJ 2010;341:c4093.

95. Jonsson B, Ohrn K, Oscarson N, et al. The effectiveness of an individually tailored oral health educational programme on oral hygiene behaviour in patients with periodontal disease: a blinded randomized-controlled clinical trial (one-year follow-up). J Clin Periodontol 2009;36:1025–34.

96. Jonsson B, Ohrn K, Oscarson N, et al. An individually tailored treatment programme for improved oral hygiene: introduction of a new course of action in health education for patients with periodontitis. Int J Dent Hyg 2009;7:166–75.

97. Preshaw PM, Alba AL, Herrera D, et al. Periodontitis and diabetes: a two-way relationship. Diabetologia 2012;55:21–31.

98. Felix DH, Luker J, Scully C. Oral medicine: 4. Dry mouth and disorders of salivation. Dent Update 2012;39:738–43.

99. Felix DH, Luker J, Scully C. Oral medicine: 7. Red and pigmented lesions. Dent Update 2013;40:231–8.

100. Naert I, Koutsikakis G, Duyck J, et al. Biologic outcome of single-implant restorations as tooth replacements: a long-term follow-up study. Clin Implant Dent Relat Res 2000;2:209–18.

101. Simonis P, Dufour T, Tenenbaum H. Long-term implant survival and success: a 10-16-year follow-up of non-submerged dental implants. Clin Oral Implants Res 2010;21:772–7.

102. Ferreira SD, Silva GL, Cortelli JR, et al. Prevalence and risk variables for peri-implant disease in Brazilian subjects. J Clin Periodontol 2006;33:929–35.

103. Koldsland OC, Scheie AA, Aass AM. Prevalence of peri-implantitis related to severity of the disease with different degrees of bone loss. J Periodontol 2010;81:231–8.

104. Tomasi C, Derks J. Clinical research of peri-implant diseases - quality of reporting, case definitions and methods to study incidence, prevalence and risk factors of peri-implant diseases. J Clin Periodontol 2012;39(Suppl 12):207–23.

105. Lindhe J, Meyle J, Group D of European Workshop on Periodontology. Peri-implant diseases: consensus report of the Sixth European Workshop on Periodontology. J Clin Periodontol 2008;35:282–5.

106. Marx RE, Sawatari Y, Fortin M, et al. Bisphosphonate-induced exposed bone (osteonecrosis/osteopetrosis) of the jaws: risk factors, recognition, prevention, and treatment. J Oral Maxillofac Surg 2005;63:1567–75.

107. Otomo-Corgel J. Osteoporosis and osteopenia: implications for periodontal and implant therapy. Periodontol 2000 2012;59:111–39.

Dermatologic Manifestations of Diabetes Mellitus: A Review

Blair Murphy-Chutorian, BA, MSIV[a], George Han, MD, PhD[b],
Steven R. Cohen, MD, MPH[c],*

KEYWORDS

- Diabetes mellitus • Bullosa diabeticorum • Necrobiosis lipoidica diabeticorum
- Granuloma annulare • Diabetic scleredema • Acanthosis nigricans • Yellow skin
- Periungual erythema

KEY POINTS

- Primer on dermatologic conditions that may serve as markers of impaired glucose metabolism, emphasizing their role in the early identification and management of diabetes mellitus.
- Understand the epidemiology, pathogenesis and treatment of diabetes-associated skin disorders.

INTRODUCTION

Diabetes mellitus is a heterogeneous group of disorders associated with abnormal carbohydrate metabolism. Diabetes affects an estimated 26 million people in the United States, including an estimated 7 million undiagnosed cases.[1] The epidemic is rapidly growing and has been projected to double by 2050.[2] Worldwide, the prevalence of diabetes is approximately 350 million.[3]

Complications of diabetes are the result of metabolic, hormonal, environmental, and genetic factors, manifesting in every organ system. According to various studies, 30% to 91% of diabetic patients experience at least 1 dermatologic complication.[4–6] The numerous cutaneous manifestations of diabetes range widely in severity (from mundane cosmetic concerns to life threatening), in prevalence (relatively common to rare), and in treatment response (responsive to refractory). Many skin manifestations disproportionately affect patients with type 1 or type 2 diabetes mellitus (**Table 1**).

Certain skin manifestations, considered specific cutaneous markers, should prompt studies of glucose metabolism because the risk of diabetes mellitus is high; other

[a] University of California, Irvine, Irvine, CA 92697, USA; [b] Albert Einstein College of Medicine, Bronx, NY 10461, USA; [c] Division of Dermatology, Albert Einstein College of Medicine, Montefiore Medical Center, 111 East 210th Street, Bronx, NY 10467, USA
* Corresponding author.
E-mail address: steven.cohen@einstein.yu.edu

Endocrinol Metab Clin N Am 42 (2013) 869–898
http://dx.doi.org/10.1016/j.ecl.2013.07.004
0889-8529/13/$ – see front matter © 2013 Elsevier Inc. All rights reserved.

Table 1
Skin manifestations demonstrating a disproportionately increased association among 1 of the 2 major types of diabetes

Type 1 Diabetes Mellitus	Type 2 Diabetes Mellitus
Necrobiosis lipoidica diabeticorum	Generalized granuloma annulare
Diabetic bullae	Scleredema diabeticorum
Vitiligo vulgaris	Diabetic dermopathy
Periungual telangiectasia	Acanthosis nigricans
	Acrochordons
	Psoriasis
	Yellow skin and nails

markers are nonspecific for diabetes but are more prevalent among diabetic patients than the general population. Skin findings may be the first sign of a metabolic disturbance caused by undiagnosed diabetes, suboptimal management of known disease, or even a prediabetic state. Skin complications of diabetes can provide clues to current and past metabolic status. Recognition of cutaneous markers enables earlier diagnosis and treatment, which may slow disease progression and ultimately improve the overall prognosis.

This review explores the acute and chronic dermatologic manifestations of diabetes according to the following categories: (1) specific cutaneous markers; (2) nonspecific skin conditions associated with diabetes (**Table 2**); and (3) other dermatologic considerations in the diabetic patient, including complications, primary skin disease associations, infections, and reactions to therapy. The focus is on clinical and histologic presentations, epidemiology, causes, and treatment options.

SPECIFIC CUTANEOUS MARKERS OF DIABETES MELLITUS
Necrobiosis Lipoidica Diabeticorum

Necrobiosis lipoidica (NL) is a chronic, necrotizing, granulomatous skin disease that occurs primarily in individuals with diabetes. It is one of the most disfiguring, disabling, and refractory cutaneous complications of diabetes.[7] NL lesions begin as small, firm, erythematous papules that gradually evolve and enlarge. Typical lesions are well-demarcated, indurated, annular plaques that contain characteristic yellow-brown atrophic centers studded with prominent ectatic vessels, and delimited by narrow, granulomatous, reddish-brown, or violaceous margins (**Fig. 1**). Solitary or

Table 2
Dermatologic manifestations of diabetes by category

Specific Cutaneous Markers	Nonspecific Conditions
Necrobiosis lipoidica	Acrochordons
Generalized granuloma annulare	Yellow skin and nails
Diabetic bullae	Generalized pruritus
Scleredema diabeticorum	Thick skin
Acanthosis nigricans	Rubiosis faciei
Eruptive xanthomatosis	Palmar erythema
Acquired perforating dermatoses	Nailbed erythema
Diabetic dermopathy	Pigmented purpuric dermatoses

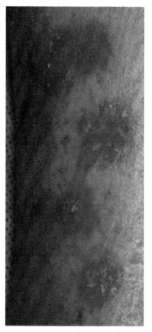

Fig. 1. Necrobiosis lipoidica diabeticorum on the pretibial leg.

multiple lesions are most commonly distributed bilaterally on the lower extremities, particularly the pretibial areas, but may occur on the face, trunk, and upper extremities as well. Distinctive necrobiosis surrounded by palisading granulomas are seen on histopathology.[8]

Although only a small proportion (0.3%–1.6%) of diabetic patients develop NL, it has long been believed that most patients with NL meet criteria for diabetes at some point in their lives.[9,10] In the 1966 seminal study of Muller and Winkelmann,[11] 60% of 171 subjects with NL were found to be diabetic, and another 20% were either glucose intolerant or reported at least 1 parent with diabetes. A strong correlation is consistently reported between NL and diabetes mellitus, although to what degree this association exists has become less clear. A retrospective review in 1999 found only 22% of 65 patients with NL to have or develop diabetes over a 15-year period.[12] Future investigations of a large sample biopsy-proven NL cases are necessary to clarify the relationship.

Diabetes precedes the onset of NL by a mean of 10 years,[9] but can develop concurrently with or later than NL. Therefore, patients with NL with normal glucose metabolism should be closely monitored over time for diabetes or insulin resistance.[10] NL in the setting of diabetes is called necrobiosis lipoidica diabeticorum (NLD).

NLD can be asymptomatic or painful and/or pruritic, especially when ulcerated. The sensation of involved skin is often reduced. The reduced innervation of NL lesions raises the possibility that local inflammation causes nerve damage and sensory loss.[13] Ulceration occurs in approximately 35% of lesions, either spontaneously or secondary to trauma.[14,15] Ulcerative lesions may be complicated by secondary infection and, rarely, by development of squamous cell carcinoma.

NLD occurs more frequently in type 1 diabetes but is associated with both types.[7] There is a female predominance (75%–80% of cases) with typical onset in the third to fourth decades of life.[4,14,16] Shall and colleagues[9] found NLD occurred significantly earlier in insulin-dependent patients (mean 22 years) compared with the non–insulin-dependent group (mean 49 years).

The cause of NLD is unknown. Vasculopathy, collagen alterations, immune complex deposition, and inflammatory mechanisms have all been implicated in the pathogenesis of NLD, and may each play a role.[17] Ngo and colleagues[18] challenged the theory that diabetic vascular disease with resulting ischemia was the main causal factor by demonstrating increased blood flow in NLD, including chronic lesions. The investigators suggest that significant evidence points to an inflammatory process, such as an antibody-mediated vasculitis, as a central cause of NLD.

The association between NL and glycemic control is unclear.[19] Until future studies clarify the relationship, tighter glucose control in NLD management is recommended. Treatment of NL is well recognized as problematic and challenging. Responses to therapy vary widely and refractory cases are the rule. There is no satisfactory universal approach to treatment. Topical and intralesional steroids, calcineurin inhibitors, compression therapy, and psoralen with ultraviolet A (PUVA) are the most frequently used modalities.[14]

There are seemingly endless reports describing successful treatments for NLD in isolated cases or case series, including. antithrombotics and platelet inhibitors (pentoxyfilline, dipyridamole, acetylsalicylic acid), heparin, topical tretinoin, topical tacrolimus, cyclosporine, systemic glucocorticoid, ticlopidine, nicotinamide, clofazimine, mycophenalate mofetil, fumaric acid esters, antimalarials, local excision with skin grafting, compression, photodynamic therapy, and CO_2 laser therapy.[7,8,15,20–31] In addition, topical granulocyte colony-stimulating factor,[32] intralesional tumor necrosis factor (TNF)-alpha inhibitors (infliximab[33] and etanercept[27]), intravenous infliximab,[22,34] and systemic colchicine[35] have demonstrated efficacy in severe refractory cases of ulcerative NL.

No single drug has shown consistent efficacy, and regardless of the modality, NL lesions tend to relapse on cessation of therapy. Without intervention, spontaneous resolution is observed in about 13% to 19% of cases of NL after 6 to 12 years.[10] Healing with persistent scarring, atrophy, and disfigurement is customary.[21] The physical and emotional toll of NLD all too frequently translates as disability and decreased quality of life.[20]

Generalized Granuloma Annulare

Granuloma annulare (GA) is a rare, necrobiotic, inflammatory disorder of unknown cause. Five clinical variants of GA include localized, subcutaneous, perforating, generalized, and arcuate dermal erythema forms. The association between GA and diabetes has been controversial because so many studies have combined data from all clinical variants. It is now accepted that only the generalized form shows consistent and significant correlation with diabetes across most studies.[36–38] Like NLD, the prevalence of GA among diabetics is only 0.3%; however, 21% to 77% of patients with generalized GA have diabetes (predominantly type 2 diabetes).[36,37] All other variants of GA, including the most common, localized GA, are not associated with diabetes.[10,39,40]

Generalized GA initially appears as multiple, small, firm, skin-colored or red dermal papules that tend to be symmetrically distributed on the distal extremities and sun-exposed areas of the trunk.[39,41] Individual lesions gradually expand and centrally involute, forming annular rings with raised borders (**Fig. 2**). The resemblance to NLD is striking but GA lacks epidermal atrophy and yellow discoloration.[42] The eruption is typically asymptomatic but can be pruritic. It is curious that up to 33% of cases of

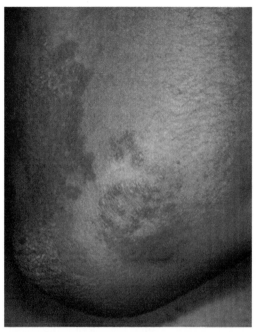

Fig. 2. Generalized granuloma annulare with involvement of upper and lower extremities bilaterally.

generalized GA are atypical presentations with nonannular, mostly coalescing papules.[43]

Generalized GA is twice as common among women and occurs at any age with an approximate mean of 50 years.[43,44] Postulated to be an immunologic disorder, GA is most likely a type IV delayed hypersensitivity reaction.[36,45] Prolonged exposure to high glucose levels may contribute to the development of generalized GA.[39,44]

The histopathology shows lymphohistiocytic granulomatous inflammation of the dermis and collagen degeneration. Colloidal iron stain reveals abundant deposition of mucin. The presence of mucin and the absence of increased plasma cells helps to histologically distinguish GA from NL.

Unlike localized disease, the course of generalized GA is often protracted and seldom resolves spontaneously. Diabetic patients in particular suffer persistent and relapsing courses, with poor long-term outcomes.[36] Although there are no standard treatment guidelines, first-line options comprise ultraviolet A-1 (UVA-1), oral psoralen (8-methoxypsoralen) and PUVA, systemic retinoids, and dapsone. By comparison, second-line therapies rely mostly on anecdotal reports and small case series that include photodynamic therapy, cryotherapy, topical, intralesional, and systemic corticosteroids, chlorambucil, pentoxifylline, antimalarials, cyclosporine, fumaric esters, potassium iodide, niacinamide, etanercept, infliximab, adalimumab, and efalizumab.[36,40,46,47] New cases of generalized GA should be screened for diabetes.

Diabetic Bullae

Diabetic bullae (DB), or bullosa diabeticorum, is a rare, noninflammatory, bullous disorder characterized by tense, painless, bullae that develop abruptly on normal-appearing skin, typically on the distal lower extremities, and less often involving the hand or forearm (**Fig. 3**).[48,49] Acute episodes are likely to occur during sleep and without preceding trauma. The blisters evolve rapidly (as quickly as 15 minutes has been reported[50]) and may become more flaccid, and sometimes uncomfortable, as they enlarge. Solitary or multiple blisters range from a few millimeters to several centimeters in diameter filled with clear, sterile, serous fluid unless complicated by secondary hemorrhage or infection.[51,52]

By definition, all patients with DB have diabetes mellitus, most commonly insulin-dependent; however the low frequency of 0.5% among diabetics may be higher than reported.[50,52] DB is most often encountered in the setting of long-standing, type 1 diabetes with late complications, such as neuropathy, nephropathy, and retinopathy.[50,53–55] DB has been described in type 2 diabetes as well. The predilection for men is reportedly 2:1. The age of onset averages 50 to 70 years, but DB has been documented in teenagers to people in their eighth decade. One study found 29 of 35 (83%) DB eruptions were correlated with highly varying blood glucose levels.[50]

Despite the poorly understood cause of DB, numerous mechanisms have been proposed, including minor trauma-induced blister formation, hypoglycemia or highly fluctuating blood glucose levels, microangiopathy, neuropathy, alterations in calcium or magnesium metabolism, UV exposure, an autoimmune phenomenon, and vascular insufficiency. None provides an adequate explanation.[40,50,53,54]

There are no specific tests for DB. The diagnosis is based on characteristic findings, clinical course, and the exclusion of other bullous disorders, such as drug eruption, immunobullous disease, and porphyria cutanea tarda. The index of suspicion should be high in the setting of negative direct immunofluorescence testing and the absence of urinary uroporphyrins. Histologic examination may aid diagnosis in certain cases.[48,50]

The microscopic findings in DB reveal 2 major groups with different levels of cleavage, suggesting different stages of development or even separate pathogenetic mechanisms.[53] The first and most common group shows intraepidermal or subepidermal cleavage at the level of the lamina lucida, without acantholysis. These lesions usually resolve spontaneously without scarring and reepithelialize early. By contrast, in the second type, cleavage is below the dermoepidermal junction with destruction of anchoring fibrils.[46,53] This type heals with scarring and atrophy.

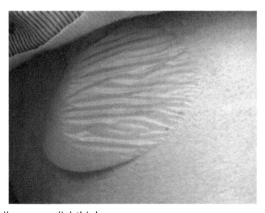

Fig. 3. Diabetic bullae on medial thigh.

Although most DB heal in 2 to 6 weeks without treatment, the course is not always smooth.[53] Secondary infection or ulceration, particularly associated with blisters on the foot, may lead to osteomyelitis, large areas of necrosis and scarring, as well as toe amputation. Healing may be as long as 2 years.[50] Surprisingly, peripheral perfusion tends to be adequate for healing, despite the occurrence of DB in diabetic patients with other late complications.[50] Even with complete resolution of DB, bullae frequently recur.[48]

Treatment of DB is focused on skin protection and preventing secondary infection. Immediate regulation of the blood glucose level has been recommended as a result of the finding that hypoglycemic episodes often precede eruptions. Uncomplicated blisters should be left intact, but sterile aspiration of fluid may prevent rupture in some cases. Ulcerated blisters should be treated with aggressive wound management.[50,53]

Scleredema Diabeticorum

Scleredema diabeticorum, or diabetic scleredema, is a rare chronic connective tissue disorder primarily associated with type 2 diabetes. The condition is characterized by impressive thickening of the reticular dermis affecting the posterior neck, upper back, and shoulders with occasional extension to the face, arms, chest, or abdomen (**Figs. 4** and **5**).[56,57] The involved skin is hard, thick, and indurated, sometimes erythematous, and may have a peau d'orange appearance (**Fig. 6**). Scleredema diabeticorum is usually asymptomatic, but pain and decreased mobility (especially of the back) may be present in severe cases. It is noteworthy that acral skin is always spared.

The prevalence of scleredema ranges from 2.5% to 14% of all diabetic patients.[56,58,59] It is most likely to develop in adults with long-standing diabetes and with poor glycemic control, occurring 10 times more frequently in men.[60]

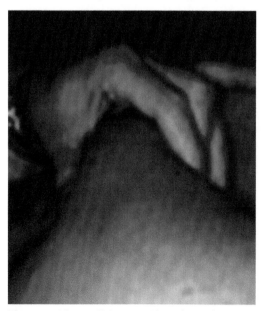

Fig. 4. A 40-year-old man without diabetes with soft easily compressible skin of the shoulder (unaffected).

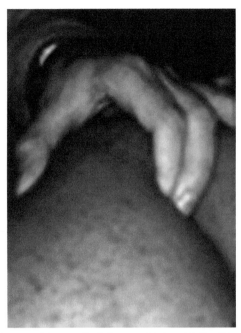

Fig. 5. A 41-year-old man with type 2 diabetes with hard inflexible skin of the shoulder, characteristic of scleredema diabeticorum.

Unequivocal diagnosis of scleredema by histologic examination requires a full thickness excisional biopsy to examine the dermis. The microscopic findings reveal a markedly thickened reticular dermis, thick collagen bundles, and mild infiltrate of mucin in the deeper dermis. Both edema and sclerosis are notably absent.[56] The diagnosis is usually based on history and physical examination.

Scleredema diabeticorum should not be confused with scleredema of Buschke or with systemic scleroderma.[56,61] Despite the similarities between the 2 names, scleredema and scleroderma are unrelated. Scleredema of Buschke and scleredema diabeticorum are frequently used interchangeably in the literature, but these disorders represent 2 distinct subtypes of scleredema. Although the clinical presentations are indistinguishable, scleredema of Buschke occurs in children after a viral or bacterial upper respiratory infection and self-resolves in months.

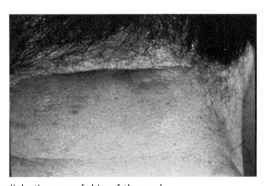

Fig. 6. Scleredema diabeticorum of skin of the neck.

There is no highly effective treatment for scleredema diabeticorum. PUVA seems most effective but other recommended therapies include strict glycemic control with an insulin pump, potent topical and intralesional steroids, penicillamine, intralesional insulin, low-dose methotrexate, prostaglandin E1, and pentoxifylline.[57,62,63] Scleredema incidentally improved in a patient treated with allopurinol for acquired reactive perforating collagenosis.[64] The combination of PUVA and physical therapy may help with mobility in patients with severe diabetic scleredema.[57] Although strict glycemic control does not show consistent therapeutic benefit in scleredema diabeticorum, it is proposed to be an effective preventive measure.

Acanthosis Nigricans

Acanthosis nigricans (AN) is characterized by diffuse, hyperpigmented, light brown to black, velvety to verrucous thickening of intertriginous and flexural areas of the body, particularly in the axilla, groin, and posterior neck (**Fig. 7**). These papillomatous plaques are poorly marginated and cause accentuation of skin markings. As a rule, AN is asymptomatic, but it may be painful, malodorous, or macerated in rare cases.[46] It occurs in all ethnicities, but disproportionately affects Native Americans, nonwhite Hispanics, and African Americans.[65] There are 2 forms of AN, benign and malignant, which share a similar clinical and histologic presentation. Unlike the benign variant, malignant AN is not associated with diabetes. Malignant AN, a rare paraneoplastic syndrome, is associated with an underlying carcinoma, most commonly adenocarcinoma of the stomach.[66,67]

Considered a marker of insulin resistance, benign AN characteristically occurs in the setting of type 2 diabetes mellitus and obesity.[10,16] In a frequently quoted study, 74% of an obese population had AN along with increased plasma insulin levels.[68] Benign AN is also associated with other endocrine abnormalities involving insulin resistance, including polycystic ovarian syndrome, lipodystrophy, acromegaly, Cushing syndrome, Addison disease, thyroid disease, and leprechaunism.[69] Nicotinic acid and other drugs are associated with benign AN, although the exact mechanism is unknown.[46] In addition, AN has been reported as a rare, local, cutaneous side effect of repeated exogenous insulin injections. It is generally accepted that injection site AN is caused by local hyperinsulinemia. Rotating injection sites may help to prevent or reverse the reaction.[70]

The histology of AN shows marked hyperkeratosis, epidermal papillomatosis, and slight, variable acanthosis.[69] There is no change in melanocyte count or melanin content. The hyperpigmentation observed mainly results from a thickened keratin-containing epithelium.[70,71] Diagnosis of AN is usually clinical and warrants screening

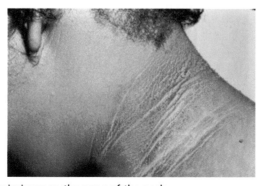

Fig. 7. Acanthosis nigricans on the nape of the neck.

for diabetes and insulin resistance. New onset of AN should prompt an evaluation for underlying malignancy.[72]

ANs is a chronic but reversible condition. Management focuses on treating the underlying cause; skin lesions are mostly of cosmetic concern. In the diabetic patient, weight control, dietary restrictions, and increased physical activity are of primary importance and have been proved to be most effective in controlling AN.[73] Lifestyle modifications may be augmented by various pharmacologic approaches to improve insulin sensitivity and reduce hyperinsulinemia. By contrast, purely dermatologic therapies that do not target hyperinsulinemia are of transient benefit at best. Nonetheless, topical keratolytics (eg, salicylic acid, retinoic acid, and ammonium lactate) and oral isotretinoin can reduce thicker plaques in areas of maceration, decreasing odor and discomfort.[46]

Diabetic Dermopathy

Diabetic dermopathy, also called shin spots or pigmented pretibial patches, is seen in 40% to 50% of diabetic patients.[46,74,75] It is characterized by the eruption of multiple asymptomatic, round, dull red to pink papules or plaques predominantly on the pretibial skin bilaterally but also occurring on the forearms, thighs, and lateral malleoli. Early lesions may be mistaken for dermatophytosis (**Fig. 8**).[76] One to 2 weeks after they appear, these lesions evolve to well-circumscribed, atrophic, brown macules often with fine scale (**Fig. 9**).[77] New lesions may emerge and older ones resolve spontaneously leaving slightly depressed, hyperpigmented areas. It is a dynamic process with lesions of varied stages present at the same time. Shin spots may occasionally be complicated by ulceration.

Diabetic dermopathy is a clinical diagnosis. Because the histopathology is relatively nonspecific, skin biopsy is best avoided. The microscopic findings in new lesions

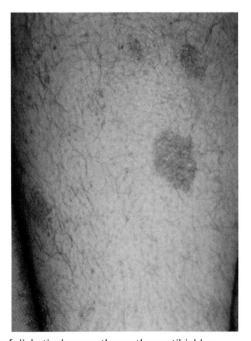

Fig. 8. Early lesions of diabetic dermopathy on the pretibial leg.

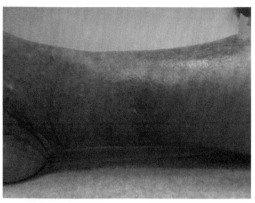

Fig. 9. Pigmented purpura with features of chronic diabetic dermopathy.

show edema of the epidermis and papillary dermis with a mild perivascular lymphohistiocytic infiltrate and hemorrhage. Older lesions feature epidermal atrophy with thickened blood vessels in the papillary dermis, no edema, and scattered hemosiderin deposits. An increase in diastase-resistant material staining positive with periodic acid-Schiff is present in the vessel walls.

Diabetic dermopathy is most commonly identified in diabetic men more than 50 years of age, especially among those with long-standing diabetes and poor glycemic control.[78] Up to 70% of diabetic men aged 60 years and older reportedly have dermopathy[16]; and many of these patients suffer from neuropathy, nephropathy, and retinopathy.[75,79] Dermopathy can also precede the onset of diabetes. Correlations between dermopathy and duration of diabetes or glycemic control have not been found.[80]

The cause of shin spots is unknown. Attempts to explain the pathogenesis have centered on trauma and on microangiopathy with associated capillary changes; however, the literature abounds with evidence to both support and refute these potential factors.[75,77,78,81] Whether dermopathy is specific for diabetes remains controversial.[78,80] It is generally agreed that 4 or more shin spots increase the probability that diabetes is present, warranting an evaluation.[82]

No medical intervention is necessary aside from prevention of secondary infection. Management should address microangiopathic complications and coronary artery disease, because of their association with diabetic dermopathy.[80]

Acquired Perforating Dermatoses

Acquired perforating dermatoses (APD) comprise a group of chronic skin disorders defined histologically by transepidermal perforation and elimination of a connective tissue component of the dermis.[83] Historically, this disorder was classified by the predominant dermal material identified microscopically (such as keratin, collagen, or elastic tissue); hence, the terminology reactive perforating collagenosis, elastosis perforans serpiginosa (EPS), as well as perforating folliculitis and Kyrle disease (**Fig. 10**). The APD group is almost exclusively associated with chronic renal failure, diabetes, and/or hemodialysis (often related to diabetic nephropathy). The skin lesions are highly pruritic, follicular, hyperkeratotic nodules and papules with a central keratin plug that may be described as umbilicated. The eruption is found primarily on the extremities

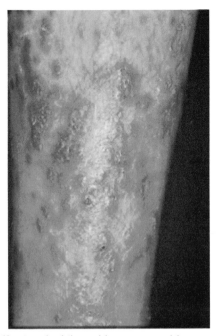

Fig. 10. Kyrle disease affecting the bilateral lower extremities.

and trunk, less often on the head. The papules of EPS are distributed in a distinctive serpiginous pattern. APD undergoes Koebnerization (the development of lesions at sites of trauma) and is typically exacerbated by excoriation.[84] The differential diagnosis of APD includes prurigo nodularis, folliculitis, arthropod bites, multiple keratoacanthomas, psoriasis, and lichen planus.[85]

In a review of 22 patients with APD, Saray and colleagues[86] found almost 73% had chronic renal failure and were on hemodialysis, and 50% had diabetes (91% of the patients with diabetes had chronic renal failure secondary to diabetic nephropathy). Yet, 13.6% of the patients were otherwise in good general health. APD has been associated with other extracutaneous diseases that include but are not limited to malignancy, hepatic disorders, hypothyroidism, AIDS, tuberculosis, atopic dermatitis, and scabies.[83,86]

The pathogenesis is poorly understood. It remains unknown whether the primary abnormality occurs in the dermis or epidermis, and whether the pruritus is an underlying cause or a resultant effect of the skin condition. Proposed theories include (1) metabolic derangements causing an epidermal or dermal alteration; (2) a deposition of some substance not removed by dialysis, which the immune system then perceives as foreign; and (3) microtrauma secondary to scratching or a manifestation of microangiopathy.[83,86–88]

APD in the setting of diabetes is relatively unresponsive to therapy. By avoiding trauma to the area, lesions may resolve slowly. Therefore, symptomatic relief of pruritus is a core treatment strategy. Varying beneficial effects are reported with topical keratolytics, topical and systemic retinoids, allopurinol, PUVA, UVB phototherapy, topical and intralesional corticosteroids, antibiotics (doxycycline), oral antihistamine, cryotherapy, and renal transplantation.[10,83,88,89] Dialysis does not improve the course of the disease.

Eruptive Xanthomatosis

Eruptive xanthomas are uncommon and virtually pathognomonic of hypertriglyceride-mia.[90] They arise suddenly in groups of multiple yellow papules, 1 to 4 mm in diameter, mainly on the extensor surfaces of the extremities and on the buttocks (**Fig. 11**). Eruptive xanthomas often arise as a Koebner phenomenon on pressure points. The papules are surrounded by erythematous halos at their base and may be tender or pruritic.[10] The histopathology shows an accumulation of lipid-laden histiocytic foam cells with a mixed infiltrate of lymphocytes and neutrophils in the dermis.

Approximately one-third of all diabetic patients have serum lipoprotein abnormalities caused by insulinopenia, but the prevalence of xanthomatosis among this population is unclear.[90] The reason for the increased frequency of eruptive xanthomatosis among individuals with diabetes has been well characterized. Because insulin is a stimulating factor critical to the normal activity of lipoprotein lipase, it plays an important role in the metabolism of serum triglycerides and triglyceride-rich lipoproteins. The insulin-deficient state of uncontrolled insulin-dependent diabetes results in the absence of lipoprotein lipase activity.[39] Consequently, the impaired clearance of very-low-density lipoproteins (VLDLs) and chylomicrons leads to a hyperlipemic syndrome, which, if severe enough, can precipitate eruptive xanthomas. Diabetic hyperlipidemia may be accelerated by polyphagia caused by glycosuria.[10,90]

As with so many of the specific cutaneous markers of diabetes, recognizing xanthomatosis may be an essential clue to deteriorating metabolic status. Thus, it cannot be overemphasized that early identification of xanthomatosis can facilitate timely treatment and possible avoidance of more serious manifestations of hyperlipidemia such as atherosclerotic complications and pancreatitis.[91] The diagnosis of eruptive xanthomatosis should prompt further investigation and treatment of hyperglycemia.[92] Xanthomatosis resolves with control of carbohydrate and lipid metabolism, therefore the diabetic patient typically requires just optimized insulin therapy. Statins or fibrates can supplement treatment as tolerated.[93]

NONSPECIFIC SKIN CONDITIONS ASSOCIATED WITH DIABETES
Acrochordons (Skin Tags)

Skin tags are soft fibromas that are particularly common in people with diabetes. These benign, asymptomatic, exophytic growths are observed on the eyelids, neck, axilla, and other skin folds. They may be flesh-colored or, less often, hyperpigmented, and can range from small papules to pedunculated polyps, typically 1 to 6 mm in diameter, with smooth or irregular surfaces.[94–97] There is a slight female predilection, and prevalence increases with age.[39] Although characteristically asymptomatic, skin tags

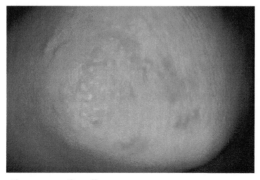

Fig. 11. Eruptive xanthomas on the elbow.

contain nerve cells and therefore may cause discomfort if irritated. Histologic features include a papillarylike dermis consisting of loose collagen fibers and supporting vasculature. The epidermis and dermis are both involved to varying degrees.[39]

Approximately 66% to 75% of patients with skin tags have frank diabetes[46] and more than 80% show impaired carbohydrate metabolism.[95] The association between diabetes and skin tags is likely related to the proliferative effect of hyperinsulinemia on keratinocytes and fibroblasts, similar to the pathogenesis of ANs. Skin tags have also been associated with colonic polyps[98] and human papillomavirus (HPV). One study found HPV DNA in 88% of skin tags.[99]

Data regarding the total number of skin tags per individual and the associated risk of diabetes is controversial.[95,97,100] In a case-control study, researchers observed a positive correlation between the incidence of diabetes or impaired glucose tolerance and the total number of skin tags,[100] however previous studies failed to find such a correlation.[95,97] The discrepancy may be accounted for by differences in the study method. For example, it is possible that a correlation exists only between a very high number of skin tags and diabetes risk. Demir and Demir[95] examined individuals with a lower mean total number of lesions. Of 120 individuals enrolled, 41% had 1 to 3 skin tags and only 31% had 10 or more. In contrast, Rasi and colleagues[100] only included individuals with a minimum of 3 skin tags, and 86.8% of the 104 case subjects had 10 or more skin tags (25.7% had 30+ skin tags). Future studies may help to determine whether there is indeed a statistically significant correlation between number of skin tags and impaired carbohydrate metabolism. Rasi and colleagues[100] found a significantly higher incidence of impaired carbohydrate metabolism in individuals with more than 30 skin tags (52%) than in those with fewer than 30 tags (27.3%).

The only correlation found between anatomic location of skin tags and impaired carbohydrate metabolism was the finding of increased risk of diabetes in inframammary skin tags in women. Treatment of skin tags is medically unnecessary, but cosmetic concerns may be addressed with snip biopsy, laser excision, cryotherapy, or electrodesiccation.[101]

Yellow Skin and Nails

Yellowish skin and nails are described with increased frequency among individuals with diabetes compared with the general population. This finding is asymptomatic and considered benign, but the exact cause has not been elucidated. Carotenoderma has traditionally been proposed as a possible cause, but supporting evidence is weak. Diabetic patients do not have increased levels of serum carotenoids (carotenemia) as previously reported,[102] and the levels of carotenoid in diabetic skin have not actually been reported in the literature. The best explanation for diabetic yellow skin is likely a discoloration caused by certain end products associated with nonenzymatic glycosylation of dermal collagen. One of these end products, 2-(2-furoyl)-4[5]-(2-furanyl)-1H-imidazole, is known to have a characteristic yellow hue.[102] Nonenzymatic glycosylation of proteins occurs only to a minor extent in nondiabetics, but it is stimulated by the hyperglycemic state in diabetes. Many of the skin manifestations of diabetes may be attributable to the glycosylation of proteins. Future biochemical analysis of diabetic skin could lead to better understanding of its yellow hue.

The increased frequency of yellow nails among diabetic patients may be at least partially attributable to an increased prevalence of onychomycosis.

Generalized Pruritus

It is widely accepted that pruritus occurs with a much higher frequency among patients with diabetes than the general population. Poor microcirculation and hypohidrosis causing xerosis were proposed as explanations. A 1986 study by Neilly and colleagues[103] investigated pruritus in diabetes by comparing 300 diabetics and 100 nondiabetic controls. Pruritus vulvae in women was the only type of localized pruritus seen more frequently in patients with diabetes. Although generalized pruritus was found to be more common among people with diabetes than a control population, most cases tended to involve an underlying illness or likely drug reaction that could better explain the itching. Otherwise, cases of generalized pruritus without such an explanation were not significantly more common among diabetics versus controls.[103] Pruritus vulvae is most frequently caused by an infectious process, particularly *Candida*. Therefore, exogenous diabetic drug therapy and pathogens may explain the increased frequency of pruritus in diabetes.[92]

Rubeosis Faciei

Rubeosis faciei has long been described as a common manifestation of diabetes mellitus. The condition is characterized by a chronically flushed face and neck. It tends to be more easily appreciated in Fitzpatrick skin types 1 and 2 because increased melanin can obscure the coloration. The reddish complexion is believed to result from microangiopathic alterations and superficial facial venous dilatation.[104]

The prevalence of rubeosis is unclear and may not be as high as previously believed, or the condition may have become less common.[105] Many review articles from the past several decades have republished data from an Israeli study that found 36 of 61 (59%) hospitalized patients with diabetes had "markedly red faces" and another 21% had "slightly red faces."[106] The only recent data on the prevalence of rubeosis are found in studies that investigated the prevalence of all cutaneous manifestations in individuals with diabetes. All these studies yielded results markedly less than 59%. In Saudi Arabia (2011)[5] and in Pakistan (2005),[6] rubeosis was observed in 3.1% and 7.1% of diabetic outpatients, respectively. Similarly, in 2007, Pavlovic and colleagues[105] reported cutaneous manifestations in 212 young (aged 2–22 years), insulin-dependent, diabetic outpatients in Serbia. Rubeosis faciei was seen in about 7% of cases, compared with none of the nondiabetic controls.

It remains to be determined whether severity of disease, inpatient status, Fitzpatrick skin type, or some other confounding factor can explain the discrepancy in the prevalence of rubeosis among diabetic patients between Gitelson and Wertheimer-Kaplinski[106] and the other studies. Gitelson and Wertheimer-Kaplinski[106] examined hospitalized patients, whereas the other studies enrolled outpatients, and none of the studies (each from different regions of the world) reported Fitzpatrick skin type.

Although rubeosis is a benign condition, it may serve as a clue to the more menacing internal processes of microangiopathy secondary to suboptimal glycemic control. Therefore, thorough patient evaluation for serious complications such as retinopathy is warranted. Treatment of rubeosis faciei is strict diabetic control and avoidance of alcohol, caffeine, and other vasodilators.

Palmar Erythema

Palmar erythema (PE) is believed to be a microvascular complication of both types 1 and 2 diabetes mellitus. This condition is a symmetric, asymptomatic, slightly warm erythema most frequently limited to the thenar and hypothenar eminences. This form of PE differs from normal physiologic mottling that involves the entire palm elicited by factors such as atmospheric temperature, emotional state, elevation of the hand, and pressure on the palm. Although similar to the palmar erythema associated with pregnancy (prevalence >30%), rheumatoid arthritis (prevalence >60%), hepatic disease, thyrotoxicosis, nutritional protein deficiency, smoking, chronic mercury poisoning, drug reactions, and neoplasms of the central nervous system,[107] it differs markedly from the more distal papular erythema of the palms and fingers of systemic lupus erythematosus.[108] The prevalence of PE among diabetic patients does not seem to have been reported in North America, but 2 observational studies in Pakistan have estimated the prevalence of palmar erythema at approximately 4%.[6,109] Like rubeosis faciei and yellow skin, diabetic PE is benign yet may signify an underlying process that calls for therapy.

Nailbed Erythema

Erythema of the proximal nailfold is another reddish color change seen in diabetic skin, and it has been attributed to dilatation of the superficial vascular plexus presenting as periungual telangiectasias (visibly dilated capillaries around the nail bed). Although classically associated with scleroderma and dermatomyositis, periungual telangiectasias are frequently observed among diabetic patients, again representing underlying diabetic microangiopathy.[110]

In 1960, Landau[111] investigated the nailbed vessels of 75 diabetic patients (>40 years of age) using a microscope with a slit lamp, and found that congestion at the venous end of nailbed capillaries was much more common in diabetes compared with healthy controls (65% vs 12%). The periungual capillaries of diabetic patients with this isolated venous portion congestion differs morphologically from those changes seen in connective tissue diseases, where the capillary loops are markedly blunted and attenuated.[110] Although it is usually asymptomatic, nailbed erythema in diabetic patients often presents with associated cuticle changes and tenderness of the fingertip. Nailbed erythema should not be confused with paronychia, which is caused by bacterial or fungal infection.

Pigmented Purpura

Pigmented purpura coexists with diabetic dermopathy (pigmented pretibial patches, shin spots) in about 50% of cases.[112] Pigmented purpura, also called pigmented purpuric dermatoses, is a heterogeneous group of uncommon, idiopathic, progressive skin conditions causing patches of orange to brown, nonblanching pigmentation speckled with 0.3 to 1.0 cm so-called cayenne pepper spots. These asymptomatic lesions are distributed mainly over the lower extremities, especially the pretibial leg (see **Fig. 9**), with occasional involvement of the ankles and dorsa of the feet,[110,112] and are caused by erythrocyte extravasation from the superficial venous plexus.[112] The deposition of hemosiderin released from red blood cells is responsible for the characteristic color. Pigmented purpura occurs most commonly in elderly diabetic patients, often precipitated by congestive heart failure and, therefore, presenting with lower extremity edema.[110] Of the 6 recognized clinical variants of pigmented purpura, the most common is progressive pigmented dermatosis or Schamberg disease.[113] In the absence of diabetic dermopathy, pigmented purpura is not considered a marker for diabetes.

OTHER DERMATOLOGIC CONSIDERATIONS IN THE DIABETIC PATIENT
Skin Manifestations of Diabetic Vascular Disease

Diabetes mellitus causes both large and small blood vessel disease. Atherosclerosis of vessels in diabetic patients often leads to ischemic changes of the lower extremities that result in classic findings: shiny, hairless, atrophic skin with cold toes and dystrophic nails, pallor on elevation, and mottling on dependence.[39] Large vessel disease contributes to poor wound healing and the frequency and recurrence of cutaneous infections in persons with diabetes, causing increased risk of gangrene and amputation.

Skin Manifestations of Diabetic Neuropathy

The neuropathic manifestations of diabetes can result in changes that affect the skin. Hypohidrosis or anhidrosis can occur as a result of autonomic neuropathy. These changes in perspiration usually affect the lower extremities. They can lead to severe xerosis as well as fissuring of the skin, which provides a portal of entry for pathogens.[92] Vascular dilatation can also result from autonomic neuropathy, manifesting as increased skin temperature and erythema.

Peripheral neuropathy is a common complication of diabetes. Loss of cutaneous sensation usually begins at the distal extremities, especially the fingers and toes. Such sensory deficits often predispose to injury, which is especially dangerous in the diabetic patient with vascular compromise and impaired healing. Chronic foot ulcers (mal perforans) often result from this combination of diabetic complications.

Skin Conditions of the Hands

Multiple skin conditions affecting the hands are seen more commonly among individuals with diabetes than among the general population. These include limited joint mobility, thick dorsal hand skin and finger pebbles, and Dupuytren contracture. Although it is possible for a patient to experience each of these 3 conditions, even concomitantly, they are considered distinct entities.

Limited joint mobility

Limited joint mobility (LJM), or diabetic cheiroarthropathy, has long been recognized as a common finding in diabetes.[114,115] Patients with LJM classically present with mildly restricted extension of the metacarpophalangeal and interphalangeal joints that generally begins with fifth finger involvement and spreads radially.[116–118] The condition is caused by thickening of periarticular connective tissue causing stiffness.[118] The prevalence of LJM in patients with diabetes is estimated to be between 30% and 40%.[116,119–122] In 2013, Rosenbloom[114] demonstrated that, over a 16-year period, LJM was associated with a nearly 4-fold increased risk of microvascular disease. Clearly this physical finding is a warning sign. Long-term diabetic control was positively correlated with LJM such that every unit increase in mean glycated hemoglobin imparted a significant increased risk of development of LJM.

Thick dorsal hand skin and finger pebbles

Nearly one-third of 309 diabetic patients found to have LJM in the study by Rosenbloom and colleagues[122] also had thick, tight, waxy skin of their dorsal hands that could not be tented on examination. Biopsies of the dermis showed marked thickening with accumulated connective tissue. Subsequent studies supported a significant correlation of thick skin with diabetes, and moderate to severe LJM with microvascular complications.[117,122,123] The relationship between thick skin and LJM is somewhat unclear; both can present independently.

A variant of thick skin manifests clinically as finger pebbles, also called pebbling or Huntley papules. These are easily recognizable, multiple, grouped, indurated, noninflammatory micropapules distributed over the extensor surfaces of the fingers and periungual region.[124] Finger papules are most prevalent in type 2 diabetes, and have been reported to affect approximately 75% of diabetics versus 12% of nondiabetic controls.[124,125] Although typically asymptomatic, finger pebbles may be associated with severe dryness and occasional pruritus. For these cases, 12% ammonium lactate reportedly provides some relief. Finger pebbles tend not to respond to topical steroids or moisturizers.[126]

Studies have shown that collagen in the skin of diabetic patients is often less soluble than the collagen of nondiabetic controls and has more ketoamine-linked glucose bound to it.[127,128] The accumulation of collagen is believed to play a major role in the pathogenesis of diabetic thick skin. Two leading theories propose explanations for the abnormal collagen build-up. Hyperglycemic states may promote nonenzymatic glycosylation of collagen, thereby causing increased cross-linking of collagen fibers, which renders the fibers resistant to collagenase degradation and results in abnormal collagen accumulation in tissue.[118,129] The other theory implicates the proliferative effect of excess insulin on collagen.[58] Tight glycemic control seems to aid resolution and prevention of thick skin.[130]

Earlier literature described LJM, diabetic scleredema, and scleredema of Buschke as synonyms. Several investigators have clarified that the 3 are not the same.[61,115]

Dupuytren contracture

Dupuytren contracture (DC), or Dupuytren disease, is a chronic and progressive fibro-proliferative disorder of palmar fascia characterized by nodules of the ventral hand that evolve to cords and fixed flexion contractures, as well as palmar skin tethering caused by shortening of skin-anchoring ligaments (**Fig. 12**).[131–133] DC is estimated to affect approximately 20% of diabetic patients; the prevalence increases with age.[121] Among patients with DC, 13% to 39% have diabetes.[134,135] The pathogenesis of diabetic DC is poorly understood, and DC seems to be independent of glycemic control.[132,136–138]

Digital sclerosis

The finding of LJM in conjunction with thick, waxy, dorsal hand skin is called digital sclerosis. Rosenbloom and Frias[139] described these findings (plus short stature) in association with insulin-dependent diabetes in 1974. A series of investigations that followed led to naming this constellation of findings Rosenbloom syndrome. Much of the literature since that time separates LJM and thick dorsal hand skin as distinct conditions, because they often do not present simultaneously.

Thick Skin

Three distinct forms of thick skin have been identified in diabetes: (1) thick waxy skin of the dorsal hand, (2) scleredema diabeticorum, and (3) subclinical, generalized, thicker-than-average skin. The first 2 have been described earlier. The third type of thick skin of diabetes is believed to be benign and is common. It is asymptomatic and usually goes unnoticed, but is apparent on ultrasonographic measurement of skin

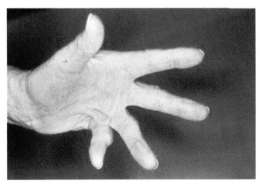

Fig. 12. Dupuytren contracture.

thickness.[140] The thickened skin may occur anywhere on the body, but the skin of the hands and feet are most commonly affected. It is unclear whether the 3 forms of thick skin share a common pathogenesis.

SELECTED CUTANEOUS DISORDERS ASSOCIATED WITH DIABETES
Psoriasis

Psoriasis is a relatively common chronic inflammatory skin disease with systemic manifestations. The worldwide prevalence of psoriasis is estimated to be 1% to 3%.[141] Inflammatory pathways and genetic susceptibility seem to be at the core of the pathologic mechanism. Many risk factors have been associated with psoriasis, including smoking, hypertension, obesity, and insulin resistance.[142] The condition is more frequent and severe in obese patients.[143]

Patients with psoriasis are believed to have a 1.5 times increased risk of developing diabetes compared with the general population, and patients with severe psoriasis may have twice the risk.[144] When adjusted for covariates, Li and colleagues[145] found psoriasis to be associated with an increased risk of type 2 diabetes among patients with psoriasis less than 60 years old.

Psoriasis and type 2 diabetes are independently known to be mediated by many major risk factors in common, such as high body mass index and smoking. Past epidemiologic studies and basic science research provide evidence of some possible links between psoriasis and type 2 diabetes: common immune-mediated inflammatory processes (specifically involving inflammatory cytokines such as interleukin [IL]-6 and TNF), an involvement of leptin and adiponectin, and environmental factors such as smoking.[145,146] The human major histocompatibility (MHC) genomic region at chromosomal position 6p21 has been associated with both psoriasis and diabetes (among 100+ other diseases).[147] Whether this contributes to the pathogenesis of diabetes and/or psoriasis is unclear.

Vitiligo

Vitiligo is an acquired, chronic, depigmenting disorder of the skin characterized by well-demarcated, achromic macules of selectively destroyed melanocytes. The exact cause of vitiligo is still debated, but either a loss of cutaneous melanocytes or a loss of melanocyte function is believed to occur, and this likely involves cell-mediated autoimmunity.[148,149] An estimated 0.1%–2.0% of people worldwide are affected with vitiligo. Dawber[150] observed that patients with type 1 diabetes were significantly more likely to have vitiligo compared with those with type 2 diabetes (3.6% vs 0.4%) and compared with the general population.[151]

CUTANEOUS INFECTIONS

Skin infections are common in those with diabetes mellitus, especially type 2 diabetes. The impaired microcirculation, sensory and autonomic neuropathy, acid-base imbalances, and impaired immune response of diabetes mellitus and its complications predispose diabetic patients to bacterial and fungal infections of the skin that may run an unusually prolonged or recurrent course. Many studies have shown the incidence of cutaneous infections is higher in people with diabetes than in the general population, and that the incidence of infection correlates with mean blood glucose levels.[4,81,152,153] Skin infections may even be the presenting feature of diabetes. The best preventive measure for all skin infections in diabetes is optimal glycemic control beginning as early as possible.

Bacterial

Staphylococcal and β-hemolytic streptococcal infections

The most common bacterial infections in diabetic patients are staphylococcal and β-hemolytic streptococcal infections, causing impetigo, erysipelas, folliculitis, carbuncles, furuncles, styes, and ecthyma.[153] Bacterial infections of the diabetic skin can progress to gangrene and even necrotizing fasciitis, a life-threatening dermatologic emergency. Depending on the severity of the infection, oral or intravenous antibiotics and diabetic control are standards of care. Tissue debridement and aggressive wound care may be required in severe cases.

Corynebacterium minutissimum

Erythrasma is a chronic superficial infection of *Corynebacterium minutissimum* and has an increased prevalence among diabetic patients, especially among obese diabetics. *C minutissimum* occurs as normal skin flora in the general population. It is believed that the increased susceptibility of diabetic patients to *C minutissimum* infection is caused by the ability of these bacteria to ferment glucose. Erythrasma presents as well-demarcated brown to red patches with fine scale, typically distributed over the inner thighs, scrotum, crural area, and fourth web space of the toes. It tends to be asymptomatic but may be pruritic. Under a Wood lamp (UV-A light), erythrasma shows a coral-red fluorescence due to the production of porphyrin by *C minutissimum*. This finding effectively distinguishes erythrasma from *Staphylococcus* intertrigo infection, which often appears identical under room light. Bacterial culture of erythrasma is known to be difficult and is not necessary for diagnosis.

Pseudomonas aeruginosa

Pseudomonas infections of the toe web spaces and colonization of the toenails are more common in diabetes than among the general population. Green discoloration may be visible under the toenail and green fluorescence can be observed under a Wood lamp. Topical antibiotics, or oral ciprofloxacin for more advanced cases, are standard therapy for these superficial infections.

Malignant otitis externa caused by *Pseudomonas aeruginosa* is a rare life-threatening skin infection of the external auditory canal that occurs most frequently in elderly patients with diabetes and is associated with high morbidity and mortality. The infection initially develops as a cellulitis that can progress to chondritis, osteomyelitis, and cerebritis.[4,154] Urgent diagnosis and treatment are essential. Antipseudomonal antibiotic therapy and necrotic tissue debridement should be initiated promptly.[154]

Fungal

Candidiasis (Moniliasis)

Recurrent candidal infections are frequently the presenting manifestation of diabetes. Patients with diabetes are believed to be particularly susceptible to *Candida* because increased glucose concentrations permit the organism to thrive. Candidal infections are often seen in the setting of diabetes include angular stomatitis (classically in young diabetic patients), paronychia of the nailfold, erosio interdigitale blastomycetica (infection of the web space between the third and fourth fingers), thrush, and intertrigo of the skinfolds. Common female-specific candidal skin infections include pruritus vulvae (often accompanying vulvovaginitis) and inframammary infection. Although much less common than female-specific infections, the male-specific infections, balanitis, balanoposthitis, and phimosis, may be an early sign of diabetes in men.[4] The pathogens most frequently implicated include *Candida albicans* and *Candida parapsilosis*.

Candidal infections should be managed with glycemic control and topical antifungals (such as nystatin, clotrimazole, and econazole) or oral fluconazole for more severe or refractory cases.

Dermatophytosis

The dermatophytes are a group of 3 genera of fungi (*Trichophyton*, *Microsporum*, and *Epidermophyton*) that cause hair, skin, and nail infections. Dermatophyte infections of the skin are most frequently caused by *Trichophyton rubrum*. Tinea pedis (dermatophytosis of the foot) is the most prevalent of these infections among both diabetic patients and the general population. Although studies show an increased prevalence of candidal infections among patients with diabetes, the data on dermatophytosis in diabetes is less clear.[155] Obesity poses an additional risk factor for dermatophyte infection of the skin, particularly of the skin folds.[94] Treatment depends on location and severity, and includes topical and systemic antifungals. Treatment of superimposed bacterial infections may be required as well.

Onychomycosis

Onychomycosis, or fungal infection of the nail, is common in diabetes, most often caused by *Candida* or *Trichophyton*. Signs of onychomychosis include yellow discoloration, subungual hyperkeratosis, distal onycholysis, and nail dystrophy (**Fig. 13**). Among 550 diabetic patients, Gupta and colleagues[152] found evidence of fungal infection in 26% versus 6.8% of nondiabetic controls. Onychomycosis has been reported in 50% of patients with type 2 diabetes.[156] The risk of onychomycosis increases with age and with male sex.[152] Nail infections are especially dangerous because they can provide a portal of entry for secondary bacterial infection at the most distal parts of the body, which are exceedingly susceptible to poor wound healing in individuals with diabetes. Patients should be educated about the importance of proper foot and nail care for prevention.

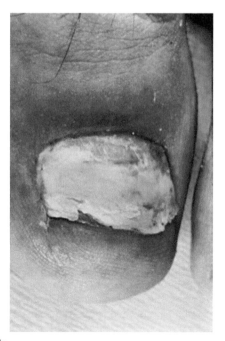

Fig. 13. Onychomycosis.

Mucormycosis

Mucormycosis is a rare life-threatening opportunistic fungal infection that occurs with increased frequency among diabetic patients. The infection is usually caused by *Rhizopus* species, or less often *Mucor* species of Zygomycetes. Typical presenting symptoms include facial or ocular pain and nasal congestion, sometimes with malaise and/or fever. Uncontrolled diabetes, especially with diabetic ketoacidosis, greatly increases the risk of mucormycosis.[157,158] It is believed that the combination of increased availability of glucose, decreased serum pH, and increased expression of host receptors that mediate epithelial cell invasion by *Rhizopus*, enables *Rhizopus* spp. to thrive.[158] Cutaneous mucormycosis begins as a cellulitis that progresses to necrosis. It occurs by introduction of the fungi through abraded skin. The infection causes tissue necrosis, infarction, and thrombosis as hyphae invade blood vessels, and is inevitably fatal without intervention.[157]

Blastomycosis

Blastomycosis, caused by *Blastomyces dermatitidis*, is another noncontagious opportunistic fungal infection that disproportionately affects patients with diabetes. It is endemic to the midwest United States and northwestern Ontario. Lung and skin involvement are most common. Infection usually occurs by inhalation of spores or, less often, by skin contact with spores. Initial symptoms include dry cough, fever, fatigue, and general malaise. Cutaneous presentations of blastomycosis vary, but small crusted pustules that rupture and ulcerate or form nonhealing abscesses are typical. Diagnosis can be achieved through identification of the organism by direct microscopy, culture, histopathology, or serologic tests. Without treatment, blastomycosis eventually causes death. Oral itraconazole or ketoconazole and intravenous amphotericin B are first-line therapies depending on severity.

Increased suspicion for the rare but urgent and life-threatening cutaneous infections of diabetes (mucormycosis, necrotizing fasciitis, and malignant otitis externa) is essential.

CUTANEOUS REACTIONS TO DIABETIC TREATMENT
Insulin

The advent of recombinant insulin preparations has largely done away with once common insulin allergies.[10] Insulin allergy is now seen in less than 1% of patients injecting insulin. Delayed hypersensitivity reactions have been the most common type of allergic reaction, but immediate-local, generalized, and biphasic reactions have also occurred. Treatment options for insulin allergies include antihistamines, the addition of steroid to insulin, desensitization therapy, rotating the injection site, or discontinuation of therapy. Anaphylaxis is extremely rare in insulin allergy.

Lipoatrophy, lipohypertrophy, or a combination of both may occur at the site of insulin injection. The exact cause of lipoatrophy is unknown, but lipohypertrophy may be caused by the lipogenic action of insulin and is best prevented by rotation of injection site.

Oral Hypoglycemic Agents

It is estimated that 1% to 5% of patients treated with a first-generation sulfonylurea, such as chlorpropamide or tolbutamide, experience a cutaneous reaction (most often a maculopapular eruption) within the first 2 months of therapy. Discontinuation usually leads to prompt resolution of the rash. Chlorpropamide causes an alcohol flush reaction, characterized by generalized warmth, erythema, headache, and tachycardia, in 10% to 30% of patients beginning about 15 minutes after consumption of alcohol and lasting for an hour. Susceptibility to this reaction may be inherited autosomal dominantly.[10]

The most common cutaneous reactions to second-generation sulfonylureas, such as glipizide (Glucotrol) and glimepiride (Amaryl), include photosensitivity, urticaria, and pruritus. Metformin (Glucophage) has been reported to cause a psoriasiform drug eruption, erythema multiforme, and leukocytoclastic vasculitis.

SUMMARY

The wide range of dermatologic conditions related to impaired glucose metabolism is important across multiple medical specialties to identify undiagnosed diabetes as early as possible and to better manage patients with known disease. Despite numerous investigations, the exact causes of many cutaneous complications of diabetes remain elusive, due in part to inherent challenges of research in diabetes, a heterogeneous group of conditions affecting patients of widely ranging demographics and often with multiple comorbidities. Much of the data has come from outdated studies and small case series. There have also been off-cited figures pertaining to diabetic skin manifestations for which no primary source seems to exist.

Better understanding of the underlying disease mechanisms, perhaps through advanced biochemical analyses and large-scale studies, could enable more tailored therapies leading to improved treatment outcomes in diabetes. Continued efforts to educate patients and encourage healthy lifestyles are of foremost importance in halting the epidemic of diabetes mellitus and its complications.

REFERENCES

1. Centers for Disease Control and Prevention. In: US Department of Health and Human Services, editor. National diabetes fact sheet: national estimates and general information on diabetes and prediabetes in the United States. Atlanta (GA): Centers for Disease Control and Prevention; 2011.
2. Boyle JP, Thompson TJ, Gregg EW, et al. Projection of the year 2050 burden of diabetes in the US adult population: dynamic modeling of incidence, mortality, and prediabetes prevalence. Popul Health Metr 2010;8:29.
3. Danaei G, Finucane MM, Lu Y, et al, Global Burden of Metabolic Risk Factors of Chronic Diseases Collaborating, Group. National, regional, and global trends in fasting plasma glucose and diabetes prevalence since 1980: systematic analysis of health examination surveys and epidemiological studies with 370 country-years and 2.7 million participants. Lancet 2011;378:31–40.
4. Perez MI, Kohn SR. Cutaneous manifestations of diabetes mellitus. J Am Acad Dermatol 1994;30:519–31 [quiz: 532–4].
5. Shahzad M, Al Robaee A, Al Shobaili HA, et al. Skin manifestations in diabetic patients attending a diabetic clinic in the Qassim region, Saudi Arabia. Med Princ Pract 2011;20:137–41.
6. Mahmood T, Bari A, Agha H. Cutaneous manifestations of diabetes mellitus. Journal of Pakistan Association of Dermatologists 2005;15:227–32.
7. Boyd AS. Tretinoin treatment of necrobiosis lipoidica diabeticorum. Diabetes Care 1999;22:1753–4.
8. Petzelbauer P, Wolff K, Tappeiner G. Necrobiosis lipoidica: treatment with systemic corticosteroids. Br J Dermatol 1992;126:542–5.
9. Shall L, Millard L, Stevens A, et al. Necrobiosis lipoidica: 'the footprint not the footstep'. Br J Dermatol 1990;123:47.

10. Ferringer T, Miller F 3rd. Cutaneous manifestations of diabetes mellitus. Dermatol Clin 2002;20:483–92.
11. Muller SA, Winkelmann RK. Necrobiosis lipoidica diabeticorum. A clinical and pathological investigation of 171 cases. Arch Dermatol 1966;93:272–81.
12. O'Toole EA, Kennedy U, Nolan JJ, et al. Necrobiosis lipoidica: only a minority of patients have diabetes mellitus. Br J Dermatol 1999;140:283–6.
13. Boulton AJ, Cutfield RG, Abouganem D, et al. Necrobiosis lipoidica diabeticorum: a clinicopathologic study. J Am Acad Dermatol 1988;18:530–7.
14. Erfurt-Berge C, Seitz AT, Rehse C, et al. Update on clinical and laboratory features in necrobiosis lipoidica: a retrospective multicentre study of 52 patients. Eur J Dermatol 2012;22:770–5.
15. Suarez-Amor O, Perez-Bustillo A, Ruiz-Gonzalez I, et al. Necrobiosis lipoidica therapy with biologicals: an ulcerated case responding to etanercept and a review of the literature. Dermatology 2010;221:117–21.
16. Sibbald RG, Landolt SJ, Toth D. Skin and diabetes. Endocrinol Metab Clin North Am 1996;25:463–72.
17. Souza AD, El-Azhary RA, Gibson LE. Does pancreas transplant in diabetic patients affect the evolution of necrobiosis lipoidica? Int J Dermatol 2009;48: 964–70.
18. Ngo B, Wigington G, Hayes K, et al. Skin blood flow in necrobiosis lipoidica diabeticorum. Int J Dermatol 2008;47:354–8.
19. Cohen O, Yaniv R, Karasik A, et al. Necrobiosis lipoidica and diabetic control revisited. Med Hypotheses 1996;46:348–50.
20. Basaria S, Braga-Basaria M. Necrobiosis lipoidica diabeticorum: response to pentoxiphylline. J Endocrinol Invest 2003;26:1037–40.
21. Rogers C. Necrobiosis lipoidica diabeticorum. Dermatol Nurs 2005;17:301, 307.
22. Kolde G, Muche JM, Schulze P, et al. Infliximab: a promising new treatment option for ulcerated necrobiosis lipoidica. Dermatology 2003;206:180–1.
23. Jelinek T, Nothdurft HD, Rieder N, et al. Cutaneous myiasis: review of 13 cases in travelers returning from tropical countries. Int J Dermatol 1995;34:624–6.
24. Binamer Y, Sowerby L, El-Helou T. Treatment of ulcerative necrobiosis lipoidica with topical calcineurin inhibitor: case report and literature review. J Cutan Med Surg 2012;16:458–61.
25. Buggiani G, Tsampau D, Krysenka A, et al. Fractional CO_2 laser: a novel therapeutic device for refractory necrobiosis lipoidica. Dermatol Ther 2012;25:612–4.
26. Kosaka S, Kawana S. Case of necrobiosis lipoidica diabeticorum successfully treated by photodynamic therapy. J Dermatol 2012;39:497–9.
27. Zeichner JA, Stern DW, Lebwohl M. Treatment of necrobiosis lipoidica with the tumor necrosis factor antagonist etanercept. J Am Acad Dermatol 2006;54: S120–1.
28. Stanway A, Rademaker M, Newman P. Healing of severe ulcerative necrobiosis lipoidica with cyclosporin. Australas J Dermatol 2004;45:119–22.
29. Handfield-Jones S, Jones S, Peachey R. High dose nicotinamide in the treatment of necrobiosis lipoidica. Br J Dermatol 1988;118:693–6.
30. Fjellner B. Treatment of diabetic nebrobiosis with aspirin and dipyridamole [letter to editor]. N Engl J Med 1978;299.
31. Unge G, Tornling G. Treatment of diabetic nebrobiosis with dipyridamole [letter to editor]. N Engl J Med 1978;299.
32. Evans AV, Atherton DJ. Recalcitrant ulcers in necrobiosis lipoidica diabeticorum healed by topical granulocyte-macrophage colony-stimulating factor. Br J Dermatol 2002;147:1023–5.

33. Barde C, Laffitte E, Campanelli A, et al. Intralesional infliximab in noninfectious cutaneous granulomas: three cases of necrobiosis lipoidica. Dermatology 2011; 222:212–6.
34. Hu SW, Bevona C, Winterfield L, et al. Treatment of refractory ulcerative necrobiosis lipoidica diabeticorum with infliximab: report of a case. Arch Dermatol 2009;145:437–9.
35. Schofield C, Sladden MJ. Ulcerative necrobiosis lipoidica responsive to colchicine. Australas J Dermatol 2012;53:e54–7.
36. Dabski K, Winkelmann RK. Generalized granuloma annulare: clinical and laboratory findings in 100 patients. J Am Acad Dermatol 1989;20:39–47.
37. Haim S, Friedman-Birnbaum R, Haim N, et al. Carbohydrate tolerance in patients with granuloma annulare. Study of fifty-two cases. Br J Dermatol 1973; 88:447–51.
38. Andersen BL, Verdich J. Granuloma annulare and diabetes mellitus. Clin Exp Dermatol 1979;4:31–7.
39. Huntley AC. The cutaneous manifestations of diabetes mellitus. J Am Acad Dermatol 1982;7:427–55.
40. Levy L, Zeichner JA. Dermatologic manifestation of diabetes. J Diabetes 2012; 4:68–76.
41. Muhlbauer JE. Granuloma annulare. J Am Acad Dermatol 1980;3:217–30.
42. Jabbour SA. Cutaneous manifestations of endocrine disorders: a guide for dermatologists. Am J Clin Dermatol 2003;4:315–31.
43. Dabski K, Winkelmann RK. Generalized granuloma annulare: histopathology and immunopathology. Systematic review of 100 cases and comparison with localized granuloma annulare. J Am Acad Dermatol 1989;20:28–39.
44. Spicuzza L, Salafia S, Capizzi A, et al. Granuloma annulare as first clinical manifestation of diabetes mellitus in children: a case report. Diabetes Res Clin Pract 2012;95:e55–7.
45. Smith MD, Downie JB, DiCostanzo D. Granuloma annulare. Int J Dermatol 1997; 36:326–33.
46. Ahmed I, Goldstein B. Diabetes mellitus. Clin Dermatol 2006;24:237–46.
47. Setterfield J, Huilgol SC, Black MM. Generalised granuloma annulare successfully treated with PUVA. Clin Exp Dermatol 1999;24:458–60.
48. Toonstra J. Bullosis diabeticorum. Report of a case with a review of the literature. J Am Acad Dermatol 1985;13:799–805.
49. Allen GE, Hadden DR. Bullous lesions of the skin in diabetes (bullosis diabeticorum). Br J Dermatol 1970;82:216–20.
50. Larsen K, Jensen T, Karlsmark T, et al. Incidence of bullosis diabeticorum–a controversial cause of chronic foot ulceration. Int Wound J 2008;5:591–6.
51. Anand KP, Kashyap AS. Bullosis diabeticorum. Postgrad Med J 2004;80:354.
52. Lopez PR, Leicht S, Sigmon JR, et al. Bullosis diabeticorum associated with a prediabetic state. South Med J 2009;102:643–4.
53. Lipsky BA, Baker PD, Ahroni JH. Diabetic bullae: 12 cases of a purportedly rare cutaneous disorder. Int J Dermatol 2000;39:196–200.
54. Bernstein JE, Levine LE, Medenica MM, et al. Reduced threshold to suction-induced blister formation in insulin-dependent diabetics. J Am Acad Dermatol 1983;8:790–1.
55. Basarab T, Munn SE, McGrath J, et al. Bullosis diabeticorum. A case report and literature review. Clin Exp Dermatol 1995;20:218–20.
56. Cole GW, Headley J, Skowsky R. Scleredema diabeticorum: a common and distinct cutaneous manifestation of diabetes mellitus. Diabetes Care 1983;6:189–92.

57. Martin C, Requena L, Manrique K, et al. Scleredema diabeticorum in a patient with type 2 diabetes mellitus. Case Rep Endocrinol 2011;2011:560273.

58. Brik R, Berant M, Vardi P. The scleroderma-like syndrome of insulin-dependent diabetes mellitus. Diabetes Metab Rev 1991;7:120–8.

59. Wilson BE, Newmark JJ. Severe scleredema diabeticorum and insulin resistance. J Am Board Fam Pract 1995;8:55–7.

60. Sattar MA, Diab S, Sugathan TN, et al. Scleroedema diabeticorum: a minor but often unrecognized complication of diabetes mellitus. Diabet Med 1988;5:465–8.

61. Hanna W, Friesen D, Bombardier C, et al. Pathologic features of diabetic thick skin. J Am Acad Dermatol 1987;16:546–53.

62. Seyger MM, van den Hoogen FH, de Mare S, et al. A patient with a severe scleroedema diabeticorum, partially responding to low-dose methotrexate. Dermatology 1999;198:177–9.

63. Ikeda Y, Suehiro T, Abe T, et al. Severe diabetic scleredema with extension to the extremities and effective treatment using prostaglandin E1. Intern Med 1998;37:861–4.

64. Lee FY, Chiu HY, Chiu HC. Treatment of acquired reactive perforating collagenosis with allopurinol incidentally improves scleredema diabeticorum. J Am Acad Dermatol 2011;65:e115–7.

65. Abraham C, Rozmus CL. Is acanthosis nigricans a reliable indicator for risk of type 2 diabetes in obese children and adolescents? A systematic review. J Sch Nurs 2012;28:195–205.

66. Torley D, Bellus GA, Munro CS. Genes, growth factors and acanthosis nigricans. Br J Dermatol 2002;147:1096–101.

67. Matsuoka LY, Wortsman J, Goldman J. Acanthosis nigricans. Clin Dermatol 1993;11:21–5.

68. Hud JA Jr, Cohen JB, Wagner JM, et al. Prevalence and significance of acanthosis nigricans in an adult obese population. Arch Dermatol 1992;128:941–4.

69. Matsuoka LY, Wortsman J, Gavin JR, et al. Spectrum of endocrine abnormalities associated with acanthosis nigricans. Am J Med 1987;83:719–25.

70. Buzasi K, Sapi Z, Jermendy G. Acanthosis nigricans as a local cutaneous side effect of repeated human insulin injections. Diabetes Res Clin Pract 2011;94:e34–6.

71. Hermanns-Le T, Scheen A, Pierard GE. Acanthosis nigricans associated with insulin resistance: pathophysiology and management. Am J Clin Dermatol 2004;5:199–203.

72. Katz RA. Treatment of acanthosis nigricans with oral isotretinoin. Arch Dermatol 1980;116:110–1.

73. Kuroki R, Sadamoto Y, Imamura M, et al. Acanthosis nigricans with severe obesity, insulin resistance and hypothyroidism: improvement by diet control. Dermatology 1999;198:164–6.

74. Fleischmajer R, Faludi G, Krol S. Scleredema and diabetes mellitus. Arch Dermatol 1970;101:21–6.

75. Shemer A, Bergman R, Linn S, et al. Diabetic dermopathy and internal complications in diabetes mellitus. Int J Dermatol 1998;37:113–5.

76. Dicken CH, Carrington SG, Winkelmann RK. Generalized granuloma annulare. Arch Dermatol 1969;99:556–63.

77. Melin H. An atrophic circumscribed skin lesion in the lower extremities of diabetics. Acta Med Scand 1964;176(Suppl 423):1–75.

78. Danowski TS, Sabeh G, Sarver ME, et al. Shin spots and diabetes mellitus. Am J Med Sci 1966;251:570–5.

79. Abdollahi A, Daneshpazhooh M, Amirchaghmaghi E, et al. Dermopathy and reti-nopathy in diabetes: is there an association? Dermatology 2007;214:133–6.
80. Morgan AJ, Schwartz RA. Diabetic dermopathy: a subtle sign with grave impli-cations. J Am Acad Dermatol 2008;58:447–51.
81. Yosipovitch G, Hodak E, Vardi P, et al. The prevalence of cutaneous manifesta-tions in IDDM patients and their association with diabetes risk factors and micro-vascular complications. Diabetes Care 1998;21:506–9.
82. Murphy R. The "spotted leg" syndrome. Am J Med Sci 1965;14:10–4.
83. Karpouzis A, Giatromanolaki A, Sivridis E, et al. Acquired reactive perforating collagenosis: current status. J Dermatol 2010;37:585–92.
84. Lynde CB, Pratt MD. Clinical Images: acquired perforating dermatosis: associ-ation with diabetes and renal failure. CMAJ 2009;181:615.
85. Rapini R. Perforating Diseases. In: Bolognia J, Jorizzo J, Rapini R, editors. Dermatology. 3rd edition. London: Mosby Elsevier; 2012. p. 1492–502.
86. Saray Y, Seckin D, Bilezikci B. Acquired perforating dermatosis: clinicopatho-logical features in twenty-two cases. J Eur Acad Dermatol Venereol 2006;20: 679–88.
87. Kawakami T, Saito R. Acquired reactive perforating collagenosis associated with diabetes mellitus: eight cases that meet Faver's criteria. Br J Dermatol 1999;140: 521–4.
88. Maurice PD, Neild GH. Acquired perforating dermatosis and diabetic nephrop-athy–a case report and review of the literature. Clin Exp Dermatol 1997;22: 291–4.
89. Farrell AM. Acquired perforating dermatosis in renal and diabetic patients. Lancet 1997;349:895–6.
90. Parker F. Xanthomas and hyperlipidemias. J Am Acad Dermatol 1985;13:1–30.
91. Kala J, Mostow EN. Images in clinical medicine. Eruptive xanthoma. N Engl J Med 2012;366:835.
92. Feingold KR, Elias PM. Endocrine-skin interactions. Cutaneous manifestations of pituitary disease, thyroid disease, calcium disorders, and diabetes. J Am Acad Dermatol 1987;17:921–40.
93. Wani AM, Hussain WM, Fatani MI, et al. Eruptive xanthomas with Koebner phe-nomenon, type 1 diabetes mellitus, hypertriglyceridaemia and hypertension in a 41-year-old man. BMJ Case Rep 2009;2009. http://dx.doi.org/10.1136/bcr.05. 2009.1871.
94. Garcia Hidalgo L. Dermatological complications of obesity. Am J Clin Dermatol 2002;3:497–506.
95. Demir S, Demir Y. Acrochordon and impaired carbohydrate metabolism. Acta Diabetol 2002;39:57–9.
96. Crook MA. Skin tags and the atherogenic lipid profile. J Clin Pathol 2000;53: 873–4.
97. Kahana M, Grossman E, Feinstein A, et al. Skin tags: a cutaneous marker for diabetes mellitus. Acta Derm Venereol 1987;67:175–7.
98. Chobanian SJ, Van Ness MM, Winters C Jr, et al. Skin tags as a marker for adenomatous polyps of the colon. Ann Intern Med 1985;103:892–3.
99. Dianzani C, Calvieri S, Pierangeli A, et al. The detection of human papillomavirus DNA in skin tags. Br J Dermatol 1998;138:649–51.
100. Rasi A, Soltani-Arabshahi R, Shahbazi N. Skin tag as a cutaneous marker for impaired carbohydrate metabolism: a case-control study. Int J Dermatol 2007; 46:1155–9.
101. Scheinfeld NS. Obesity and dermatology. Clin Dermatol 2004;22:303–9.

102. Hoerer E, Dreyfuss F, Herzberg M. Carotenemic, skin colour and diabetes mellitus. Acta Diabetol Lat 1975;12:202-7.
103. Neilly JB, Martin A, Simpson N, et al. Pruritus in diabetes mellitus: investigation of prevalence and correlation with diabetes control. Diabetes Care 1986;9: 273-5.
104. Namazi MR, Jorizzo JL, Fallahzadeh MK. Rubeosis faciei diabeticorum: a common, but often unnoticed, clinical manifestation of diabetes mellitus. ScientificWorldJournal 2010;10:70-1.
105. Pavlovic MD, Milenkovic T, Dinic M, et al. The prevalence of cutaneous manifestations in young patients with type 1 diabetes. Diabetes Care 2007;30:1964-7.
106. Gitelson S, Wertheimer-Kaplinski N. Color of the face in diabetes mellitus; observations on a group of patients in Jerusalem. Diabetes 1965;14:201-8.
107. Serrao R, Zirwas M, English JC. Palmar erythema. Am J Clin Dermatol 2007;8: 347-56.
108. Bravermen I. Skin signs of systemic disease. 3rd edition. Philadelphia: WB Saunders; 1998.
109. Ahmed K, Muhammad Z, Qayum I. Prevalence of cutaneous manifestations of diabetes mellitus. J Ayub Med Coll Abbottabad 2009;21:76-9.
110. Ngo BT, Hayes KD, DiMiao DJ, et al. Manifestations of cutaneous diabetic microangiopathy. Am J Clin Dermatol 2005;6:225-37.
111. Landau J, Davis E. The small blood-vessels of the conjunctiva and nailbed in diabetes mellitus. Lancet 1960;2:731-4.
112. Lithner F. Purpura, pigmentation and yellow nails of the lower extremities in diabetics. Acta Med Scand 1976;199:203-8.
113. Ratnam KV, Su WP, Peters MS. Purpura simplex (inflammatory purpura without vasculitis): a clinicopathologic study of 174 cases. J Am Acad Dermatol 1991; 25:642-7.
114. Rosenbloom AL. Limited joint mobility in childhood diabetes: discovery, description, and decline. J Clin Endocrinol Metab 2013;98:466-73.
115. Jelinek JE. Cutaneous manifestations of diabetes mellitus. J Am Acad Dermatol 1995;32:143-4.
116. Fitzgibbons PG, Weiss AP. Hand manifestations of diabetes mellitus. J Hand Surg Am 2008;33:771-5.
117. Fitzcharles MA, Duby S, Waddell RW, et al. Limitation of joint mobility (cheiroarthropathy) in adult noninsulin-dependent diabetic patients. Ann Rheum Dis 1984;43:251-4.
118. Otto-Buczkowska E, Jarosz-Chobot P. Limited joint mobility syndrome in patients with diabetes. Int J Clin Pract 2012;66:332-3.
119. Jennings AM, Milner PC, Ward JD. Hand abnormalities are associated with the complications of diabetes in type 2 diabetes. Diabet Med 1989;6:43-7.
120. Somai P, Vogelgesang S. Limited joint mobility in diabetes mellitus: the clinical implications. J Musculoskelet Med 2011;28:118-24.
121. Al-Matubsi HY, Hamdan F, Alhanbali OA, et al. Diabetic hand syndromes as a clinical and diagnostic tool for diabetes mellitus patients. Diabetes Res Clin Pract 2011;94:225-9.
122. Rosenbloom AL, Silverstein JH, Lezotte DC, et al. Limited joint mobility in childhood diabetes mellitus indicates increased risk for microvascular disease. N Engl J Med 1981;305:191-4.
123. Collier A, Matthews DM, Kellett HA, et al. Change in skin thickness associated with cheiroarthropathy in insulin dependent diabetes mellitus. Br Med J (Clin Res Ed) 1986;292:936.

124. Huntley AC. Finger pebbles: a common finding in diabetes mellitus. J Am Acad Dermatol 1986;14:612–7.
125. Cabo H, Woscoff A, Casas JG. Cutaneous manifestations of diabetes mellitus. J Am Acad Dermatol 1995;32:685.
126. Libecco JF, Brodell RT. Finger pebbles and diabetes: a case with broad involvement of the dorsal fingers and hands. Arch Dermatol 2001;137:510–1.
127. Schnider SL, Kohn RR. Effects of age and diabetes mellitus on the solubility and nonenzymatic glucosylation of human skin collagen. J Clin Invest 1981;67:1630–5.
128. Hamlin CR, Kohn RR, Luschin JH. Apparent accelerated aging of human collagen in diabetes mellitus. Diabetes 1975;24:902–4.
129. Seibold JR, Uitto J, Dorwart BB, et al. Collagen synthesis and collagenase activity in dermal fibroblasts from patients with diabetes and digital sclerosis. J Lab Clin Med 1985;105:664–7.
130. Lieberman LS, Rosenbloom AL, Riley WJ, et al. Reduced skin thickness with pump administration of insulin. N Engl J Med 1980;303:940–1.
131. Michou L, Lermusiaux JL, Teyssedou JP, et al. Genetics of Dupuytren's disease. Joint Bone Spine 2012;79:7–12.
132. Noble J, Heathcote JG, Cohen H. Diabetes mellitus in the aetiology of Dupuytren's disease. J Bone Joint Surg Br 1984;66:322–5.
133. Renard E, Jacques D, Chammas M, et al. Increased prevalence of soft tissue hand lesions in type 1 and type 2 diabetes mellitus: various entities and associated significance. Diabete Metab 1994;20:513–21.
134. Starkman HS, Gleason RE, Rand LI, et al. Limited joint mobility (LJM) of the hand in patients with diabetes mellitus: relation to chronic complications. Ann Rheum Dis 1986;45:130–5.
135. Lennox IA, Murali SR, Porter R. A study of the repeatability of the diagnosis of Dupuytren's contracture and its prevalence in the Grampian region. J Hand Surg Br 1993;18:258–61.
136. Arkkila PE, Kantola IM, Viikari JS. Dupuytren's disease: association with chronic diabetic complications. J Rheumatol 1997;24:153–9.
137. Arkkila PE, Kantola IM, Viikari JS, et al. Dupuytren's disease in type 1 diabetic patients: a five-year prospective study. Clin Exp Rheumatol 1996;14:59–65.
138. Sherry DD, Rothstein RR, Petty RE. Joint contractures preceding insulin-dependent diabetes mellitus. Arthritis Rheum 1982;25:1362–4.
139. Grgic A, Rosenbloom AL, Weber FT, et al. Joint contracture - Common manifestation of diabetes mellitus. J Pediatr 1976;88(4):584–8.
140. Huntley AC, Walter RM Jr. Quantitative determination of skin thickness in diabetes mellitus: relationship to disease parameters. J Med 1990;21:257–64.
141. Arunachalam M, Dragoni F, Colucci R, et al. Non-segmental vitiligo and psoriasis comorbidity - a case-control study in Italian patients. J Eur Acad Dermatol Venereol 2013. [Epub ahead of print].
142. Cohen JD, Bournerias I, Buffard V, et al. Psoriasis induced by tumor necrosis factor-alpha antagonist therapy: a case series. J Rheumatol 2007;34:380–5.
143. Farias MM, Achurra P, Boza C, et al. Psoriasis following bariatric surgery: clinical evolution and impact on quality of life on 10 patients. Obes Surg 2012;22:877–80.
144. Cheng J, Kuai D, Zhang L, et al. Psoriasis increased the risk of diabetes: a meta-analysis. Arch Dermatol Res 2012;304:119–25.
145. Li W, Han J, Hu FB, et al. Psoriasis and risk of type 2 diabetes among women and men in the United States: a population-based cohort study. J Invest Dermatol 2012;132:291–8.

146. Takahashi N, Takasu S. A close relationship between type 1 diabetes and vitamin A-deficiency and matrix metalloproteinase and hyaluronidase activities in skin tissues. Exp Dermatol 2011;20:899–904.

147. Shiina T, Inoko H, Kulski JK. An update of the HLA genomic region, locus information and disease associations: 2004. Tissue Antigens 2004;64:631–49.

148. Richetta A, D'Epiro S, Salvi M, et al. Serum levels of functional T-regs in vitiligo: our experience and mini-review of the literature. Eur J Dermatol 2013;23(2): 154–9.

149. Forschner T, Buchholtz S, Stockfleth E. Current state of vitiligo therapy–evidence-based analysis of the literature. J Dtsch Dermatol Ges 2007;5:467–75.

150. Dawber RP. Vitiligo in mature-onset diabetes mellitus. Br J Dermatol 1968;80: 275–8.

151. Gould IM, Gray RS, Urbaniak SJ, et al. Vitiligo in diabetes mellitus. Br J Dermatol 1985;113:153–5.

152. Gupta AK, Konnikov N, MacDonald P, et al. Prevalence and epidemiology of toenail onychomycosis in diabetic subjects: a multicentre survey. Br J Dermatol 1998;139:665–71.

153. Meurer M, Szeimies RM. Diabetes mellitus and skin diseases. Curr Probl Dermatol 1991;20:11–23.

154. Grandis R, Branstetter B, Yu V. The changing face of malignant (necrotising) external otitis: clinical, radiological, and anatomic correlations. Lancet Infect Dis 2004;4:34–9.

155. Lugo-Somolinos A, Sanchez JL. Prevalence of dermatophytosis in patients with diabetes. J Am Acad Dermatol 1992;26:408–10.

156. Gulcan A, Gulcan E, Oksuz S, et al. Prevalence of toenail onychomycosis in patients with type 2 diabetes mellitus and evaluation of risk factors. J Am Podiatr Med Assoc 2011;101:49–54.

157. Petrikkos G, Skiada A, Lortholary O, et al. Epidemiology and clinical manifestations of mucormycosis. Clin Infect Dis 2012;54(Suppl 1):S23–34.

158. Casqueiro J, Casqueiro J, Alves C. Infections in patients with diabetes mellitus: a review of pathogenesis. Indian J Endocrinol Metab 2012;16(Suppl 1):S27–36.

Reproductive Sequelae of Diabetes in Male Patients

Geoffrey Gaunay, MD[a], Harris M. Nagler, MD[a,b,*], Doron S. Stember, MD[a,b]

KEYWORDS

- Diabetes mellitus • Erectile dysfunction • Ejaculatory dysfunction
- Retrograde ejaculation • Anejaculation • Hypogonadism

KEY POINTS

- Diabetes mellitus (DM) is an increasingly prevalent systemic disorder.
- DM has been associated with reproductive dysfunction in men.
- DM exerts deleterious effects in reproductive potential via multiple pathways, including erectile dysfunction, ejaculatory dysfunction, and alterations of the hypothalmic-pituitary axis.
- Increased recognition of the mechanisms of reproductive impact of DM should allow physicians to help their patients improve fertility potential.

INTRODUCTION

Diabetes mellitus (DM) is an increasingly prevalent public health concern. A recent study projected the number of people worldwide with DM to increase from 171 million in 2000 to 366 million in 2030.[1] Although DM is a systemic disease that often leads to end-organ dysfunction of multiple body systems, the effects of the condition on male fertility are often not fully appreciated. DM is associated with multiple risk factors for reduced male fertility potential: erectile dysfunction (ED), various types of ejaculatory dysfunction (EjD), and hypogonadism (HG).

Mechanism of Normal Erection

Tumescence

A normal penile erection is physiologically composed of a complex cascade of events involving the coordination of the somatic and autonomic nervous systems, the endocrine system, and the pelvic and penile vasculature.[2] With sexual arousal or physical stimulation, the molecule nitric oxide (NO) is released from parasympathetic nerves

[a] Sol and Margaret Berger Department of Urology, Beth Israel Medical Center, Phillips Ambulatory Care Center, 10 Union Square Suite 3A, New York, NY 10003, USA; [b] Albert Einstein College of Medicine of Yeshiva University, Bronx, NY 10461, USA
* Corresponding author.
E-mail address: hnagler@chpnet.org

Endocrinol Metab Clin N Am 42 (2013) 899–914
http://dx.doi.org/10.1016/j.ecl.2013.07.003
0889-8529/13/$ – see front matter © 2013 Elsevier Inc. All rights reserved.

endo.theclinics.com

through the action of the enzyme nitric oxide synthase (NOS). Endothelial NOS, stimulated by the shear stress of increased blood flow and neurohumoral factors, is also responsible for the increase in penile NO with erection.[3] The expression of NOS within the penis has been shown to be testosterone dependent.[4] On release in the cavernosal tissue, NO then stimulates the production of cyclic guanosine monophosphate (cGMP) from cyclic guanosine triphosphate via the enzyme guanylate cyclase that is located within smooth muscle cells.[5] The resultant increase in cGMP leads to a decrease in intracellular calcium that results, in turn, in relaxation in smooth muscle within the corporal cavernosum.

As smooth muscle within the corporal vessels begins to relax, the lacunar spaces within the erectile tissue dilate and fill with blood. Penile arterial inflow is also increased due to relaxation of smooth muscle lining the vessel walls. The rapid increase in arterial blood volume within a relatively fixed space generates an intracavernosal pressure up to 100 mm Hg for typical erections.[6] The increased pressure also results in compression of the subtunical veins between the tough tunical layer and the high-pressure, dilated lacunar spaces. Mechanical compression of the veins sharply limits venous outflow from the corpora cavernosa. The combined effect of increased arterial inflow and decreased venous outflow maintains the rigidity of the erection.[7]

Detumescence

Detumescence, the process by which the penis returns to a flaccid state after erection, is primarily controlled by the sympathetic nervous system mediator, norepinephrine. Norepinephrine release is increased at the time of orgasm. Stimulation of α-adrenergic receptors on corporal smooth muscle causes vasoconstriction leading to a reduced arterial inflow. Subtunical veins, previously compressed, are now able to drain the lacunar spaces of the corporal body. As this process proceeds, the penis assumes a more flaccid appearance.[2]

ERECTILE AND REPRODUCTIVE DYSFUNCTION AND DM

ED is defined as the inability to achieve or maintain an erection sufficient for satisfactory sexual performance.[8] Normal sexual reproduction depends on erectile rigidity sufficient for vaginal penetration and subsequent deposition of ejaculate. In 2010, the International Consultation Committee for Sexual Medicine reported the prevalence and incidence of risk factors for ED.[9] Increasing age was identified as the primary risk for ED. DM type 2 was identified as the second most common factor. The report estimated that ED develops in 50% to 75% of diabetic men. Furthermore, ED occurs nearly 3 times as often in men with DM compared with those without the condition,[10] and difficulty in initiation or maintaining erections has been identified as an early sign of eventual DM in up to 12% of patients with DM.[11] Diabetic ED tends to occur 10 to 15 years earlier than in the general populace.[12] Poor control of blood glucose may hasten the development of ED, imparting a 2 to 5 times greater risk of developing of organic impotence.[13,14]

The effects of DM are not limited to the reproductive organs. Diabetes may affect a host of other illnesses, including coronary artery disease (CAD), peripheral vascular disease, stroke, hypertension, hyperlipidemia, and the metabolic syndrome.[15–19]

Neurologic Pathophysiology

Intact neurologic functioning is critical for normal erectile physiology. Sensory nerves to the penis relay impulses related to sexual stimulation mainly via the pudendal nerves (S2–S4) that branch into the penile dorsal nerve. Autonomic nerves are supplied by the inferior hypogastric plexus that then branches into cavernous nerves.

The paired cavernous nerves release a neurotransmitter, NO, that triggers a cascade culminating in relaxation of erectile chambers and arterial dilation, thereby allowing the penis to become engorged with blood, as discussed previously. (See later in this article for discussion of vascular pathophysiology.)

DM also contributes to ED via nerve damage. In addition to direct neurologic injury secondary to hyperglycemia, DM is associated with the increased production of inflammatory cytokines, free radicals, and oxidative stress, all of which have been shown to cause nerve fiber degeneration and impaired axonal transport.[20] Multiple neurophysiologic changes resulting in neuropathies have been demonstrated in diabetic patients. Both motor and sensory neuropathic changes, either of which can contribute to ED, have been found specifically to occur in prediabetic as well as frankly diabetic men.[21] Peripheral neuropathy is, in fact, an overwhelmingly common complication of DM, with a prevalence of 45% to 50%.[22]

Reduced or absent parasympathetic input to the penis is the main mechanism of autonomic nervous system dysfunction causing ED in diabetic men.[23] Relaxation of corporal cavernosal smooth muscle is dependent on parasympathetic tone causing the release of NO from noncholinergic neurons and a decrease in circulating norepinephrine, a product of sympathetic neurons. Men with autonomic neuropathy affecting other organ systems are especially prone to the development of ED.[23] Autonomic dysfunction may also be an independent risk factor for cardiovascular disease[24] and, indeed, ED is increasingly recognized as an early warning sign that should prompt a thorough cardiovascular evaluation.

Vascular Pathophysiology

The penis is an end organ that is particularly susceptible to diabetic microvasculopathy and macrovasculopathy. Endothelial dysfunction, or damage to the inner lining of penile vasculature, is thought to play a major role in diabetic ED.[6] Increased circulating serum glucose in diabetic individuals has been shown to induce the formation of advanced glycation end products (AGEs). AGEs form due to noncatalyzed reactions between glucose, fats, proteins, and other circulating substrates.[25] Accumulation of AGEs has been shown to lead to increased oxidative stress, as well as impaired axonal and intracellular signaling.[20,26] Enhanced glycation at tissue levels has been shown to increase expression of endothelial adhesion molecules ICAM-1 and VCAM-1. Low-density lipoprotein oxidation, contributing to the formation of free radicals, is also increased in diabetic patients. Both of these findings have been correlated with glycemic control, using hemoglobin A1C (HbA1c) as a surrogate measure, and are thought to contribute to the vasculopathy of the penile erectile chambers.[6,25] In a study of diabetic men with and without ED, patients with ED experienced a lower drop in blood pressure and a greater platelet aggregation response when infused with L-arginine, a precursor of NO. These findings support the concept of endothelial dysfunction playing a major role in ED.[27] Impairment in the production of NO through suppression of NOS has also been implicated as a factor underlying ED in diabetic men.

Studies have shown increased circulating levels of the vasoconstrictor endothelin-1 (ET-1) in patients with DM, possibly secondary to endothelial cell damage.[28] Endothelin exerts influence through an Rho-kinase–dependent cascade leading to smooth muscle contraction and vasoconstriction. Antagonism of this Rho-kinase has shown some effectiveness in animal studies as a target for pharmacologic intervention to enhance vasodilatation and erection.[29] Endothelial dysfunction underlying ED is not limited to diabetic individuals. In fact, the obese and first-degree relatives of diabetic patients have shown signs of endothelial dysfunction even when they exhibit normal glucose tolerance.[30,31]

Clinical evidence of impaired penile vascular hemodynamics in diabetic patients compared with age-matched controls has been demonstrated with duplex Doppler sonographic studies. In the flaccid state, diabetic patients, in particular those with HG, had lower mean peak systolic velocities. Similarly, after intracavernosal injection (ICI) of prostaglandin E1, diabetic men were found to have lower mean peak systolic velocities compared with healthy controls.[32]

Treatment of ED

Treatment options for men with ED and DM are similar to those available to all men with ED. Some special considerations, however, apply to diabetic men. These are summarized in **Table 1**. The first-line treatment for patients with ED is oral phosphodiesterase (PDE5) inhibitors. PDE5 inhibitors work by preventing the breakdown of cGMP within smooth muscle of the corpora cavernosa and thus potentiate rigidity and duration of erections, as well as decreasing latency time between erections.[33] This class of medication is generally safe and effective,[34] with 57% to 74% of men experiencing a degree of improvement.[35,36] A significant reduction in the efficacy of PDE5 inhibitors, however, has been reported in diabetic men versus nondiabetic controls.[35,37,38] Diabetic men, in addition, typically require higher dosing to achieve results similar to men without DM.[39] Unfortunately no "head-to-head trials" comparing the available various PDE5 inhibitors in diabetic patients exist. Double-blind randomized control trials of each PDE5 inhibitor (vardenafil, sildenafil, and tadalafil) have shown, however, to provide significant improvement in men with DM compared with placebo.[35,36,40–46] These medications are usually well tolerated in diabetic patients and

Table 1
Treatment options for erectile dysfunction in men with DM

Therapy	Special Considerations in Men with DM
Lifestyle modification (exercise, healthy diet, improved glycemic control)	Recommended for systemic health in diabetic patients as well as prevention of worsening ED; unfortunately, ED due to DM is considered irreversible and would not be expected to be improved by behavioral modification alone
Oral phosphodiesterase inhibitor (sildenafil, tadalafil, vardenafil)	Many diabetic patients have comorbid coronary artery disease; PDE5 inhibitors are strictly contraindicated for patients who carry nitrates for possible angina
Intraurethral alprostadil (MUSE)	Penile diabetic neuropathy is associated with increased incidence of penile pain in the presence of alprostadil
Intracavernosal injection	Penile diabetic neuropathy is associated with increased incidence of penile pain in the presence of alprostadil
Semirigid penile prosthesis implantation	Diabetic men with poor glycemic control may be at increased risk for urethral perforation with semirigid prostheses, which exert more pressure on the urethral lining than inflatable devices
IPP	Although published data are inconclusive, poorly controlled DM is widely considered a risk factor for IPP infection

Abbreviations: DM, diabetes mellitus; ED, erectile dysfunction; IPP, inflatable penile prosthesis implantation; MUSE, Medicated Urethral System for Erection; PDE5, phosphodiesterase.

adverse effects are usually mild, including headache, dizziness, facial flushing, and visual disturbances. Care must be taken in prescribing to patients with CAD, which is particularly prevalent in the diabetic population. Although most patients with stable CAD may use PDE5 inhibitors safely,[47] concomitant use of nitrates is a contraindication to avoid potentially fatal hypotension.[48,49]

Even for men who have not been diagnosed with CAD, ED should still be considered a potential manifestation of systemic cardiovascular disease. This is particularly true in men who do not exercise on a continual basis. A 2011 meta-analysis of 10 studies demonstrated that sexual activity is associated with acute cardiac events in men who engage in little physical activity, and also that fewer cardiac events occurred with sexual activity in men who exercise regularly.[50] The Princeton Consensus Conference is an interdisciplinary expert panel that has made recommendations regarding preservation of sexual and cardiac health. The most recent meeting produced a statement focusing on evaluation of cardiac risk in men with ED to identify those men in whom sexual activity represents a risk for an acute cardiac event.[51] The Consensus states that men with ED should have exercise ability evaluated before prescribing treatment for ED. The exertion of sexual activity is roughly equivalent to climbing 2 flights of stairs in 10 seconds. Men who are able to accomplish this without significant difficulty are considered low risk for cardiac complications and treatment should focus on ED, with optional further cardiac evaluation (as ED is itself considered to be a cardiac risk factor). Men with moderate stair-climbing ability are at indeterminate risk and should undergo a stress test. Those who pass are then considered low risk. Those who fail are considered to be at high risk of a cardiac event. These men should consult with a cardiologist, as should those with marked difficulty or shortness of breath climbing 2 flights of stairs briskly.

Even if cardiovascular risk has been assessed and determined to be acceptable to allow sexual activity and medications, not all men respond to (or tolerate the side effects of) first-line oral medications. The next line of therapy used is typically intraurethrally or intracavernosally injected vasoactive mediators. The 3 common agents used are alprostadil or prostaglandin E1 (PGE1), an activator of adenylate cyclase leading to an intracellular increase in cAMP; papaverine, a nonspecific inhibitor of phosphodiesterase; and phentolamine, which inhibits detumescense by blocking α-adrenergic receptors. Medicated Urethral System for Erection (MUSE) is a urethral suppository form of alprostadil that exerts its effect after diffusion through the urethral mucosa. A multi-institutional study of 996 men, approximately 20% of whom had DM, showed an efficacy of 65% with no significant difference between diabetic patients and nondiabetic patients.[52] ICIs are often more effective than PDE5 inhibitors. Diabetic patients have been shown to tolerate and have greater treatment compliance with ICIs than nondiabetic patients, despite typically requiring steadily increasing doses over time.[53]

It should be noted that intraurethral and ICI of alprostadil have been associated with penile pain in the setting of nerve damage, such as occurs with DM or following radical prostatectomy (RP).[54] Alprostadil is the most common component of injectable compounds, which also frequently include the off-label use of papaverine and phentolamine to increase treatment efficacy.[55] For diabetic patients who experience pain throughout the entire penis following ICI (as opposed to at the injection site), consideration should be given to a compound that does not include alprostadil. Response rates to ICI of approximately 70% have been reported among diabetic patients.[56] The major risk of ICI is priapism, or a prolonged (>4 hours) duration erection that occurs in the absence of sexual stimulation. Priapism is a medical emergency that requires treatment with intracavernosal phenylephrine, aspiration of clots, and, occasionally, bedside or operating room (OR) procedures to restore normal penile blood flow. The ultimate result is long-term severe ED that is unresponsive to ICI. It is therefore critically important to titrate the patient's ICI dose in the office before prescribing it for at-home use. The technique for ICI is depicted in **Fig. 1**.

For diabetic men in whom oral medication and ICI are ineffective, contraindicated, or intolerable, penile prostheses represent an effective treatment option. Penile prostheses are surgically implanted under strict sterile conditions in the OR and are available in 2 basic forms. Semirigid, or malleable, implants are simply bendable rods (**Fig. 2**). A total of 2 rods are placed, one each traversing the length of left and right penile erectile body. The advantage of the semirigid device is simplicity of use for the patient. The rods are flexible enough to be pointed downward when wearing clothes, but rigid enough to allow for sexual penetration when the rods are bent into the erect position. The major complaint regarding semirigid devices is, not surprisingly, that they do not provide optimal rigidity or flaccidity when each is desired. They are usually reserved for men who do not have the ability to manipulate the more sophisticated multicomponent inflatable penile prostheses (IPPs) (**Fig. 3**). IPPs consist of 3 components: paired penile cylinders, a scrotal pump, and an abdominal reservoir. The components are connected to one another by tubing and sterile water is contained within the system. The scrotal pump is compressed several times to transfer water stored in the reservoir to the cylinders. As the reservoir empties, the cylinders become engorged with water and the resulting rigidity provides an erection with a natural appearance that is capable of penetration. The erection will be maintained (regardless of whether the patient has an orgasm) until he decides to squeeze the release valve on the scrotal pump. The release valve allows water to transfer from the cylinders to the reservoir again.

Prevention of implant infection is of paramount concern, as removal of the entire device is required. Although the data are equivocal regarding whether diabetic patients are at an increased risk of infection with penile implant placement, most surgeons exercise great caution regarding implant surgery in poorly controlled diabetic

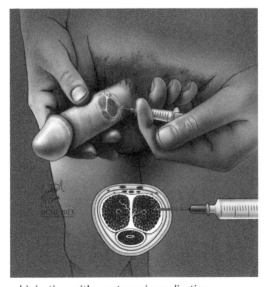

Fig. 1. Intracavernosal injection with erectogenic medication.

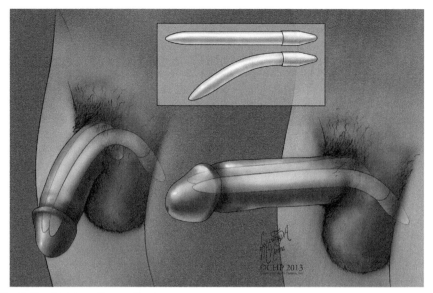

Fig. 2. Semirigid penile prosthesis.

patients because of the perceived or real increased risks.[57–61] In diabetic men, additionally, the constant low pressure associated with semirigid devices is relatively likely to lead to erosion of the device through the penile skin or urethra. IPPs provide lower pressure when in the flaccid state and are therefore the better choice for diabetic individuals who are physically able to use the pump mechanism.

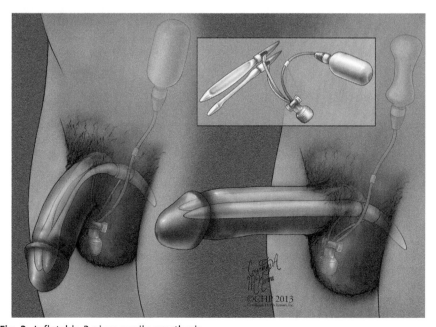

Fig. 3. Inflatable 3-piece penile prosthesis.

EJACULATORY DYSFUNCTION AND DM
Normal Ejaculatory Physiology

Sexual stimulation eventually brings about the climatic synchronization of neurologic and muscular response known as ejaculation.[62] Both central and peripheral nervous system integration is necessary for this complex process. A spinal ejaculatory center integrates the cognitive arousal signals from central nervous system centers with that of peripheral sensory stimulus and generates the autonomic and somatic motor response of ejaculation.[63]

Sympathetically generated smooth muscle contraction in the male reproductive system creates peristalsis in the reproductive tract, propelling sperm forward through the vas and toward the urethra. Concurrent sympathetic contraction of seminal vesicles forces seminal fluid through the ejaculatory ducts into the urethra, where it mixes with sperm and prostatic secretions.[7]

Somatically generated, involuntary rhythmic contraction of the bulbospongiosus and ischiocavernosus muscles mediated by the pudendal nerve causes the expulsion of semen from the urethra.[64] This rhythmic contraction of the muscles of the pelvic floor is pleasurable and generates the sensation of orgasmic climax. Although the terms orgasm and ejaculation frequently are used interchangeably, they are actually 2 different phenomena that happen to occur simultaneously in the normal state. The sensation of orgasm, however, can occur without ejaculation.

EjD is a common form of male sexual disorder that is associated with severe distress and can affect men of all ages. EjD is a broad term that encompasses premature ejaculation (PE), delayed or retarded ejaculation (DE), anejaculation (AE), and retrograde ejaculation (RE). In a recent multinational survey with nearly 13,000 respondents, 46% of men reported reduced ejaculate volume and 5% reported total absence of ejaculate within the previous month.[65] Intact ejaculatory function is particularly important to men interested in reproduction for the purpose of intromission of ejaculate into the female genital tract.

Although PE and DE are prevalent sexual disorders that are associated with a significantly impaired quality of life, they are not typically associated with fertility issues. AE and RE, on the other hand, are conditions that represent serious barriers to normal fertility. Both AE and RE are strongly associated with DM but may be caused by other conditions as well.

AE and RE

AE is defined as the complete absence of emission of semen into the posterior portion of the urethra. The most common causes, accounting for nearly 90% of AE cases, are spinal cord injury and retroperitoneal lymph node dissection surgery.[66] Most of the remaining cases occur in men with autonomic neuropathy associated with DM, although DM-related neuropathic EjD more commonly results in RE. With AE, failure of peristalsis of the vasal and seminal vesicle muscular lining prevents urethral deposition of ejaculate.

RE is characterized by ejaculate that is deposited into the posterior urethra but propelled backward into the bladder rather than forward toward the distal penis. In the normal state, the bladder neck (BN) closes with high pressure during orgasm and the seminal bolus takes the route of least resistance, which is antegrade. Closure of the BN is under sympathetic control. Diabetic neuropathy can interfere with the sympathetic fibers that provide for normal high-pressure BN closure, resulting in a relatively low-pressure route into the bladder for semen. RE can be partial or complete and the diagnosis is often suggested by patient report of cloudy urine following orgasm. The diagnosis is confirmed by postejaculatory urinalysis that reveals sperm, seminal fluid, or fructose.

One study of a young male diabetic population (mean age 36 years) found AE or RE in 6% of subjects.[67] In a review of more than 400 men who presented with infertility, only 3 (0.7%) patients had DM.[68] A more recent report of nearly 500 consecutive men presenting with infertility found that only 5 (1.1%) had type 1 DM.[69] The true incidence of AE and RE is associated with DM is unknown, however, as many elderly diabetic men likely are not interested in fertility and therefore do not seek treatment for these conditions.

Treatment of Diabetes-associated EjD

Treatment for RE and AE is initially alpha-1-adrenoreceptor antagonists (α-blockers), often prescribed for lower urinary tract symptoms associated with benign prostatic hyperplasia, which can inadvertently cause or contribute to absence of antegrade ejaculation. Therefore, diabetic men on α-blockers should have these medications at least temporarily discontinued. Drugs such as α-agonists, anticholinergics, or antihistamines have been shown to improve antegrade propulsion of semen by either increasing sympathetic or decreasing parasympathetic tone to the BN and may be given to increase the likelihood of antegrade ejaculation.[66,70] If medical therapy fails to restore antegrade ejaculation, and complete RE is demonstrated by postorgasmic urinalysis, then sperm may be harvested from the bladder, treated, and subsequently used for vaginal or intrauterine insemination or in vitro fertilization (IVF).[70] A suggested protocol for performing this procedure is outlined in **Box 1**.

Men with AE failing to respond to medications may be candidates for more invasive methods to harvest sperm. Penile vibratory stimulation (PVS), electroejaculation (EEJ), or testicular sperm extraction (TESE) may be attempted. PVS involves placing a vibratory stimulator on the ventral aspect of the glans penis for 2 to 3 minutes or until antegrade ejaculation. Successful PVS requires that the ejaculatory reflex arc, including peripheral sympathetic outflow, to be intact.[7] The best candidates with AE for this procedure are selected patients with spinal cord injury. No study has ever documented the efficacy of PVS in diabetic men with sympathetic pelvic neuropathy; although, based on the mechanism of action of PVS, they would not be expected to respond well.

Box 1
Instructions for collection of sperm in men with retrograde ejaculation

1. Patient abstains from ejaculation for 2–4 days before collection

2. Limit fluid intake for 12 hours before collection to minimize urine dilution

3. Patient takes potassium citrate or sodium bicarbonate 12 and 2 hours before collection (to counteract urine acidity that is inhospitable to sperm)

4. Patient voids immediately before self-stimulation for collection (alternatively, bladder may be drained with red rubber catheter; if catheter is used, then sperm transport medium should be inserted via catheter immediately before removal)

5. Patient ejaculates into sterile collection cup (if antegrade ejaculate present)

6. After 15 minutes, patient voids into second sterile collection cup (alternatively, bladder is recatheterized and additional sperm transport medium is used to irrigate bladder before removal)

7. Collection cups are immediately sent to the laboratory for semen analysis and/or processing; technician should be made aware to survey urine for sperm as well as urine

EEJ involves placing a specifically designed metal probe into the rectum with the patient under general anesthesia. The probe is connected to an adjustable power source and rhythmic current delivery is increased in voltage until ejaculation occurs.[63] The current induces contraction of pelvic floor and periurethral muscles, potentially providing emission to the posterior urethra. Ejaculate may be immediately seen exiting from the urethral meatus and may also travel retrograde into the bladder. Therefore, following removal of the EEJ probe, a red rubber catheter should always be placed into the bladder and flushed with sperm transport medium to drain any potential sperm into a sterile collection receptacle. EEJ does not require an intact ejaculatory reflex, unlike PVS, and has been shown to be effective in men with diabetic neuropathy.[71]

An alternative approach to retrieving sperm is to retrieve it from the testicles directly, either via office-based biopsy or TESE under general anesthesia. Sperm harvested from the testes is typically cryopreserved and can then be used for IVF.

HG AND DM
Sex Hormones

Diabetic men frequently exhibit low serum testosterone (T) levels and many are symptomatically hypogonadal.[72] Poor glycemic control (HgbA1c >7%) and hyperinsulinemia have been linked to lower circulating levels of testosterone and dehydroepiandrosterone sulfate.[73] Higher body mass index (BMI), greater visceral adiposity, and obesity have all been positively correlated with lower testosterone levels and symptomatic HG.[32,73,74]

Recent studies have revealed a significantly lower mean testis size and serum luteinizing hormone (LH) levels among diabetic, hypogonadal men.[32] Increased visceral adiposity, frequently found in diabetic men, may be to blame. In HG, reduced T levels have been shown to lead to increased uptake of free fatty acids through the action of lipoprotein lipase, thereby promoting adipose cell proliferation.[75] Aromatase activity in adipose cells causes conversion of T to estradiol (E2). Obese individuals tend to exhibit lower serum T and higher serum E2 concentrations, likely explained by increased aromatase activity in large quantities of visceral adipose tissue. These findings are supported by the increase in T and decrease in E2 noted after administration of testolactone, a potent inhibitor of aromatase.[76] Increased E2 levels contribute to the previously noted reduction in levels of LH through feedback inhibition on gonadotropin release, which can also result in testicular atrophy.[76]

Leptin, a potent adipose-derived hormone, is found in plasma at levels proportional to the degree of adiposity and regulates energy intake and use.[77] Rat studies have revealed the inhibitory effect of leptin on T production.[78] Leptin has also been shown to inhibit basal and LH-stimulated release of T from Leydig cells in obese men,[79] further linking excess adipose tissue and HG.

An additional mechanism leading to hypogonadotrophic HG in diabetic men may be based on the interaction between hypothalamic neurons and insulin. Insulin receptors have been shown to mediate action of anterior preoptic hypothalamic neurons involved in the production of gonadotropin-releasing hormone (GnRH). In cases of insulin resistance, this process is perturbed, impairing secretion of GnRH and its downstream effectors.[80]

Impaired libido is common among men suffering from HG,[32] and may impair erectile function directly or due to a lack of sexual desire. However, the role of T in erectile function and its impairment are unclear. Studies have shown a definitive link between ED and T, revealing a rate of ED in 58%[81] to 100%[82,83] of patients after castration. Testosterone replacement therapy (TRT) has shown promise in ameliorating ED, but only when HG is the only detectable causative factor.[72] Lack of T may contribute to physiologic changes in the penis, which may contribute to ED. Corporal smooth muscle has been shown to undergo apoptosis when deprived of T.[84] Research suggests that penile parasympathetic fibers are dependent on T for proper function.[85] The expression of NOS in corporal vessels also may be dependent on circulating T.[86]

Not unexpectedly, the metabolic syndrome is likewise associated with male HG.[87] Many of the postulated mechanisms for the generation of HG in patients with metabolic syndrome mirror those discussed for DM alone. In addition, the metabolic syndrome is considered an inflammatory condition and it is thought that the increased circulating levels of cytokines may impair the production of T.[88]

Testosterone Supplementation

Unfortunately, there is a scarcity of randomized data regarding the use of T supplementation in hypogonadal diabetic men. General recommendations include a workup for HG in a patient with ED when suggestive symptoms (ie, low libido, fatigue, depressed mood) exist. TRT may be considered when low morning serum T (<300 ng/dL) is detected with concurrent symptoms.[89] Additional guidelines encourage exogenous treatment for T levels lower than 8 nmol/L and its consideration for levels 8 to 12 nmol/L, if the patient in question is symptomatically hypogonadal.[90]

Exogenous T supplementation is contraindicated in hypogonadal men who are interested in fertility. T replacement will impair sperm production via feedback inhibition on the anterior pituitary and interfere with follicle-stimulating hormone and LH release. Although circulating serum T levels may be increased to normal levels, the intratesticular T levels, which are normally several hundred-fold higher than serum levels, will drop to far below the levels needed to support spermatogenesis.

Antiestrogens including clomiphene citrate and tamoxifen citrate may be used to stimulate steroidogenesis in hypogonadal men who seek fertility. These agents block the estrogen receptors in both the hypothalamus and pituitary, thereby minimizing negative feedback of estrogen on gonadatropin release.[89] The result is increased gonadotropin levels with increased intratesticular T levels (in contradistinction to the decreased levels that occur with exogenous T administration). Although serum T levels can be increased without threatening sperm production, the actual benefits regarding fertility are unclear. A Cochrane meta-analysis of 10 randomized controlled studies that involved estrogen receptor blockers failed to demonstrate improved pregnancy rates.[91] Other trials have failed to convincingly demonstrate even improved semen parameters.[92]

An alternative medical therapy for patients with both HG and elevated serum estradiol levels is an oral aromatase inhibitor (anastrazole 1 mg daily, testalactone 100–200 mg daily, or letrazole 2.5 mg daily). This class of medications prevents the peripheral conversion of T to E2. Optimal candidates for aromatase inhibition have serum T:E2 ratios less than 10.

SUMMARY

DM and its associated complications represent an enormous public health challenge. A relatively underrecognized aspect of this complicated disease process is the impact on male sexual function and fertility potential. Traditionally, the prevalence of DM among male patients undergoing evaluation for infertility has been low, ranging from 0.7% to 1.1%.[68,69] This can likely be attributed to the older age of men acquiring type 2 DM who, in most cases, are beyond their desired reproductive years. The obesity epidemic facing the United States today, however, has involved increasingly greater numbers of children and young adults who are being diagnosed with DM. According to the American Diabetes Association 2011 National Diabetes Fact Sheet, 8.3% of the population and approximately 11.8% of all men older than 20 have DM.[93] Perhaps most striking, about 1 in every 400 children has been diagnosed with DM.[93] Many more have yet to be diagnosed or have evidence of prediabetes. The higher prevalence of DM in younger patients will ultimately result in more DM-associated infertility as this population reaches the typical reproductive years. It is critically important for patients and relevant clinicians to recognize the severe potential effects of DM on male sexual function and fertility, as well as to be familiar with the appropriate treatment modalities.

REFERENCES

1. Wild S, Roglic G, Green A, et al. Global prevalence of diabetes: estimates for the year 2000 and projections for 2030. Diabetes Care 2004;27(5):1047–53.
2. Prieto D. Physiological regulation of penile arteries and veins. Int J Impot Res 2008;20:17–29.
3. Busse R, Fleming I. Regulation of endothelium-derived vasoactive autacoid production by hemodynamic forces. Trends Pharmacol Sci 2003;24(1):24–9.
4. Traish AM, Munarriz R, O'Connell L, et al. Effects of medical surgical castration on erectile function in an animal model. J Androl 2003;24:381–7.
5. Cellek S, Rodrigo J, Lobos E, et al. Selective nitrergic neurodegeneration in diabetes mellitus—a nitric oxide-dependent phenomenon. Br J Pharmacol 1999; 128:1804–12.
6. Solomon H, Man JW, Jackson G. Erectile dysfunction and the cardiovascular patient: endothelial dysfunction is the common denominator. Heart 2003;89: 251–3.
7. Barazani S, Nagler S. Management of ejaculatory disorders in infertile men. Asian J Androl 2012;14(4):525–9.
8. Impotence. NIH Consens Statement 1992;10:1.
9. Lewis RW, Fugl-Meyer KS, Corona G, et al. Definitions/epidemiology/risk factors for sexual dysfunction. J Sex Med 2010;7:1598–607.
10. Ponholzer A, Temml C, Mock K, et al. Prevalence and risk factors for erectile dysfunction in 2869 men using a validated questionnaire. Eur Urol 2005;47(1): 80–5 [discussion: 85–6].
11. Gatti A, Mandosi E, Fallarino M, et al. Metabolic syndrome and erectile dysfunction among obese non-diabetic subjects. J Endocrinol Invest 2009;32(6):542–5.
12. Feldman HA, Goldstein I, Hatzichristou DG, et al. Impotence and its medical and psychosocial correlates: results of the Massachusetts Male Aging Study. J Urol 1994;151:54–61.
13. Esposito K, Giugliano F, Martedi E, et al. High proportions of erectile dysfunction in men with the metabolic syndrome. Diabetes Care 2005;28:1201–3.
14. Gündüz MI, Gümüs BH, Sekuri C. Relationship between metabolic syndrome and erectile dysfunction. Asian J Androl 2004;6:355–8.
15. Inman BA, Sauver JL, Jacobson DJ, et al. A population-based, longitudinal study of erectile dysfunction and future coronary artery disease. Mayo Clin Proc 2009;84:108–13.
16. Thompson IM, Tangen CM, Goodman PJ, et al. Erectile dysfunction and subsequent cardiovascular disease. JAMA 2005;294:2996–3002.
17. Clark NG, Fox KM, Grandy S, for the SHIELD Study Group. Symptoms of diabetes and their association with the risk and presence of diabetes: findings

from the Study to Help Improve Early evaluation and management of risk factors Leading to Diabetes (SHIELD). Diabetes Care 2007;30:2868–73.

18. Ponholzer A, Gutjahr G, Temml C, et al. Is erectile dysfunction a predictor of cardiovascular events or stroke? A prospective study using a validated questionnaire. Int J Impot Res 2010;22:25–9.

19. Chung SD, Chen YK, Lin HC, et al. Increased risk of stroke among men with erectile dysfunction: a nationwide population-based study. J Sex Med 2011;8:240–6.

20. Yagihashi S, Yamagishi S, Wada R. Pathology and pathogenetic mechanisms of diabetic neuropathy: correlation with clinical signs and symptoms. Diabetes Res Clin Pract 2007;77(Suppl 1):S184–9.

21. Singleton JR, Smith AG, Bromberg MB. Painful sensory polyneuropathy associated with impaired glucose tolerance. Muscle Nerve 2001;24:1225–8.

22. Shaw JE, Zimmet PZ. The epidemiology of diabetic neuropathy. Diabetes Rev 1999;7:245–52.

23. Hecht MJ, Neundörfer B, Kiesewetter F, et al. Neuropathy is a major contributing factor to diabetic erectile dysfunction. Neurol Res 2001;23:651–4.

24. Vinik AI, Maser RE, Mitchell BD, et al. Diabetic autonomic neuropathy. Diabetes Care 2003;26:1553–79.

25. Wen Y, Skidmore JC, Porter-Turner MM, et al. Relationship of glycation, antioxidant status and oxidative stress to vascular endothelial damage in diabetes. Diabetes Obes Metab 2002;4:305–8.

26. Sima AA, Sugimoto K. Experimental diabetic neuropathy: an update. Diabetologia 1999;42:773–88.

27. Angelis LD, Marfella MA, Siniscalchi M, et al. Erectile and endothelial dysfunction in type II diabetes: a possible link. Diabetologia 2001;44:1155–60.

28. Takahashi K, Ghatei MA, Lam HC, et al. Elevated plasma endothelin in patients with diabetes mellitus. Diabetologia 1990;33:306–10.

29. Rees RW, Ziessen T, Ralph DJ, et al. Human and rabbit cavernosal smooth muscle cells express Rho-kinase. Int J Impot Res 2002;14:1–7.

30. Steinberg HO, Chaker H, Leaming R, et al. Obesity/insulin resistance is associated with endothelial dysfunction. Implications for the syndrome of insulin resistance. J Clin Invest 1996;97:2601–10.

31. Caballero AE, Arora S, Saouaf R, et al. Microvascular and macrovascular reactivity is reduced in subjects at risk for type 2 diabetes. Diabetes 1999;48:1856–62.

32. Corona G, Mannucci E, Petrone L, et al. Association of hypogonadism and type II diabetes in men attending an outpatient erectile dysfunction clinic. Int J Impot Res 2006;18:190–7.

33. Wallis RM, Corbin JD, Francis SH, et al. Tissue distribution of phosphodiesterase families and the effects of sildenafil on tissue cyclic nucleotides, platelet function, and the contractile responses of trabeculae carneae and aortic rings in vitro. Am J Cardiol 1999;83:3C–12C.

34. Vardi M, Nini A. Phosphodiesterase inhibitors for erectile dysfunction in patients with diabetes mellitus. Cochrane Database Syst Rev 2007;(1):CD002187.

35. Goldstein I, Young JM, Fischer J, et al. Vardenafil, a new phosphodiesterase type 5 inhibitor, in the treatment of erectile dysfunction in men with diabetes: a multicenter double-blind placebo-controlled fixed-dose study. Diabetes Care 2003;26:777–83.

36. Rendell MS, Rajfer J, Wicker PA, et al. Sildenafil for treatment of erectile dysfunction in men with diabetes: a randomized controlled trial. Sildenafil diabetes study group. JAMA 1999;281:421–6.

37. Ng KK, Lim HC, Ng FC, et al. The use of sildenafil in patients with erectile dysfunction in relation to diabetes mellitus—a study of 1,511 patients. Singapore Med J 2002;43:387–90.

38. Padma-Nathan H. Efficacy and tolerability of tadalafil, a novel phosphodiesterase 5 inhibitor, in treatment of erectile dysfunction. Am J Cardiol 2003;92: 19M–25M.

39. Malavige LS, Levy JC. Erectile dysfunction in diabetes mellitus. J Sex Med 2009; 6:1232–47.

40. Ishii N, Nagao K, Fujikawa K, et al. Vardenafil 20-mg demonstrated superior efficacy to 10-mg in Japanese men with diabetes mellitus suffering from erectile dysfunction. Int J Urol 2006;13:1066–72.

41. Ziegler D, Merfort F, van Ahlen H, et al. Efficacy and safety of flexible-dose vardenafil in men with type 1 diabetes and erectile dysfunction. J Sex Med 2006;3: 883–91.

42. Stuckey BG, Jadzinsky MN, Murphy LJ, et al. Sildenafil citrate for treatment of erectile dysfunction in men with type 1 diabetes: results of a randomized controlled trial. Diabetes Care 2003;26:279–84.

43. Safarinejad MR. Oral sildenafil in the treatment of erectile dysfunction in diabetic men: a randomized double-blind and placebo-controlled study. J Diabet Complications 2004;18:205–10.

44. Boulton AJ, Selam JL, Sweeney M, et al. Sildenafil citrate for the treatment of erectile dysfunction in men with Type II diabetes mellitus. Diabetologia 2001; 44:1296–301.

45. Sáenz de Tejada I, Anglin G, Knight JR, et al. Effects of tadalafil on erectile dysfunction in men with diabetes. Diabetes Care 2002;25:2159–64.

46. Hatzichristou D, Gambla M, Rubio-Aurioles E, et al. Efficacy of tadalafil once daily in men with diabetes mellitus and erectile dysfunction. Diabet Med 2008; 25:138–46.

47. Jackson G, Betteridge J, Dean J, et al. A systematic approach to erectile dysfunction in the cardiovascular patient: a consensus statement—update 2002. Int J Clin Pract 2002;56:663–71.

48. Kostis JB, Jackson G, Rosen R, et al. Sexual dysfunction and cardiac risk (the Second Princeton Consensus Conference). Am J Cardiol 2005;96:313–21.

49. Cheitlin MD. Should the patient with coronary artery disease use sildenafil? Prev Cardiol 2003;6:161–5.

50. Dahabreh IJ, Paulus JK. Association of episodic physical and sexual activity with triggering of acute cardiac events: systematic review and meta-analysis. JAMA 2011;305(12):1225–33.

51. Nehra A, Jackson G, Miner M, et al. The Princeton III Consensus recommendations for the management of erectile dysfunction and cardiovascular disease. Mayo Clin Proc 2012;87(8):766–78.

52. Padma-Nathan H, Hellstrom WJ, Kaiser FE, et al. Treatment of men with erectile dysfunction with transurethral alprostadil. Medicated Urethral System for Erection (MUSE) Study Group. N Engl J Med 1997;336:1–7.

53. Perimenis P, Gyftopoulos K, Athanasopoulos A, et al. Diabetic impotence treated by intracavernosal injections: high treatment compliance and increasing dosage of vaso-active drugs. Eur Urol 2001;40:398–402 [discussion: 403].

54. Yiou R, Cunin P, de la Taille A, et al. Sexual rehabilitation and penile pain associated with intracavernous alprostadil after radical prostatectomy. J Sex Med 2011;8(2):575–82.

55. Phé V, Rouprêt M. Erectile dysfunction and diabetes: a review of the current evidence-based medicine and a synthesis of the main available therapies. Diabete Metab 2012;38:1–13.
56. Moore CR, Wang R. Pathophysiology and treatment of diabetic erectile dysfunction. Asian J Androl 2006;8:675–84.
57. Montague DK, Angermeier KW, Lakin MM. Penile prosthesis infections. Int J Impot Res 2001;13:326–8.
58. Wilson SK, Carson CC, Cleves MA, et al. Quantifying risk of penile prosthesis infection with elevated glycosylated haemoglobin. J Urol 1998;159:1537–9 [discussion: 1539–40].
59. Wilson SK, Delk JR 2nd. Inflatable penile implant infection: predisposing factors and treatment suggestions. J Urol 1995;153(3 Pt 1):659–61.
60. Jarow JP. Risk factors for penile prosthetic infection. J Urol 1996;156(2 Pt 1): 402–4.
61. Bishop JR, Moul JW, Sihelnik SA, et al. Use of glycosylated haemoglobin to identify diabetics at high risk for penile periprosthetic infections. J Urol 1992; 147:386–8.
62. Rowland D, McMahon CG, Abdo C, et al. Disorders of orgasm and ejaculation in men. J Sex Med 2010;7:1668–86.
63. Calabrò RS, Polimeni G, Ciurleo R, et al. Neurogenic ejaculatory disorders: focus on current and future treatments. Recent Pat CNS Drug Discov 2011;6:205–21.
64. Hershlag A, Schiff SF, DeCherney AH. Retrograde ejaculation. Hum Reprod 1991;6:255–8.
65. Rosen R, Altwein J, Boyle P, et al. Lower urinary tract symptoms and male sexual dysfunction: the multinational survey of the aging male (MSAM-7). Eur Urol 2003;44:637–49.
66. Kiamischke A, Nieschlag E. Update on medical treatment of ejaculatory disorders. Int J Androl 2002;25:222–44.
67. Dinulovic D, Radonjic G. Diabetes mellitus/male infertility [review]. Arch Androl 1990;25:277–93.
68. Greenberg SH, Lipshultz LI, Wein AJ. Experience with 425 subfertile male patients. J Urol 1978;119:507–10.
69. Sexton WJ, Jarow JP. Effect of diabetes mellitus upon male reproductive function. Urology 1997;49:508–13.
70. Fode M, Krogh-Jespersen S, Brackett NL, et al. Male sexual dysfunction and infertility associated with neurological disorders. Asian J Androl 2011;14:61–8.
71. Ohl DA, Quallich SA, Sonksen J, et al. Anejaculation: an electrifying approach. Semin Reprod Med 2009;27:179–85.
72. Kapoor D, Aldred H, Clark S, et al. Clinical and biochemical assessment of hypogonadism in men with type 2 diabetes: correlations with bioavailable testosterone and visceral adiposity. Diabetes Care 2007;30:911–7.
73. El-Sakka AI, Sayed HM, Tayeb KA. Type 2 diabetes-associated androgen alteration in patients with erectile dysfunction. Int J Androl 2008;31:602–8.
74. Kapoor D, Clarke S, Channer KS, et al. Erectile dysfunction is associated with low bioactive testosterone levels and visceral adiposity in men with type 2 diabetes. Int J Androl 2007;30:500–7.
75. Kapoor D, Malkin CJ, Channer KS, et al. Androgens, insulin resistance and vascular disease in men. Clin Endocrinol 2005;63:239–50.
76. Cohen PG. The hypogonadal-obesity cycle: role of aromatase in modulating the testosterone estradiol shunt—a major factor in the genesis of morbid obesity. Med Hypotheses 1999;52:49–51.

77. Lee MJ, Fried SK. Integration of hormonal and nutrient signals that regulate leptin synthesis and secretion. Am J Physiol Endocrinol Metab 2009;296:E1230.

78. Tena-Sempere M, Pinilla L, Gonzalez LC, et al. Leptin inhibits testosterone secretion from adult rat testis in vitro. J Endocrinol 1999;161:211–8.

79. Isidori AM, Caprio M, Strollo F, et al. Leptin and androgens in male obesity: evidence for leptin contribution to reduced androgens levels. J Clin Endocrinol Metab 1999;84:3673–80.

80. Brüning JC, Gautam D, Burks DJ, et al. Role of brain insulin receptor in control of body weight and reproduction. Science 2000;289:2122–5.

81. Ellis WJ, Grayhack JT. Sexual function in aging males after orchiectomy and estrogen therapy. J Urol 1963;89:895–9.

82. McCullagh EP, Renshaw JF. The effects of castration in the adult male. JAMA 1934;103:1140–3.

83. Greenstein A, Plymate SR, Katz PG. Visually stimulated erection in castrated men. J Urol 1995;153:650–2.

84. Hartmut Porst JB, editor. Standard practice in sexual medicine. 1st edition. Oxford (United Kingdom): Blackwell; 2007.

85. Baba K, Yajima M, Carrier S, et al. Effect of testosterone on the number of NADPH diaphorase-stained nerve fibers in the rat corpus cavernosum and dorsal nerve. Urology 2000;56:533–8.

86. Reilly CM, Zamporano P, Stopper VS, et al. Androgenic regulation of NO availability in rate penile erection. J Androl 1997;18:110.

87. Corona G, Mannucci E, Ricca V, et al. The age-related decline of testosterone is associated with different specific symptoms and signs in patients with sexual dysfunction. Int J Androl 2009;32:720.

88. Kalyani RR, Dobs AS. Androgen deficiency, diabetes, and the metabolic syndrome in men. Curr Opin Endocrinol Diabetes Obes 2007;14:226.

89. Bhasin S, Cunningham GR, Hayes FJ, et al. Testosterone therapy in men with androgen deficiency syndrome: an Endocrine Society clinical practice guideline. J Clin Endocrinol Metab 2010;95(6):2536–59.

90. Nieschlag E, Swerdloff R, Behre HM, et al. Investigation, treatment and monitoring of late-onset hypogonadism in males. ISA, ISSAM, and EAU recommendations. Eur Urol 2005;48:1–4.

91. Vandekerckhove P, Lilford R, Vail A, et al. Clomiphene or tamoxifen for idiopathic oligo/astheno-spermia. Cochrane Database Syst Rev 2000;(2):CD000151.

92. Torok L. Treatment of oligozoospermia with tamoxifen (open and controlled studies). Andrologia 1985;17(5):497–501.

93. Centers for Disease Control and Prevention. National diabetes fact sheet: national estimates and general information on diabetes and prediabetes in the United States, 2011. Atlanta (GA): U.S. Department of Health and Human Services, Centers for Disease Control and Prevention; 2011.

Diabetes and the Female Reproductive System

Anindita Nandi, MD, Leonid Poretsky, MD*

KEYWORDS

- Diabetes in pregnancy • Insulin and the ovary • PCOS

KEY POINTS

- Insulin and IGF-1 pathways are important in the development and maintenance of the female reproductive system.
- Insulin resistance is linked to varying degrees of ovulatory dysfunction, hyperandrogenism, and infertility.
- Aggressive treatment of hyperglycemia in pregnancy is important in optimizing maternal and fetal outcomes.

INTRODUCTION

The importance of insulin action in maintaining female reproductive function was suggested as early as 1925, with observations of ovarian hypofunction in patients with insulin-dependent diabetes mellitus (type 1 diabetes mellitus). Joslin and colleagues[1] reported that girls with type 1 diabetes mellitus failed to develop menarche.[2] Within 2 months to 1 year of insulin administration, however, menarche was observed in some of the girls. States of insulin resistance or hyperinsulinemia have also been associated with female reproductive abnormalities. In 1765, a description of females with signs of androgen excess and obesity (*valde obesa et virili*) was put forth by Morgagni.[3] In 1921, Archard and Thiers described the plight of *diabete des femmes a barbe* (diabetes of the bearded woman).[4] Since then, identification of altered menstruation, decreased fertility, and hirsuitism in women with syndromes of severe insulin resistance, such as Rabson-Mendenhall syndrome, type A insulin resistance syndrome, or type B insulin resistance syndrome, have linked insulin resistance with hyperandrogenism and abnormalities of female reproduction.[5,6] Recently, the more prevalent condition of polycystic ovarian syndrome (PCOS) has supported this correlation.[7]

Disclosure: The authors have no conflict of interest to disclose.
Division of Endocrinology and Metabolism, Beth Israel Medical Center, Albert Einstein College of Medicine, 317 East 17th Street, 7th Floor, New York, NY 10003, USA
* Corresponding author.
E-mail address: lporetsk@chpnet.org

Endocrinol Metab Clin N Am 42 (2013) 915–946
http://dx.doi.org/10.1016/j.ecl.2013.07.007
0889-8529/13/$ – see front matter © 2013 Elsevier Inc. All rights reserved.

INSULIN ACTION IN THE FEMALE REPRODUCTIVE SYSTEM
Insulin and the Ovary

The insulin receptor is a heterotetramer consisting of 2 α subunits and 2 β subunits.[8] Insulin binds to the extracellular α subunit. Subsequently, the β subunit becomes phosphorylated on tyrosine residues and acquires kinase activity. This phosphorylation initiates activation of a series of intracellular proteins, including insulin receptor substrate (IRS) proteins, phosphatidylinositide-3 kinase (PI3K), and mitogen-activated protein kinase (MAPK).[8,9] The activation of this signaling cascade acts as an effector for insulin's many metabolic effects in protein synthesis, lipogenesis, and carbohydrate metabolism. Perhaps the most important effect is facilitation of glucose transport through the plasma membrane mediated by translocation of intravesicular glucose transporter proteins (GLUTs) from the cytoplasm to the cell membrane. This process is mediated by the PI3K pathway. MAPK activation is thought to mediate the growth-promoting effects of insulin.[8,9]

An alternative signaling pathway for insulin action has been described. Insulin binding to the α subunit, independent of β-subunit activation, leads to the generation of inositol-glycan second messengers at the cell membrane. The role of this pathway in traditional metabolic effects of insulin has not been identified. It has been suggested that this alternative pathway may participate in regulation of ovarian steroidogenesis mediated by insulin. Definitive evidence for this, however, is lacking (**Fig. 1**).[9]

The classical target organs for insulin action are the muscle, liver, and adipose tissue. Demonstration of insulin receptor expression, however, in ovaries from both humans and animals supports a role for insulin action in the ovary. Insulin receptors are widely distributed throughout all ovarian components, including the granulosa, thecal, and stromal compartments.[10,11] Studies of normal ovarian tissue have shown

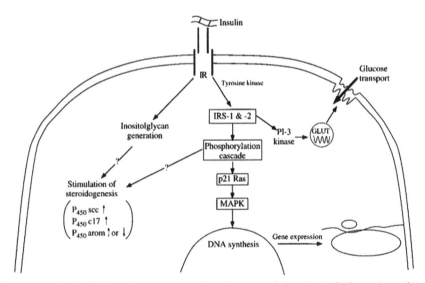

Fig. 1. Once insulin binds to its receptor, a signaling cascade is activated. The main pathway involves binding to the insulin receptor α-subunit and activation of the β-subunit tyrosine kinase activity. This, in turn, leads to IRS-1 and IRS-2 phosphorylation and PI3K activation. Subsequently, GLUT are translocated to cell membranes to allow influx of glucose. An alternate pathway leads to generation of inositol glycans after insulin binding to its own receptor. This second pathway may be important in mediating steroidogenic effects of insulin action.

that insulin binds to its receptor in stromal and follicular components of the ovary. Complete inhibition of insulin binding by specific anti-insulin receptor antibodies and lack of such an effect with antibodies to the type 1 insulinlike growth factor (IGF-1) receptor demonstrate that insulin binds to its ovarian receptors. Moreover, insulin receptors extracted from ovarian stromal tissues were shown to be autophosphorylated by incubation with insulin, similar to insulin receptor activation in classic target tissues.[11] Insulin has also been shown to bind to stromal tissues in ovaries from women with PCOS. Complete inhibition by anti-insulin receptor antibodies demonstrates the specificity of this interaction. Insulin binding to ovarian cell membranes from the luteal phase is similar to that in the follicular phase.[10]

Although it was shown that insulin specifically binds to its own receptor in the ovary, the question arose whether ovarian insulin receptor function and regulation were similar to those in classical target organs. Hyperinsulinemia is known to down-regulate insulin receptor expression in classical target tissues.[12-14] In vitro, exposure of stromal ovarian tissue to high-dose insulin eliminates specific insulin binding, whereas termination of exposure leads to the recovery of this activity within 4 hours.[12] In vivo, induction of hyperinsulinemia is accompanied by decreased insulin binding in the ovary, indicating the down-regulation of insulin receptors. Labeled IGF-1 binding was increased, suggesting up-regulation of IGF-1 receptors by hyperinsulinemia.[15] Therefore, in settings of insulin resistance, alternate pathways may become important players in the ovary. In human studies, a correlation has been seen in insulin binding to ovarian stromal tissue and circulating leukocytes in postmenopausal women. This relationship was not consistent in premenopausal women.[9,12] It is plausible that in premenopausal women, other factors, such as circulating gonadotropins, gonadal steroids, and autocrine regulators (such as IGFs), may influence insulin receptor expression.

Insulin effects on ovarian steroidogenesis have been studied both in vitro and in vivo. In vitro, insulin increases production of androgens, estrogens, and progesterone by granulosa and thecal cells.[1,16] Because, in some studies, hyperinsulinemia is required to stimulate steroidogenesis, it has been debated whether this action is modulated through IGF-1 receptors. The ability to block steroidogenesis from both granulosa cells and theca cells obtained from women with PCOS with anti-insulin receptor antibodies but not with antibodies against IGF-1 receptors, however, indicates that insulin mediates these actions through its own receptor.[17,18] It is possible that insulin's effect on steroidogenesis is mediated through stimulation of aromatase activity.[19] Insulin in some studies has also been shown to activate 17α-hydroxylase and enhance forskolin stimulation of 3β-hydroxysteroid dehydrogenase.[20,21] It has not been clearly demonstrated that insulin acutely stimulates steroidogenesis in vivo. In some studies of PCOS patients, insulin levels have been correlated with testosterone levels. Other studies, however, have not consistently supported this relationship.[22-24] Similarly, discrepant results in effect on androgen production have been noted with insulin infusion studies that have maintained euglycemic hyperinsulinemia for several hours.[25-28]

Studies suggest that insulin acts as a co-gonadotropin at the level of the ovary. It enhances steroidogenic responses to gonadotropins both in vivo and in vitro.[19,29-31] Insulin also enhances human chorionic gonadotropin (hCG)-induced ovarian growth and cyst formation in experimental animals.[8] In vivo, the degree of hyperinsulinemia in women with PCOS has been correlated with ovarian volume.[32] Moreover, with gonadotropin hyperstimulation, the increase in ovarian dimensions is greater in hyperinsulinemic PCOS patients than in normoinsulinemic PCOS women.[32]

Insulin has been shown to decrease hepatic sex hormone–binding globulin (SHBG) production. This suppressive action may be an important player in increasing free testosterone in patients with hyperinsulinemia. An increase in SHBG can be seen in women with PCOS who are treated with insulin sensitizers.[33,34] Another protein that is under the regulatory control of insulin is IGF binding protein (IGFBP)-1. Insulin inhibits production of this protein by the liver, thereby resulting in reduced circulating levels of IGFBP-1. Insulin also inhibits IGFBP-1 production by ovarian granulosa cells through activation of the insulin receptor. Decreased IGFBP-1 may increase circulating free IGF-1 levels.[9]

IGF Proteins

Insulin and IGF-1 are closely related peptides. They share sequence homology and have nearly identical 3-D structures.[35] The hormone receptors also have significant homology, featuring a heterotetrameric structure where 2 α subunits serve as the hormone binding site and 2 β subunits become autophosphorylated and acquire tyrosine kinase activity. Insulin binds to the IGF-1 receptor with lower affinity than to its intrinsic receptor. Although insulin shares significant homology with IGF-2, it does not bind the IGF-2 receptor. IGF-1 is not able to propagate phosphorylation of the insulin receptor, which maintains its specificity for insulin.[36]

Unlike insulin receptor, IGF and IGF receptor expression shows a cell-specific and stage-specific distribution in the human ovary. IGF peptides enter the ovarian follicular fluid (FF) both from the general circulation and intraovarian production. IGF-1 is largely released from the circulation, however, whereas IGF-2 is obtained mainly from local ovarian cells. IGF-2 levels in FF are 8 times higher than IGF-1 levels.[9] IGF-1 mRNA is barely detected in the adult ovary and excluded from the granulosa cell lineage. IGF-2 mRNA and protein are noted in thecal cells and perifollicular vessels in all follicles. In small antral follicles, it is detected in both granulosa and thecal cells. IGF-2 mRNA is secreted by the granulosa cells of preovulatory follicles and of those extracted after ovarian hyperstimulation.[37,38]

IGF-1 receptor expression is predominantly in granulosa cells and oocytes in dominant antral follicles. IGF-2 receptors are also expressed in the dominant follicles, localized to both the granulosa and thecal layers.[37] By reverse transcription–polymerase chain reaction analysis, both types of receptors are also noted in the stromal components of the ovary.[38] Growth hormone receptor deficiency does not interfere with abilιty to ovulate, maintain fertility, and respond to superovulation, suggesting that IGF-1 action is not necessary for the ovulatory process in women.[39]

The predominant ligand produced by the human ovary is IGF-2. Most of the studies of IGF effects on ovarian function and steroidogenesis, however, have been done with IGF-1. IGF-1 stimulates DNA synthesis and estrogen secretion by granulosa and luteal cells. Like insulin it inhibits IGFBP-1 production and acts synergistically with gonadotropins to augment estrogen and progesterone production.[38,39] In more recent studies, IGF-2 stimulates basal progesterone and estrogen secretion as well as aromatization of androgens. Similar to insulin and IGF-1, IGF-2 has been shown to inhibit IGFBP-1 production. Both IGF-1 and IGF-2 act on human thecal cells in vitro to enhance androgen production.[9,40]

IGFBPs are a family of homologous proteins that regulate bioavailability of the IGFs and, therefore, play an important role in regulating their actions. There are 6 IGFBPs, IGFBP-1 through IGFBP-6. Although all of the IGFBPs have been shown to inhibit IGF action by limiting their bioavailability, IGFBP-1 and IGFBP-3 can also have a stimulatory effect by forming a pool of slow-release IGFs. A subset of the IGFBPs also has IGF-independent actions, such as inhibition of DNA synthesis and alteration of cellular motility.[41]

IGFBPs are expressed by granulosa and thecal cells and are present in FF in most species. In situ hybridization studies have shown distinct patterns of IGFBP mRNA expression in the ovary.[42] For example, IGFBP-1 is expressed only in granulosa cells of dominant follicles; IGFBP-2 is expressed in granulosa cells of small antral follicles; and IGFBP-3 is expressed in the theca layer of all follicles and the granulosa layer of dominant follicles. Furthermore, production of each IGFBP by granulosa cells is uniquely regulated. IGFBP-1 is inhibited by follicle-stimulating hormone (FSH), insulin, IGF-1, and IGF-2 and increased by luteinizing hormone (LH), epidermal growth factor, prostaglandins, and phorbol esters. IGFBP-2 production, however, is negatively regulated by LH.[40,43–45]

IGFBPs that are found in FF may be produced locally in the ovary or may have originated in other organs, such as the liver. There are differential patterns of IGFBP levels in FF in androgen-dominant and estrogen-dominant FF.[46,47] FF obtained after hyperstimualtion with menopausal gonadotropins followed by hCG has demonstrated a distinct pattern of IGFBP production, suggesting that the hormonal milieu regulates the pattern of IGFBP expression.[48]

IGFBP proteases are a superfamily of proteins that regulate IGFBP levels. They include several classes of proteases, including metalloproteinases, kallikreins, and cathepsins. IFGBP proteases are specific for IGFBP substrates. IGFBP-3 is most susceptible to proteolysis whereas IGFBP-1 is most resistant.[49] IGFBP proteases activate partial degradation of the IGFBPs, leading to affinity for IGF proteins. This, in turn, allows increased binding to and activation of the IGF receptors. The relationships between the various components of the insulin-related ovarian regulatory system is shown in **Fig. 2**.

Reproductive Phenotypes with Altered Insulin Signaling

The importance of insulin action in female reproductive function is suggested by the preservation of this effect in various species. Mutations in the insulin and the related

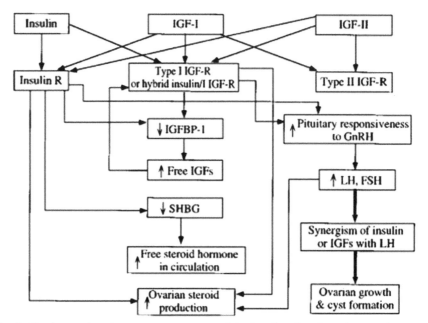

Fig. 2. The interactions between components of the insulin-related ovarian regulatory system, which involves insulin, IGF-I, IGF-II, and their receptors and IGFBPs.

IGF-1 pathways have repeatedly resulted in alterations of the female hypothalamic-pituitary-gonadal axis. In *Caenorhabditis elegans*, mutations in the insulin/IGF-1 receptor homolog, DAF-2, induce developmental arrest in the dauer stage with reduced fertility.[50] Mutations in the *Drosophila* IRS protein, CHICO, cause female sterility accompanied by reduced growth and increased lipid storage.[51] In mammals, female IRS-2 null mice are sterile. They have small anovulatory ovaries. The ovaries are resistant to superovulation with gonadotropins, suggesting an intrinsic ovarian defect. In addition, there seem be central abnormalities, because the pituitary size is decreased and expression of LH is low in these animals.[52] Female mice with neuron-specific insulin receptor knockout have impaired follicular maturation secondary to altered hypothalamic control of LH secretion.[53] Reconstitution of the brain, liver, and pancreas insulin signaling in insulin receptor knockout mice rescues the mice from neonatal death, prevents diabetes, and restores reproductive function.[54] Despite this evidence that insulin/IGF-1 is important in the proper development and functioning of the reproductive system, the exact mechanism by which these pathways regulate gonadal function remains elusive.

OVULATORY FUNCTION IN TYPE 1 DIABETES MELLITUS AND TYPE 2 DIABETES MELLITUS
Type 2 Diabetes Mellitus

Given the role of insulin in ovarian physiology (discussed previously), it is not surprising that irregular menstrual cycles or anovulatory cycles have been associated with both type 1 diabetes mellitus and type 2 diabetes mellitus. In type 2 diabetes mellitus, it is difficult to dissect how much the confounding obesity or insulin resistance contributes to development of oligomenorrhea. Pima Indians have one of the highest rates of type 2 diabetes mellitus and obesity among ethnic populations. A cross-sectional study in nonpregnant women showed a significantly higher prevalence of type 2 diabetes mellitus in women with menstrual irregularities. When adjusted for body mass index (BMI), however, this difference was no longer significant. A higher rate of diabetes was most strongly correlated in the least obese quartile of women with anovulatory cycles. This relationship persisted with adjustment for age and BMI but was no longer significant when adjusted for waist-to-hip ratio.[55] Thus, the presence of obesity or abnormal fat distribution makes it difficult to assess the true relationship between ovulation and type 2 diabetes mellitus. The importance of insulin resistance, independent of obesity and hyperglycemia, in ovulatory function has also been shown. Lean, euglycemic mice with varying degrees of hyperinsulinemia demonstrate abnormal estrous cycles and follicular development in comparison with wild-type counterparts.[56]

The prospective Nurses Health Study II showed an increased risk of developing type 2 diabetes mellitus in women with irregular menstrual cycles. The relative risk was greater in women with higher BMI but was also persistent in nonobese women.[57] A large prospective study in the Netherlands similarly demonstrated increased prevalence of hyperglycemia in women with menstrual irregularities but no increase in risk of hypertension, hyperlipidemia, or inflammatory markers. This cohort was also shown to have 28% increased risk of developing coronary heart disease in comparison with women with regular cycles.[58]

Until recently, adolescents were not commonly diagnosed with type 2 diabetes mellitus and insulin resistance. Studies have shown, however, that those who have a history of premature puberty are at higher risk of ultimately developing hyperinsulinemia and type 2 diabetes mellitus. They are also at higher risk of developing truncal and general obesity.[59–62] Additionally, the earliest clinical change in patients who develop

PCOS may be premature puberty. It is important, therefore, to serially assess the metabolic status of these patients.[63]

Type 1 Diabetes Mellitus

Menstrual dysfunction has been extensively studied in patients with type 1 diabetes mellitus. Historically, before the discovery of insulin (discussed previously), young girls with type 1 diabetes mellitus failed to develop menarche. Early studies after insulin became more widely available, continued to report delays in the age of onset of menstruation in comparison with nondiabetic girls. Bergqvist and colleagues[64] in 1954 reported an average age of menarche of 13.9 years in nondiabetic patients versus 15.0 in diabetic girls. In 1982, Djursing and colleagues[65] reported that menarche occurred 1 year later in diabetic girls. This difference, however, was not found statistically significant.

Since the introduction of intensive diabetes treatment after the Diabetes Control and Complications Trial, such differences have been greatly reduced. Recent studies, however, indicate a persistent delay in age of menarche in adolescents with type 1 diabetes mellitus despite the advancements in diabetes treatment. A large cross-sectional study showed a later age of menarche in girls with type 1 diabetes mellitus than in normoglycemic peers (12.92 ± 0.09 vs 12.32 ± 0.18; $P = .0062$). Although those with higher BMI had earlier onset of menarche, there was no correlation with hemoglobin A_{1C} (HbA_{1c}) level. Similarly, there was no association of delayed menarche with episodes of diabetic ketoacidosis or hypoglycemia in the 2 years preceding menarche.[66] Similar delays in the age of menarche (12.6 ± 1.5 years vs 12.25 ± 1.4; $P = .01$) were noted in a case control study with type 1 diabetic adolescents. This delay was not influenced by BMI or HbA_{1c}.[67]

Maintenance of a functional reproductive system is reflected in the presence of regular ovulatory cycles. Menstrual irregularities, however, are common in women with type 1 diabetes mellitus. Approximately, one-third of these women have irregular cycles during their reproductive years.[66] A higher prevalence of oligomenorrhea is seen in women with poor metabolic control as indicated by HbA_{1c}.[68] Other studies in adolescents, however, have not shown an increased effect of type 1 diabetes mellitus on ovulatory function.[69] Women with type 1 diabetes have also been shown to have an earlier age of menopause in comparison to nondiabetic sisters and controls. The presence of type 1 diabetes mellitus, menstrual irregularity before the age of 30, and unilateral oophorectomy seem to independently affect age of menopause.[70]

There are many theories as to the cause of ovulatory dysfunction in women with type 1 diabetes mellitus. The data (discussed previously) suggest that although hyperglycemia likely contributes to these manifestations, other factors may be involved in the pathophysiology. States of chronic disease and physiologic stress, such as malnutrition, are associated with delayed puberty and menarche. It is possible that the metabolic stress of the onset of type 1 diabetes mellitus affects age of menarche in the girls.[66] Increased catecholamine and dopamine release during periods of hyperglycemia may also suppress LH levels. Additionally, in mice with streptozotocin-induced diabetes, there is a hypogonadotrophic supresssion of LH and FSH. The mechanism for this effect is believed to involve abnormal gonadotropin-releasing hormone (GnRH) secretion.[71]

A subset of women with type 1 diabetes mellitus also seems to develop a hyperandrogenic state with oligomenorrhea similar to PCOS, a disease typically associated with insulin resistance. Clinical hyperandrogenism is noted in as many as 30% to 40% women with type 1 diabetes mellitus. Moreover, ultrasonographic evidence of polycystic ovaries is seen in 40% to 50% of adult type 1 diabetic women but only in

13% of age-matched nondiabetic controls. The number of women using intensive in-sulin treatment was higher in women with evidence of PCOS.[72,73] It is hypothesized that this syndrome results from exogenous hyperinsulinemia due to intensive glucose control regimens. Under physiologic conditions, the insulin produced by the pancreas undergoes first-pass metabolism through the liver. This eliminates 50% to 70% of insulin secreted by the pancreas. Type 1 diabetic patients do not experience this first-pass metabolism and thus have higher systemic insulin levels for similar glucose control. This may explain the high prevalence of the syndrome in type 1 diabetic women.[72,73]

The PCOS in type 1 diabetic women, however, differs from that in nondiabetic patients. There is a less pronounced hirsuitism and, although total testosterone and androstenedione levels are increased, SHBG, gonadotropin, estradiol and dehydro-epiandrosterone sulfate (DHEAS) levels remain within the normal range. Portal insulin levels are important in down-regulation of SHBG synthesis. Because exogenous insu-lin does not reach high levels in the portal circulation, SHBG levels are not suppressed and, thus, free testosterone levels are not elevated. These changes are not associated with degree of glucose control. Therefore, it is unlikely that hyperglycemia plays a causative role in the PCOS presentation. Moreover, during adolescence, there is an increased degree of weight gain, fat mass, and insulin resistance that may also play a role in development of hyperandrogemia and oligomenorrhea in this age group.[71,73] There are to date no conclusive studies as to the best modality of treatment of the PCOS presentation in type 1 diabetic women.

SYNDROMES OF EXTREME INSULIN RESISTANCE

As discussed previously, syndromes of insulin resistance spanning the gamut of mild to severe have been associated with both hyperandrogenism and female reproductive abnormalities and infertility. Some of the rare forms of extreme insulin resistance/hyperinsulinemia are reviewed first. Severe insulin resistance is defined as fasting plasma insulin levels above 50 µU/mL to 70 µU/mL or peak (post–oral glucose toler-ance test [OGTT]) insulin levels above 350 µU/mL.[74] Some of the hyperinsulinemic dis-orders that report insulin levels in this range are due to genetic mutations in the insulin receptor gene, such as type A syndrome, leprechaunism, and Rabson-Mendenhall syndrome. In other syndromes, antibodies against the insulin receptor can be detected as in the type B syndrome.[75]

Despite the differing mechanisms of decreased insulin action, these syndromes of severe insulin resistance share similar clinical manifestations. There are both symp-toms resulting from deficiency of insulin action at target organs and those resulting from high levels of circulating insulin. Insulin resistance at traditional target organs, such as the liver, and fat can lead to impaired glucose homeostasis and varying de-grees of lipoatrophy. The diabetes in these patients can often be resistant to insulin action, requiring at times thousands of units of insulin daily to lower glucose levels. In syndromes that result from autoantibodies to the insulin receptor, however, hypo-glycemia can result from activation of the insulin receptor by a stimulating antibody clone.[74,75]

The presence of acanthosis nigricans and ovarian hyperandrogenism has been attributed to the severe hyperinsulinemia. Acanthosis nigricans is a hyperpigmented lesion that usually occurs in the back of the neck and in the axilla. It is characterized by hyperkeratosis and epidermal papillomatosis. Acanthosis is present in all congenital syndromes of severe insulin resistance and is correlated with the degree of hyperinsu-linemia. The exact mechanism leading to acanthosis nigricans has not been fully delineated. It is attributed in part to insulin binding to IGF-1 receptors.[75] Hyperandrogenism is a common feature in women with extreme insulin resistance syndromes. Studies suggest an ovarian source of hyperandrogenism rather than an adrenal source. Taylor and coworkers reported that only premenopausal women with type B syndrome develop hyperandrogenism.[76,77] Subsequently, selective catheterization of the adrenal and ovarian veins showed significantly higher androgen levels in ovarian veins than in adrenal veins. Fasting insulin levels are correlated with ovarian volume. High levels of insulin have also been shown to stimulate androgen-producing cells in the ovary.[75,78]

Although a correlation between insulin resistance and hyperandrogenism has been established, it is debated which of these states develops first. Several studies support the hypothesis that hyperandrogenism leads to insulin resistance.[75] Givens and associates[79] reported that resection of a luteoma in a PCOS patient led to the regression of acanthosis nigricans, a marker of insulin resistance. Shoupe and Lobo[80] showed that antagonism of androgens with spironolactone leads to decreased fasting insulin levels in patients with PCOS. Insulin resistance is a common occurrence during puberty, suggesting that sex hormones contribute to this state.[81] Other studies, however, fail to support the role of hyperandrogenism in the development of insulin resistance. Administration of androgens does not affect insulin sensitivity in normal men.[82] Billiar and colleagues[83] demonstrated that sustained levels of hyperandrogenism in female monkeys did not alter insulin sensitivity. The effect of insulin resistance on development of hyperandrogenism is discussed later in the section on PCOS.

Because of the presence of extreme insulin resistance, it is a challenge to successfully treat these patients. Diet and exercise have less efficacy in patients with extreme insulin resistance than in typical type 2 diabetes mellitus patients. Insulin sensitizers, including metformin and thiazolidinediones, have been shown to improve glycemia in type B syndrome and lipoatrophic diabetes.[74,75] Insulin, despite use of high doses, often fails to provide adequate glycemic control. Similarly, sulfonylureas have shown limited benefit in this patient population.[74] A few studies have looked at the effects of IGF-1 administration on glycemic control. Although short-term improvements in metabolic parameters were seen in several syndromes of severe insulin resistance, longer-term trials failed to show sustained improvements. Additionally, IGF-1 administration can be associated with side effects, such as fluid retention, carpal tunnel syndrome, and jaw pain. There is also some concern that IGF-1 may increase the risk of retinopathy and breast and prostate cancers.[84] In patients with autoantibody-mediated insulin resistance, such as type B syndrome, immunomodulation has been explored as a modality of treatment. One suggested combination is short-term suppression with plasmapheresis and cyclophosphamide, with longer-term maintenance using cyclosporin A and azathioprine.[74,75]

POLYCYSTIC OVARY SYNDROME

Milder states of insulin resistance have also been associated with abnormalities of female fertility. The Stein-Leventhal syndrome was described as a combination of "enlarged sclerotic ovaries" associated with obesity, hirsuitism, irregular menstruation, and infertility.[7,85] PCOS may be defined by 1 of 3 sets of criteria. Of the 3, the definition most commonly used was adapted by the National Institutes of Health (NIH), which defines PCOS by the presence of (1) hyperandrogenism, (2) ovulatory dysfunction, and (3) exclusion of disorders, such as hyperprolactinemia, thyroid disorders, and congenital adrenal hyperplasia. The Rotterdam criteria, alternatively, require the presence of 2 of the 3 following conditions: hyperandrogenism, ovulatory dysfunction, and polycystic ovaries on ultrasound. In 2005, the Androgen Excess and PCOS Society put forth a third set of consensus criteria that define PCOS as the presence of hyperandrogenism, along with either or both ovarian dysfunction and polycystic ovaries.[86,87]

Prevalence

The prevalence of PCOS ranges from 4% to 10% of the female population. The differences in criteria used to diagnose PCOS likely account for the variability in analyzing studies related to PCOS. Use of the Rotterdam criteria rather than the NIH criteria leads to the identification of 2 to 5 times larger cohort of women with this diagnosis.[7] It is intriguing that a disease that actually decreases female fertility would have such a high prevalence rate within the general population. In genome-wide searches, many of the genes associated with or linked to PCOS fall within the category of metabolism and downstream targets of insulin action. Some of these genes lead to the thrifty phenotype, a group of cellular and physiologic changes that gear the body to conserve energy. This may have provided survival advantage during periods of famine, flooding, or other conditions that decrease food sources.[88] The PCOS phenotype may also have conferred economic and health advantages by providing fewer family members to feed at a time of contraceptive unavailability and by spacing children to ease the burden on the mother's health.

Clinical Presentation

The clinical signs and symptoms of PCOS are varied; 60% of women have evidence of hirsuitism (increased hair growth), acne, and alopecia. Clinically, this syndrome is accompanied by oligomenorrhea or anovulatory cycles and signs of insulin resistance, such as acanthosis nigricans. These velvety hyperkeratotic plaques are directly correlated with the degree of insulin resistance.[7] PCOS is strongly associated with metabolic and cardiovascular diseases outside of the reproductive axis. Obesity is strongly correlated with PCOS, with prevalence ranging between 30% and 75 % in some series.[89,90] Women in the United States tend to have higher body weight than European counterparts. Visceral adiposity, as measured by increased waist circumference or waist-to-hip ratio, has been linked to hyperandrogenism, insulin resistance, and glucose intolerance; 30% to 40 % of women with PCOS have impaired glucose tolerance and as many as 10% have type 2 diabetes mellitus by their fourth decade. Dunaif and colleagues[91] demonstrated that women with PCOS have greater insulin resistance than normal women, even when matched for BMI and body fat distribution.[89]

Hypertension develops in some women with PCOS early during the reproductive years. This is often accompanied by reduced vascular compliance and endothelial dysfunction.[92] Insulin-lowering therapy seems to improve endothelial function.[93] Women with PCOS also have an increased prevalence of macrovascular disease and thrombosis. Lipid changes reflect increased triglycerides and decreased high-density lipoprotein, the pattern most frequently seen in insulin resistance and type 2 diabetes mellitus.[89] Women with PCOS additionally have an increased risk of endometrial hyperplasia and cancer. This is likely due to prolonged stimulation of endometrial tissue by estrogen without opposing progesterone effects. Breast and ovarian cancer have also been variably associated with PCOS.[94]

Biochemical and Laboratory Testing

Biochemically PCOS is associated with elevated androgens (total and free testosterone) in 80% to 90% of cases. DHEAS can also be elevated in 25% of women with polycystic ovaries. These biochemical changes are frequently associated with decreased SHBG levels, resulting in elevated free testosterone with normal to mildly elevated total testosterone levels. Changes in steroid hormone levels are accompanied by alterations in gonadotropins. It is believed that increased responsiveness of gonadotropins to GnRH leads to increased amplitude and pulse frequency of LH secretion. This effect is independent of obesity in PCOS patients. Increased LH levels lead to ovarian thecal hypertrophy and subsequently increased androgen production. FSH levels, alternatively, are normal to low, resulting in an increased LH-to-FSH ratio. This phenomenon is due to negative feedback from estrogen, aromatized from increased amounts of testosterone.[87,95,96]

Pathophysiology

Insulin resistance is strongly correlated with PCOS. Euglycemic hyperinsulinemic glucose clamp studies have demonstrated significant reduction in insulin mediated glucose disposal in PCOS subjects, independent of obesity.[87] Thus, lean PCOS patients have greater insulin resistance than lean normal counterparts. Increased body fat has a synergistic negative effect on insulin sensistivity.[90] Insulin reistance may influence PCOS pathology through insulin's direct actions on the ovary. As discussed previously, in vitro studies have shown stimulation of androgen production by incubation of ovarian thecal cells with insulin.[16] Moreover, exposure of ovaries to insulin and hCG synergistically leads to ovarian growth and cyst formation (**Fig. 3**).[87,97]

Hyperinsulinemia and obesity are both also associated with a state of low-grade inflammation.[98] Elevations are noted in cytokines (interleukin [IL]-6 and tumor necrosis factor [TNF]-α), chemokines (IL-18 and monocyte chemoattractant protein [MCP]-1) and adipokines (leptin and resistin). Systematic inflammation is believed to lead to recruitment of macrophages to the adipose tissue.[99] Long-term consequences of the increased inflammatory state include increased risk of development of hypertension, dyslipidemia, and endothelial dysfunction. Endothelial dysfunction is partially due to inhibitory effects of cytokines on expression and activity of *endothelial nitric oxide synthase*, decreasing *nitric oxide* synthesis and vasodilation.[98]

Insulin resistance is noted in 50% to 70% of PCOS patients. It is not surprising, then, that positive correlations have also been noted between PCOS and elevated cytokines, such as C-reactive protein, IL-18, and TNF-α. Markers of lymphocytic and monocytic activation, such as IL-6, MCP-1, and *migration inhibitory factor*, have also been correlated with PCOS. Moreover, insulin sensitizer use has decreased these inflammatory markers.[100] PCOS has also been associated with adhesion molecules and markers of endothelial dysfunction, such as soluble intercellular adhesion molecule 1 and soluble vascular adhesion molecule 1. These markers have been correlated with both the degree of insulin resistance and hyperandrogenemia.[98]

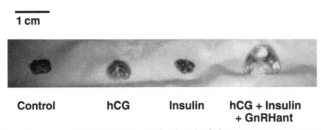

1 cm

| Control | hCG | Insulin | hCG + Insulin + GnRHant |

Fig. 3. Insulin acts as a co-gonadotropin at the level of the ovary. Greater ovarian growth and cyst formation is seen after 23 days of combined hCG, insulin, and GnRH antagonist (GnRHant) injections than insulin or hCG alone in Sprague-Dawley rats. Normal saline served as the control injection.

In vitro data show that TNF-α stimulates proliferation and androgen production by thecal cells. TNF-α has also been shown to be synergistic with similar effects of insulin and IGF-1.[101,102] II-6, another cytokine, stimulates adrenal cells in vitro, increasing adrenal androgen steroidogenesis.[103] Alternatively, androgens may stimulate low-grade inflammation through their effects on adipocyte biology. Androgens stimulate adipocyte hypertrophy and differentiation of preadipocytes into mature adipocytes.[104] Androgens also increase lipolysis, leading to increased flux of free fatty acids into circulation.[105]

Insulin may directly affect the pituitary gland by increasing gonadotroph sensitivity to GnRH. This has been demonstrated in several in vitro studies with cultured pituitary cells.[106,107] Moreover, treatment of PCOS with insulin sensitizers decreases LH levels. Insulin also alters several key regulators of signal transduction and function in the ovary. Studies in hyperinsulinemic experimental animals and women with PCOS show decreased insulin receptors, but increased IGF-1 receptors in the ovary.[108,109] As discussed previously, insulin additionally inhibits IGFBP-1 production, leading to higher circulating and intraovarian levels of free IGF-1. Furthermore, insulin not only increases the expression of peroxisome-proliferator-activated receptor γ (PPAR-γ) in vitro in ovarian cells but also activates the steroidogenic acute regulatory protein (StAR) protein, through which PPAR-γ enhances steroidogenesis (**Fig. 4**).[87]

Treatment of PCOS

PCOS is manifested by a conglomeration of symptoms that have been previously reviewed. These include hyperandrogenism, anovulation or oligomenorrhea, infertility,

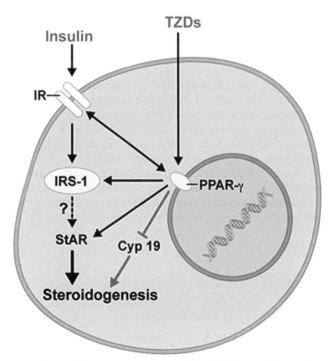

Fig. 4. After interaction with its own receptor, insulin stimulates StAR protein expression via activation of insulin signaling cascade protein, IRS-1. Insulin can also amplify StAR protein expression by activation of PPAR-γ expression. StAR protein expression leads to steroidogenesis in human ovarian cells.

and insulin resistance or elevations of glucose. The treatment armamentarium for PCOS addresses one or more of these manifestations of PCOS; they are reviewed sequentially. Because of the complexity of the topic of ovulation induction, however, it is reviewed separately in this article.

One of the defining clinical signs of PCOS is hyperandrogenism. Hirsuitism can be addressed with depilatories, shaving, waxing, and electrolysis. Antiandrogenic agents can also be utilized. The most commonly used agent is spironolactone, an antimineralocorticoid with antiandrogenic activity. Others in this category include cyproterone acetate (a competitive inhibitor of testosterone and 5α-dihydrotestosterone binding to the androgen receptor), flutamide (a nonsteroidal antiandrogen), and finasteride (a 5α-reductase activity inhibitor). These agents can have feminizing effects on the male fetus and thus should be avoided in pregnancy.[89,110]

Oral contraceptives (OCPs) can also reduce hyperandrogenism by direct negative feedback on LH secretion, resulting in reduced androgen production by thecal cells. OCPs also stimulate the production of SHBG by the liver, leading to decreased free testosterone levels.[89,110] In choosing an OCP, it is advisable to select a progestin with low androgenic potential, such as norethindrone, desogestrel, norgestimate, and drosperinone. There are conflicting data as to whether drospirenone is associated with increased risk of venous thromboembolism.[111–114]

Insulin sensitizers, such as metformin and thiazolidinediones, are effective agents in reducing circulating androgen levels. Metformin is a biguanide that functions by activating adenosine monophosphate–activated protein kinase. This results in decreased hepatic gluconeogenesis and increased insulin sensitivity.[115,116] Metformin's effect on hormonal changes in PCOS is mediated through its systemic effects on hyperinsulinemia and insulin sensitivity.[87] Thiazolidinediones are PPAR-γ agonists. They improve insulin sensitivity at the level of the skeletal muscle and adipocytes. Thiazolidinediones also have direct effects on ovarian steroid production, independent of improvement in insulin resistance.[79]

Several of these agents, in addition to lowering androgen levels, have greater metabolic and hormonal effects that decrease insulin resistance and improve ovulation rates in women. Prior to prescribing medications, however, a trial of lifestyle changes and weight management is an acceptable option. Reductions of 5% to 10% in weight can improve hyperinsulinemia, circulating androgens, ovulation, and pregnancy rate. Even more modest weight loss of 2% to 5% can restore ovulation. Very low calorie diets (350 kcal/d) for 4 weeks can reduce fasting insulin and free testosterone levels.[117,118] Surgical weight loss with gastric banding, gastroplasty, or Roux-en-Y gastric bypass can also be considered. In a group of 12 patients with PCOS, bariatric surgery restored regular menstrual cycles in all patients. In a group of 17 patients with PCOS, weight loss surgery led to improvement in ovulation rates, insulin resistance, and hyperandrogenism in 12 months.[110,119] It is postulated that the primary mechanism by which weight loss improves reproductive outcomes is by reduction of circulating insulin levels.[118]

Insulin sensitizers are not only important in improving hyperinsulinemia, insulin sensitivity, glucose dysregulation, and dyslipidemia but also in ameliorating the low-grade inflammatory state seen in insulin resistance and PCOS.[98,100] Changes in systemic metabolic parameters and direct insulin effects in the ovary lead to improved ovulation rates and normalization of hormonal changes with the use of metformin.[120] A study comparing pioglitazone and metformin in obese PCOS patients showed similar improvements in insulin resistance.[121]

Thiazolidinediones have also been shown to improve dyslipidemia and have beneficial effects on proinflammatory and prothrombotic markers, such as TNF-α, plasminogen activator inhibitor type 1, and IL-6.[122] Thiazolidinediones have both direct ovarian effects, mediated through the PPAR-γ and the StAR protein, and indirect effects, mediated via insulin-independent action on the ovary (**Table 1**). Insulin-independent effects result in increased progesterone production and lower testosterone and estradiol levels. Decreased total and free testosterone with increased SHBG levels result from systemic changes in insulin levels induced by thiazolidinediones.[87,123,124] In comparison with metformin, thiazolidinediones have similar effects on ovulation rates.[121] There are caveats with the use of thiazolidinediones, however. Rosiglitazone has been reported to be associated with increased risk of myocardial infarction.[125] There may be an increased risk of bladder cancer with the use of pioglitazone.[126] Moreover, thiazolidinediones are linked to increased bone loss and risk of fractures in women with diabetes.[127] Pioglitazone and rosiglitazone may affect bone metabolism by inhibiting osteoblast growth, increasing precursor differentiation into adipocytes, increasing fatty acid uptake, and reducing both alkaline phosphatase and osteocalcin activity.[128]

Glucagon-like peptide-1 (GLP-1) agonists are also being studied in PCOS patients. These agents enhance glucose-dependent insulin secretion, delay gastric emptying, and reduce appetite. A recent study compared exenatide versus metformin versus combination therapy in obese PCOS patients for 24 weeks. Higher ovulation rates were seen in the exenatide and combination groups: exenatide (50%), metformin (29%), and combination (86%). Greater weight loss was also noted in the exenatide and combination groups.[129]

When monotherapy is not effective, combination therapies can be considered. Comparison of metformin and OCP (ethinyl estradiol–cyproterone acetate) versus OCP showed greater decrease in androstenedione and increase in SHBG levels. There was, however, greater increase in cholesterol with the OCP alone group.[86,130] Similarly, rosiglitazone and OCP showed greater decrease in androgen levels and increase in SHBG. Here, combination therapy resulted in higher decreased high-density lipoprotein levels than monotherapy.[87,131]

Ovulation Induction in PCOS

PCOS is a major cause of subfertility in the United States. To conceive, many women require ovulation induction or in vitro fertilization (IVF). The treatment options for induction of ovulation are reviewed. Clomiphene citrate is a synthetic triphenylethyne, a

Table 1	
Effects of thiazolidinediones in ovarian function	
Direct: Can be Observed in Vitro; may be Present in Vivo	**Indirect: Observed in Vivo; are due to Systemic Insulin-sensitizing Action and Reduction of Hyperinsulinemia**
Insulin independent	
↑ Progesterone	↓ Testosterone
↓ Testosterone	↑ IGFBP-1
↓ Estradiol	↑ SHBG
↑ IGFBP-1 (in the absence of insulin)	↓ Free testosterone
Insulin sensitizing (enhanced insulin effect)	
↓ IGFBP-1 production	
↑ Estradiol production (in vivo, in a setting of high-dose insulin infusion)	

partial estrogen receptor antagonist with antiestrogenic effects in the hypothalamus that interfere with the negative feedback from estrogen resulting in increased FSH levels, which in turn lead to follicular growth.[87,132] Because of the high rate of successful ovulation and cost effectiveness of this treatment, it is considered first-line treatment of ovulation induction. The live birth rate after 6 months of clomiphene citrate treatment ranges from 20% to 40%. There is a discrepancy between ovulation rate (60%–85%) and pregnancy rate (30%–40%). This may be due to clomiphene's antiestrogenic effects on the uterus. The risks associated with clomiphene citrate use include multiple pregnancies and ovarian hyperstimulation syndrome (OHSS).[132] In 2007, a large prospective randomized controlled trial in 626 anovulatory, infertile women with PCOS showed higher rates of live birth in the clomiphene (22.5%) or combined metformin and clomiphene group (26.8%) compared with the metformin alone group (7.2%). Currently combination therapy is recommended in the subset of patients with BMI greater than 35, glucose intolerance, and clomiphene citrate resistance.[133]

Thus, although improved pregnancy rates are seen with metformin versus placebo, no improvement is seen with live birth rates. In clomiphene-resistant patients, a combination of metformin and clomiphene citrate significantly improves ovulation and pregnancy rates but, importantly, not the rate of live births. Metformin as a single agent does not show any benefit in clomiphene-resistant patients.[110,134] Metformin, however, may improve oocyte and embryo quality in clomiphene citrate patients undergoing in IVF.[135] Thiazolidinediones enhance spontaneous and clomiphene-induced ovulation. Fetal safety for these agents has not been established, however. Thus, they should be stopped in case of pregnancy.[121]

If patients are clomiphene-resistant, in addition to insulin sensitizers several other agents can be considered for fertility treatment. Administration of exogenous FSH can be effective but is an expensive treatment option that requires frequent monitoring with estradiol levels and ultrasound.[110,118] The addition of clomiphene citrate to gonadotropins and GnRH antagonists leads to decreased rates of OHSS without evidence of effect on live birth and pregnancy.[136] Aromatase inhibitors block peripheral conversion of androgens to estrogens. This reduction in estrogens increases FSH production and optimizes ovulation. In a prospective randomized trial, no difference in pregnancy rates between letrozole and clomiphene citrate was noted. Despite concern for teratogenicity, there was no increase in incidence of malformations.[135] Another study comparing anastrazole and clomiphene citrate demonstrated thicker endometrium, fewer mature follicles, and a higher rate of pregnancy (nonsignificant) in the aromatase inhibitor arm.[137] The efficacy and safety of these agents in comparison with clomiphene citrate in achieving live births may be more definitively answered in an ongoing trial, Pregnancy in Polycystic Ovary Syndrome II (PPCOS II).[138]

If treatment with clomiphene citrate, gonadotropins, and aromatase inhibitors is not successful, in vitro fertilization is recommended. There is an increased risk of multiple gestations with this treatment. The risk decreases, however, with single embryo transfer. A meta-analysis in 2006 showed that women with PCOS undergo greater numbers of cycle cancellations and increased duration of stimulation cycle compared with the general IVF population.[139] Addition of clomiphene citrate may improve IVF outcomes.[140] Coincident use of metformin increases viable pregnancy rates and decreases OHSS.[118] Glucocorticoids, such as prednisone and dexamethasone, can suppress adrenal androgens and thus have been used to induce ovulation in women with PCOS.[110,118] Although a trial of dexamethasone use in 230 clomiphene-resistant women showed efficacy in ovulation and pregnancy rates, glucocorticoids are currently not recommended for treatment of infertility.[118,141] Surgical intervention with laparoscopic ovarian drilling (LOD) can restore ovulation in 50% of women. In clomiphene-resistant women, LOD is associated with higher pregnancy and ovulation rates that metformin. There is, however, no difference in live birth rates between LOD and either clomiphene citrate combined with metformin or gonadotropin treatment.[110,118] In addition, there is risk of developing pelvic adhesions with this procedure.

Pregnancy Complications in PCOS

Even after pregnancy is achieved, women with PCOS face greater challenges in achieving a successful outcome from the pregnancy. Rates of early pregnancy loss or miscarriage have been reported as high as 40% in these women compared with 14.3% in normal fertile women.[142,143] Possible culprits for this high rate of pregnancy loss include the use of ovulation inducing agents, elevated LH levels, increased androgen levels, insulin resistance, and obesity. Several studies also suggest poor folliculogenesis, resulting in compromised oocyte quality, as a cause for failed pregnancies.[144,145] The complex process of follicular and oocyte maturation involves cross-talk between cumulus cells and the oocyte. Gradually this develops the microenvironment that allows the oocyte to gain competence to undergo fertilization and embryogenesis. It is believed that the regulatory system governing follicular development and oocyte maturation may be altered in the setting of PCOS.

Pregnancy outcomes in PCOS are also affected by increased risk of late gestational complications. A meta-analysis showed a significantly higher rate of gestational diabetes mellitus (GDM) in women with PCOS. These women, however, also had a higher rate of obesity, which may contribute to the increased risk. Most studies indicate a higher risk of preeclampsia or hypertensive disorders in PCOS pregnancies. Many of these studies, however, are limited by small numbers of subjects. Insulin resistance in the first trimester seems to be associated with an increased risk of preeclampsia. Whether PCOS is associated with preterm birth and low birth weight in infants is unclear. These complications are associated with increased neonatal morbidity and 2.3 times higher rate of admission to the neonatal ICU for PCOS offspring. A meta-analysis indicates a 3-times higher incidence of perinatal mortality due to causes, such as cervical insufficiency, sepsis, and placental abruption.[142,143] These complications, however, are also noted with obesity, which often coexists with PCOS. No significant differences have been noted in neonatal malformations from these pregnancies.

Because diabetes and obesity often accompany PCOS, it is difficult to dissect the effects of hyperglycemia and adiposity from that of insulin resistance on follicular development and pregnancy outcomes. A recent study, however, in mouse models of varying degrees of insulin resistance in lean, euglycemic mice showed increased antral follicles, abnormal oocyte morphology, increased early pregnancy loss, and low embryonic birth weights in the insulin-resistant mice in comparison with wild type.[56] This suggests that insulin resistance or hyperinsulinemia independently affects parameters of female reproduction and gestation. It is, thus, not surprising that the insulin sensitizer, metformin, has been offered as an agent to minimize pregnancy complications. Thus far, studies and meta-analyses have not shown any adverse effects or increased risk of malformations from the use of metformin throughout pregnancy.[142] Metformin use during early pregnancy seems to decrease the rate of miscarriages and GDM in women with PCOS.[146,147] Use of metformin throughout pregnancy also reduces first-trimester miscarriages and development of diabetes in gestation.[148,149]

DIABETES IN PREGNANCY

Diabetes in pregnancy remains a significant contributor to maternal and fetal morbidity—affecting 6% to 7% of all pregnancies in the United States.[150,151] Pregnancy-related diabetes falls into 2 categories—GDM and pre-GDM. GDM, representing 85% of the cases, manifests in the second to third trimesters of pregnancy. Late gestation is a period of metabolic stress and increased insulin resistance, challenging those with susceptibility to the development of diabetes. This effect is largely attributed to placental secretion of diabetogenic hormones, including growth hormone, corticotropin-releasing hormone, placental lactogen, and corticotropin. Diabetes develops when pancreatic insulin secretion fails to overcome the physiologic insulin resistance.[150,151] This subcategory of maternal diabetes is more prevalent in certain ethnic groups, such as Asians, African Americans, Native Americans, and Hispanic individuals compared with the non-Hispanic white population. The category of pre-GDM includes preexisting type 1 diabetes mellitus and type 2 diabetes mellitus. Here, hyperglycemia is seen prior to and throughout the pregnancy. Hyperglycemia typically worsens as pregnancy progresses due to the increasingly insulin-resistant hormonal milieu (described previously).

If women do not carry the diagnosis of type 1 diabetes mellitus or type 2 diabetes mellitus, they are screened for diabetes at their first prenatal visit. If the fasting plasma glucose level is greater than 126 mg/dL or HbA_{1c} is greater than 6.5, patients are diagnosed with diabetes and managed accordingly. If the random glucose level exceeds 200 mg/dL, the diagnosis of diabetes is confirmed with an abnormal fasting glucose or HbA_{1c} level. If the initial results are negative, both the American Diabetes Association (ADA) and American Congress of Obstetricians and Gynecologists (ACOG) recommend a 2-step approach to the diagnosis of GDM. A 50-g OGTT at weeks 24 to 28 of gestation is followed by a 100-g, 3-hour OGTT if the 1-hour glucose value is greater than 140 mg/dL during the glucose challenge. Glucose values exceeding the recommended levels at 2 or more time points of the 3-hour test signify a positive result. Two different sets of diagnostic criteria for GDM with the 100-g 3-hour glucose tolerance test have been proposed. The Expert Committee on the Diagnosis and Classification of Diabetes Mellitus and the National Diabetes Data Group (NDDG) have proposed threshold values of 105 mg/dL, 190 mg/dL, 165 mg/dL, and 140 mg/dL at baseline and the hourly testing time points, respectively. The Fourth International Workshop-Conference on Gestational Diabetes has proposed lower threshold values based on the Carpenter and Coustan modifications: 95 mg/dL, 180 mg/dL, 155 mg/dL, and 140 mg/dL at baseline, 1, 2, and 3 hours after glucose challenge.[152] Internationally, however, a 1-step approach is widely practiced using a 75-g OGTT with 2-hour venous sampling. The World Health Organization (WHO) recommends a diagnosis of diabetes if the fasting glucose level is greater than 125 mg/dL or the 2-hour value is greater than 140 mg/dL. The International Association of Diabetes and Pregnancy Study Groups (IADPSG) and the ADA present slightly different cutoff values at fasting, 1-hour, and 2-hour time points (**Table 2**). Early screening for GDM is recommended in women with strong risk factors, including obesity, family history of diabetes, personal history of GDM, prior stillbirth, and neonate weight greater than 4500 g.[150,151]

Once a diagnosis of diabetes is ascertained, it is important to counsel those with both GDM and pre-GDM about the increased risk of adverse outcomes for both mother and fetus. Pre-GDM, both type 1 and type 2, can lead to difficulties with fertilization and progression of early pregnancy. Diabetes may affect development of oocyte competence by altering mitchondrial function and altering cell-to-cell interactions between the cumulus cells and the oocyte.[153] Periconceptional hyperglycemia

Table 2				
Positive screening criteria for gestational diabetes mellitus				
	2-h 75-g WHO	OGTT IADPSG	3-h 100-g Carpenter/Couston	OGTT NDDG
Fasting	125 mg/dL	92 mg/dL	95 mg/dL	105 mg/dL
1 h		180 mg/dL	180 mg/dL	190 mg/dL
2 h	140 mg/dL	153 mg/dL	155 mg/dL	165 mg/dL
3 h			140 mg/dL	145 mg/dL

can significantly alter organogenesis and lead to malformations in the fetus.[154] Congenital malformations have a 4-fold to 10-fold higher incidence in diabetic pregnancies. The most common abnormalities are found in the cardiovascular, central nervous system, gastrointestinal system, urinary tract, caudal regression syndrome, and cleft and palate deformities.

Both gestational and pre-GDM conveys an increased risk of developing preeclampsia, miscarriage, and cesarean delivery. Miscarriage occurs at a 3-fold to 5-fold higher rate in diabetic pregnancies than in normal gestations. Fetal outcomes show increased risk of macrosomia, organomegaly, and neonatal respiratory and metabolic complications, such as hypoglycemia, hypocalcemia, and hyperbilirubinemia.[155,156] Longer-term effects on the children from diabetic pregnancies may include increased risk of childhood obesity and development of diabetes (**Table 3**).[157–159]

The precise mechanism by which hyperglycemia exerts its teratogenic effects is not fully known. Several theories have been proposed. First, glucose is freely transportable

Table 3				
Effects of glucose dysregulation on female reproductive function				
	Insulin Resistance	Type 1 Diabetes Mellitus	Type 2 Diabetes Mellitus	Gestational Diabetes Mellitus
Puberty	Premature menarche	Delayed menarche	Premature menarche	
Ovulation	Anovulatory cycles Hyperandrogenism Acanthosis nigricans	Anovulatory cycles Hyperandrogenism	Anovulatory cycles Hyperandrogenism Acanthosis nigricans	
Pregnancy	Decreased fertility	Decreased fertility	Decreased fertility	
Maternal	Preeclampsia Miscarriage Cesarean delivery GDM	Preeclampsia Miscarriage Cesarean delivery	Preeclampsia Miscarriage Cesarean delivery	Preeclampsia Miscarriage Cesarean delivery
Fetal	Preterm birth Low birth weight Neonatal mortality	Macrosomia Organomegaly Respiratory complications Hypoglycemia Hyperbilirubinemia Shoulder dystocia Congenital anomalies Malformations	Macrosomia Organomegaly Respiratory complications Hypoglycemia Hyperbilirubinemia Shoulder dystocia Congenital anomalies Malformations	Macrosomia Organomegaly Respiratory complications Hypoglycemia Hyperbilirubinemia Shoulder dystocia

across the placenta. Hyperglycemia or the resultant hyperinsulinemia in the embryo may mediate some of these effects. For example, the heart has high levels of insulin receptors. Hypertrophic myopathy can be seen in newborns from diabetic mothers that, at times, regresses after birth. Excess insulin can also delay pulmonary maturation by decreased surfactant production. A second theory suggests that generation of reactive oxygen species leads to damage of the developing yolk sac. Epigenetic changes in diabetic pregnancies may also affect organogenesis and fetus viability.

Because of the high rate of complications in the setting of hyperglycemia, the ADA currently recommends stricter glycemic control, with an HbA_{1c} goal of less than 6.0%, prior to conception and throughout pregnancy. The importance of glucose control in improving pregnancy outcomes was demonstrated in 2 large prospective randomized controlled trials.[151] The Australian Carbohydrate Intolerance Study in Pregnant Women is a multicenter, 10-year study conducted in 14 sites in Australia, evaluating the benefits of glucose control in mild GDM in 1000 women.[160] Treatment was associated with a significant reduction in the primary outcome of perinatal complications (including perinatal death, shoulder dystocia, and birth trauma), with an adjusted relative risk of 0.33% and 95% CI of 0.14–0.75. In secondary outcomes, treatment did reduce the rate of large for gestational age neonates and maternal preeclampsia but failed to show differences in rates of neonatal hypoglycemia, jaundice, or respiratory difficulties. A second study evaluating treatment of mild GDM in 958 women was conducted by the National Institute of Child Health and Human Development Maternal-Fetal Medicine Units. The primary outcomes of perinatal death, neonatal hypoglycemia, and elevated cord C-peptide did not show any significant differences between the 2 groups. There was an improvement in secondary outcomes, however, including lower frequency of fetal overgrowth, development of neonatal fat, risk of shoulder dystocia, cesarean delivery, and preeclampsia.[161]

The initial approach to treatment of diabetes in pregnancy consists of lifestyle counseling and dietary changes. The recommendations include a diet of 2000 kcal to 2500 kcal daily intake, with carbohydrates comprising 33% to 40% of calories.[162,163] Three meals and 2 to 3 snacks allow distribution of glucose intake without significant elevations in postprandial glucose excursions. The Institute of Medicine recommends a weight gain of 5 kg to 19 kg dependent on the maternal pregestational BMI.[164] Although regular exercise improves insulin resistance and is recommended as an adjunct to dietary changes, studies evaluating exercise in GDM have shown mixed results.[165]

Daily self–glucose monitoring is an important component of diabetes management in pregnancy. The ADA recommends target glucose values of fasting less than 95 mg/dL, 1-hour postprandial less than 140 mg/dL, and 2-hour postprandial less than 120 mg/dL. The ACOG recommends fasting glucose less than 95 mg/dL, 1-hour postprandial less than 130 mg/dL to 140 mg/dL, and 2-hour postprandial less than 120 mg/dL. Approximately 25% of women with GDM require medication. The mainstay of treatment has been the use of neutral protamine Hagedorn (NPH) and regular insulin to provide basal and bolus dosing. The newer classes of insulin analogs, although widespread in practice in the general population, must be used with caution in the pregnant diabetic woman. The insulin analogs have alterations in the amino acid sequence or post-translational modification that lead to decreased or increased affinity for the IGF-1 receptor. IGF-1 is a critical player in embryo maturation, implantation, and pregnancy progression. Therefore, well-controlled, randomized, and long-term studies are needed to assure the safety of using insulin analogs in pregnancy.[166]

The first study to indicate the safety and efficacy of insulin lispro was published in 1999.[167] Lispro was successful in lowering postprandial glucose excursions and

HbA$_{1c}$ levels similar to regular insulin while producing fewer episodes of hypoglycemia. Similarly, in a large clinical trial with 213 patients randomized to receive either lispro or regular insulin, no significant differences were noted in maternal or fetal outcomes.[168,169] There is some concern that although insulin does not seem to cross the placental barrier, insulin bound to immunoglobulin can do so and potentially lead to diabetic fetopathy. In both of these studies, however, lispro was not associated with a greater increase in anti-insulin antibody levels. Short-acting insulin aspart was introduced in 1999. Initial studies suggest the safety and efficacy of this insulin analog for use in women with GDM.[170–172] Higher patient satisfaction was noted with the short-acting insulin analogs in comparison with regular insulin use.

Insulin detemir and insulin glargine are long-acting insulin analogs, the latter with a 6-fold increase in affinity for IGF-1 receptor in comparison with human insulin.[166] There have not yet been extensive randomized controlled trials in pregnant women with either of these agents. A meta-analysis of observational studies, including 331 pregnancies with use of glargine during the first, second, or third trimester, did not show any increase in adverse fetal and maternal outcomes with glargine versus NPH insulin. The number of women in these studies using glargine in the first trimester was, however, too small to assess an effect on congenital malformations.[173] In 2012, insulin detemir was revised as a category B pregnancy therapeutic from pregnancy category C. This reclassification was based on a large ramdomized trial in women with type 1 diabetes mellitus given either NPH or insulin detemir treatment. Insulin detemir and NPH achieved similar HbA$_{1c}$ and hypoglycemia rates. No increase in adverse maternal or fetal health events has been noted.[174] One limiting factor, however, with basal insulin is the steady rate of insulin release. It may be more difficult to mimic the diurnal variations in glucose range, with increased insulin resistance and hyperglycemia occurring in the morning hours.

Insulin pump device as a modality for insulin delivery is increasingly used to treat pregnant women. Theoretically, this approach may allow more rapid adjustments in basal as well as bolus insulin regimen as insulin needs change throughout the pregnancy. A review of 6 randomized trials comparing the use of the traditional multiple daily injections versus continuous subcutaneous insulin infusion, however, found no significant differences between the 2 groups in terms of glucose control or maternal and fetal outcomes.[175]

It is important to be aware of the variations in insulin requirement throughout gestation. Observational studies suggest an early rise in insulin needs in weeks 3 to 7, followed by a decrease in insulin requirements in the second trimester. The increased production of placental hormones as the pregnancy progresses, however, increases gestational hyperglycemia. The average insulin requirement in type 1 diabetes mellitus progresses from 0.7 U/kg in the first trimester to 0.8 U/kg in the second trimester, 0.9 U/kg in weeks 29 to 34, and 1.0 U/kg after week 35. These ratios should be individualized. Obese insulin-resistant women may require up to 1.5 U/kg to 2.0 U/kg in initial dosing.[176] At times, glucose values can decrease after week 35, especially in women with type 1 diabetes mellitus. A fall in insulin dosing of 5% to 10% should instigate a review of fetal health. Up to 30% reduction in insulin requirements, however, can also be seen in healthy pregnancies.[177]

Oral hypoglycemic agents, such as glyburide and metformin, have traditionally been excluded from the treatment armamentarium for diabetes in pregnancy because of concern regarding fetal teratogenicity and neonatal hypoglycemia. These concerns stem from the lack of certainty about crossing the placental barrier. In a recent meta-analysis reviewing randomized controlled trials comparing oral hypoglycemic agents with insulin use in diabetes of pregnancy, few differences were noted in both fetal and maternal outcomes. There were no significant differences in glucose control between the 2 groups, either in fasting glucose or postprandial glucose excursion. There was no increase with use of an oral hypoglycemic agent in neonatal hypoglycemia, birthweight, admission to neonatal ICU, respiratory distress, preterm births, congenital anomalies, or intrauterine fetal death. With maternal complications, there was no significant difference in the rate of cesarean sections, but there was a lower rate of hypoglycemia and gestational hypertension in the oral hypoglycemic cohorts.[178] A second systematic review by Nicholson and colleagues[179] of randomized controlled trials and observational studies confirmed these results. Differences in study design and lack of long-term outcome data make it difficult, however, to endorse the use of oral hypoglycemic agents in the treatment of diabetes in pregnancy.

Glyburide, a second-generation sulfonylurea, is the oral antidiabetic agent most commonly used in diabetic pregnancies. Langer and colleagues[180] conducted a large randomized trial with 404 women who received insulin or glyburide. Similar improvements were noted in hyperglycemia, whereas there were no differences seen in macrosomia, neonatal hypoglycemia, neonatal morbidities, or cord insulin concentrations. Of note, 4% of the women treated with glyburide ultimately needed insulin in the treatment of maternal diabetes. A smaller study, however, demonstrated higher mean glucose levels in women treated with glyburide versus insulin.[181]

Metformin, a biguanide, has also been used in the treatment of diabetes in pregnancy. Although metformin is able to cross the placenta, it does not seem to have teratogenic effects. The largest study assessing the use of metformin in 751 Australian women given biguanide or insulin at weeks 20 to 33 of gestation reported similar perinatal morbidity in the 2 groups. No serious adverse outcomes were found in the metformin group. However, 46% of women receiving metformin required supplemental insulin to achieve glycemic control.[181] A randomized controlled trial comparing metformin with glyburide use in GDM suggests that glyburide is more effective in achieving adequate glycemic control—16% of the glyburide group and 35% of the metformin group required supplemental insulin.[182] The ADA and the ACOG, however, do not endorse the use of either of these agents in the treatment of diabetes in pregnancy. There are currently no controlled trials using other hypoglycemic agents, such as thiazolidinediones, α-glucosidase inhibitors, glitinides, or GLP-1 agonists in pregnancy.

Women with GDM have a high risk of recurrence in subsequent pregnancies, as high as 41.3%.[180] There seems to be an increased risk in women with increased age, multiparous state, greater prepregnancy weight, and higher infant birth weight.[183] One third of women with GDM continue to have overt diabetes, impaired fasting glucose, or impaired glucose tolerance during the postpartum period. Both the ADA and ACOG recommend screening with fasting plasma glucose and 2-hour, 75-g OGTT at 6 to 12 weeks postpartum.[180] If this screening is found negative, assessment of glycemic status is recommended every 3 years. The relative risk of developing type 2 diabetes mellitus is 4.69 within the first 5 years after gestation and 9.34 more than 5 years after delivery.[184] The presence of islet cell antibodies, specific HLA alleles (DR3 or DR4), and development of diabetic ketoacidosis predisposes the mother to development of type 1 diabetes mellitus postpartum.[185,186] Careful postpartum monitoring in GDM is important in decreasing maternal morbidity.

SUMMARY

In summary, the insulin/IGF pathways and glucose metabolism act as key mediators of human ovarian function and female fertility. In the setting of normal insulin action, insulin binds to its own receptors in the ovary to mediate steroidogenesis and act as a co-gonadotropin. Insulin in synergy with other factors, such as hCG, may also influence ovarian growth and cyst formation. The IGF pathway also seems to influence normal ovarian function. Insulin signaling affects reproductive function through brain-specific or central action as well as direct gonadal action.

The importance of insulin/IGF action in female reproductive function is conserved throughout various species. Dysregulation of this pathway leads to altered puberty, ovulation, and fertility. When fertility is achieved, there remain risks to both maternal health and fetal development (see **Table 3**). Better understanding of the normal physiology and pathophysiology of insulin, IGF, and glucose effects on the human reproductive system will allow for better outcomes in affected women.

REFERENCES

1. Joslin EP. The growth, development, and prognosis of diabetic children. JAMA 1985;85:420.
2. Poretsky L, Kalin MF. The gonadotropic function of insulin. Endocr Rev 1987; 8(2):132.
3. Morgagni J, editor. De sedibus et causis morborum per anatonem indagata (The seats and causes of diseases investigated by anatomy), Tomus primus, 2nd edition. Patavii (Italy): sumptibus remondiniaris; 1765.
4. Achard EC, Thiers J. Le virilisme et son association a l'insuffisnace glycolytique (diabete des femme a barbe). Acad Natl Med 1921;86:51.
5. Kahn CR, Flier JS, Bar RS, et al. The syndromes of insulin resistance and acanthosis nigricans: insulin receptor disoreders in man. N Engl J Med 1976;294(14): 739.
6. Flier JS, Kahn CR, Roth J, et al. Antibodies that impair insulin receptor binding in an unusual diabetic syndrome with severe insulin resistance. Science 1975; 190(4209):63.
7. Diamanti-Kandarakis E, Dunaif A. Insulin resistance and the polycystic ovary syndrome revisited: an update on mechanisms and implications. Endocr Rev 2012;33(6):981–1030.
8. Benito M. Tissue specificity on insulin action and resistance: past to recent mechanisms. Acta Physiol (Oxf) 2011;201(3):297.
9. Poretsky L, Cataldo NA, Rosenwales Z, et al. The insulin-related ovarian regulatory system in health and disease. Endocr Rev 1999;20(4):535.
10. Poretsly L, Smith D, Seibel M, et al. Specific insulin binding sites in human ovary. J Clin Endocrinol Metab 1984;59(4):809.
11. Poretsky L, Bhargava G, Kalin MF, et al. Distribution and characterization of insulin and insulin-like growth factor I receptors in normal human ovary. J Clin Endocrinol Metab 1985;61(4):728.
12. Poretsky L, Bhargava G, Kalin MF, et al. Regulation of insulin receptors in the human ovary: in vitro studies. J Clin Endocrinol Metab 1988;67(4):774.
13. Poretsky L, Bhargava G, Saketos M, et al. Regulation of human ovarian insulin receptors in vivo. Metabolism 1990;39(2):161.
14. Nandi A, Kitamura Y, Kahn CR, et al. Mouse models of insulin resistance. Physiol Rev 2004;84(2):623.
15. Poretsky L, Glover B, Laumas V, et al. The effects of experimental hyperinsulinemia on steroid secretion, ovarian (^{125}I) insulin binding, and ovarian (^{125}I) insulin-like growth factor I binding in the rat. Endocrinology 1988;122(2):581.
16. Barbieri RL, Makris A, Ryan KJ, et al. Effects of insulin on steroidogenesis in cultured porcine ovarian theca. Fertil Steril 1983;40(2):237.

17. Willis D, Frank S. Insulin action in human granulosa cells from normal and polycystic ovaries is mediated by the insulin receptor and not the type-1 insulin-like growth factor receptor. J Clin Endocrinol Metab 1995;80(12):3788.
18. Nestler JE, Jakubowicz DJ, de Vargas AF, et al. Insulin stimulates testosterone biosynthesis by human thecal cells from women with polycystic ovary syndrome by activating its own receptor and usng inositolglycan mediators as the signal transduction system. J Clin Endocrinol Metab 1998;83(6):2001.
19. Garzo VG, Dorrington JH. Aromatase activity in human granulosa cells during follicular development and the modulation by follicle-stimulating hormone and insulin. Am J Obstet Gynecol 1984;148(5):657.
20. Nestler JE, Jakubowicz DJ. Decreases in ovarian cytochrome P450c17a activity and serum free testosterone after reduction of insulin secretion in polycystic ovary syndrome. N Engl J Med 1996;335(9):617.
21. McGee E, Sawetawan C, Bird I, et al. The effects of insulin on 3 beta-hydroxysteroid dehydrogenase expression in human luteinized granulosa cells. J Soc Gynecol Investig 1995;2(3):535.
22. Falcone T, Finegood DT, Fantus IG, et al. Androgen response to endogenous insulin secretion during the frequently sampled intravenous glucose tolerance test in normal and hyperandrogenic women. J Clin Endocrinol Metab 1990;71(6): 1653.
23. Toscano V, Blanchi P, Balducci R, et al. Lack of linear relationship between hyperinsulinemia and hyperandrogenism. Clin Endocrinol 1992;36(2):197.
24. Sharp PS, Kiddy DS, Reed MJ, et al. Correlation of plasma insulin and insulin-like growth factor-1 with indices of androgen transport and metabolism in women with polycystic ovary syndrome. Clin Endocrinol 1991;35(3):253.
25. Stuart CA, Nagamani M. Acute augmentation of plasma androstenedione and dehydroepiandrosterone by euglycemic insulin infusion: evidence for a direct effect of insulin on ovarian steroidogenesis. In: Dunaif A, et al, editors. Polycystic ovary syndrome. Boston: Blackwell Scientific Publications; 1992. p. 279–88.
26. Stuart CA, Prince MJ, Peters EJ, et al. Hyperinsulinemia and hyperandrogenism: in vivo androgen response to insulin infusion. Obstet Gynecol 1987; 69(6):921.
27. Stuart CA, Nagamani M. Insulin infusion acutely augments ovarian androgen production in normal women. Fertil Steril 1990;54(5):788.
28. Micic D, Popovic V, Nesovic M, et al. Androgen levels during sequential insulin euglycemic clamp studies in patients with polycystic ovary disease. J Steroid Biochem 1988;31(6):995.
29. Willis D, Mason H, Gilling-Smith C, et al. Modulation by insulin of follicle-stimulating hormone and luteinizing hormone actions in human granulosa cells of normal and polycystic ovaries. J Clin Endocrinol Metab 1996;81(1): 302.
30. Cara JF, Rosenfield RL. Insulin-like growth factor I and insulin potentiate luteinizing hormone-induced androgen synthesis. Endocrinology 1988;123(2):733.
31. Davoren JB, Hsueh AJ. Insulin enhances FSH-stimulated steroidogenesis by cultured rat granulosa cells. Mol Cell Endocrinol 1984;35(2–3):97.
32. Markussis V, Goni MH, Tolis G, et al. The role of insulin in ovarian size in patients with polycystic ovary syndrome. Gynecol Endocrinol 1994;8(3):197.
33. Velazquez EM, Mendoza S, Hamer T, et al. Metformin therapy in polycystic ovary syndrome reduces hyperinsulinemia, insulin resistance, hyperandrogenemia, and systolic blood pressure, while facilitating normal menses and pregnancy. Metabolism 1994;43(5):647.

34. Dunaif A, Scott D, Finegood D, et al. The insulin-sensitizing agent troglitazone improves metabolic and reproductive abnormalities in the polycystic ovary syndrome. J Clin Endocrinol Metab 1996;81(9):3299.

35. Zapf J, Schmid C, Froesch ER, et al. Biological and immunological properties of insulin-like growth factors (IGF) I and II. Clin Endocrinol Metab 1984;13(1):3.

36. Kahn CR, Crettaz M. Insulin receptors and the molecular mechanism of insulin action. Diabetes Metab Rev 1985;1(1–2):5.

37. El-Roeiy A, Chen X, Roberts VJ, et al. Expression of insulin-like growth factor-1 (IGF-1) and IGF-II and the IGF-I, IGF-II, and insulin receptor genes and localization of the gene products in the human ovary. J Clin Endocrinol Metab 1993; 77(5):1411.

38. Voutilainen R, Frank S, Mason HD, et al. Expression of insulin-like growth factor (IGF), IGF binding protein, and IGF receptor messenger ribonucleic acids in normal and polycystic ovaries. J Clin Endocrinol Metab 1996;81(3):1003.

39. Rosenfeld RG, Rosenbloom AL, Guevara-Aguire J, et al. Growth hormone (GH) insensitivity due to primary GH receptor deficiency. Endocr Rev 1994;15(3):369.

40. Poretsky L, Chun B, Liu HC, et al. Insulin-like growth factor II (IGF-II) inhibits insulin-like growth factor binding protein I (IGFBP-1) production in luteinized human granulosa cells with a potency similar to insulin-like growth factor I (IGF-I). J Clin Endocrinol Metab 1996;81(9):3412.

41. Collett-Solberg PF, Cohen P. The role of the insulin-like growth factor binding proteins and the IGFBP proteases in modulating IGF action. Endocrinol Metab Clin North Am 1996;25(3):591.

42. El-Roeiy A, Chen X, Roberts VJ, et al. Expression of the genes encoding the insulin-like growth factors (IGF-I and II), the IGF and insulin receptors, and IGF-binding proteins 1-6 and the localization of their gene products in normal and polycystic ovary syndrome ovaries. J Clin Endocrinol Metab 1994;78(6): 1488.

43. Poretsky L, Chandrasekher VA, Bai C, et al. Insulin receptor mediates inhibitory effect of insulin, but not of insulin-like growth factor (IGF-I), on IGF binding protein (IGFBP-1) production on human granulosa cells. J Clin Endocrinol Metab 1996;81(2):493.

44. Adachi T, Iwashita M, Kuroshima A, et al. Regulation of IGF binding proteins by FSH in human luteinizing granulosa cells. J Assist Reprod Genet 1995;12(9): 639.

45. Holst N, Kierulf KH, Sepala M, et al. Regulation of insulin-like growth factor-binding protein-1and progesterone secretion by cultured human granulosa-luteal cells: effects of octreotide and insulin. Fertil Steril 1997;68(3):478.

46. San Roman GA, Magoffin DA. Insulin-like growth factor-binding proteins in healthy and atretic follicles during natural menstrual cycles. J Clin Endocrinol Metab 1993;76(3):625.

47. Cataldo NA, Giudice LC. Insulin-like growth factor binding protein profiles in human ovarian follicular fluid correlate with follicular functional status. J Clin Endocrinol Metab 1992;74(4):821.

48. Giudice LC, Farrell EM, Pham H, et al. Identification of insulin-like growth factor-binding protein-3 (IGFBP-3) and IGFBP-2 in human follicular fluid. J Clin Endocrinol Metab 1990;71(5):1330.

49. Lamson G, Giudice LC, Cohen P, et al. Proteolysis of IGFBP-3 may be a common regulatory mechanism of IGF action in vivo. Growth Regul 1993;3(1):91.

50. Hsin H, Kenyon C. Signals from the reproductive system regulate the lifespan of C. Elegans. Nature 1999;399(6734):362.

51. Bohni R, Riesgo-Escobar J, Oldham S, et al. Autonomous control of cell and organ size by CHICO, a Drosophila homolog of vertebrate IRS 1-4. Cell 1999; 97(7):865.
52. Withers DJ. Insulin receptor substrate proteins and neuroendocrine function. Biochem Soc Trans 2001;29(Pt 4):525.
53. Bruning JC, Gautam D, Burks DJ, et al. Role of brain insulin receptor in control of body weight and reproduction. Science 2000;289(5487):2122.
54. Okamoto H, Nakae J, Kitamura T, et al. Transgenic rescue of insulin receptor-deficient mice. J Clin Invest 2004;114(2):214.
55. Roumain J, Charles MA, de Courten MP, et al. The relationship of menstrual irregularity to type 2 diabetes in Pima Indian Women. Diabetes Care 1998;21(3):346.
56. Nandi A, Wang X, Accili D, et al. The effect of insulin signaling on female reproductive function independent of adiposity and hyperglycemia. Endocrinology 2010; 151(4):1863-71.
57. Solomon CG, Huf B, Dunaif A, et al. Long or highly irregular menstrual cycles as a marker for risk of type 2 diabetes mellitus. JAMA 2001;286(19):2421.
58. Gast GC, Grobbee DE, Smith HA, et al. Menstrual cycle characteristics and risk of coronary heart disease and type 2 diabetes. Fertil Steril 2010;94(6):2379.
59. Stockl D, Meisinger C, Peters A, et al. Age at menarche and its association with the metabolic syndrome and its components: results from the KORA F4 Study. PLoS One 2011;6(10):e26076.
60. Chen L, Zhang C, Yeung E, et al. Age at menarche and metabolic markers for type 2 diabetes in premenopausal women: the Biocycle Study. J Clin Endocrinol Metab 2011;96(6):E1007-12.
61. Stockl D, Doring A, Peters A, et al. Age at menarche is associated with prediabetes and diabetes in women (age 32-81) from the general population: the KORA F4 Study. Diabetologia 2012;55(3):681.
62. Pierce MB, Kuh D, Hardy R, et al. The role of BMI across the life course in the relationship between age at menarche and diabetes in a British Birth Cohort. Diabet Med 2012;29(5):600-3.
63. Kent SC, Legro RS. Polycystic ovary syndrome in adolescents. Adolesc Med 2002;13(1):73-88.
64. Bergqvist N. The gonadal function in female diabetics. Acta Endocrinol Suppl (Copenh) 1954;19:1.
65. Djursing H, Nyholm HC, Hagen C, et al. Clinical and hormonal characteristics in women with anovulation and insulin-treated diabetes mellitus. Am J Obstet Gynecol 1982;143(8):876.
66. Schweiger BM, Snell-Bergeon JK, Roman R, et al. Menarche delay and menstrual irregularities persist in adolescents with type 1 diabetes. Reprod Biol Endocrinol 2011;9:61.
67. Picardi A, Cipponeri E, Bizzarri C, et al. Menarche in type 1 diabetes is still delayed despite good metabolic control. Fertil Steril 2008;90(5):1875.
68. Gaete X, Vivanco M, Eyzaguirre FC, et al. Menstrual cycle irregularities and their relationship with HbA1c and insulin dose in adolescents with type 1 diabetes mellitus. Fertil Steril 2010;94(5):1822.
69. Codner E, Eyzaguirre FC, Iniguez G, et al. Ovulation rate in adolescents with type 1 diabetes mellitus. Fertil Steril 2011;95(1):197.
70. Dorman JS, Steenkiste AR, Foley TP, et al. Menopause in type 1 diabetic women: is it premature? Diabetes 2001;50(8):1857.
71. Codner E, Cassorla F. Puberty and ovarian function in girls with type 1 diabetes mellitus. Horm Res 2009;71:12.

72. Codner E, Soto N, Lopez P, et al. Diagnostic criteria for polycystic ovary syndrome and ovarian morphology in women with type 1 diabetes mellitus. J Clin Endocrinol Metab 2006;91(6):2250.

73. Codner E, Escobar-Morreale HF. Clinical review: hyperandrogenism and polycystic ovary syndrome in women with type 1 diabetes mellitus. J Clin Endocrinol Metab 2007;92(4):1209.

74. Tritos NA, Mantzoros CS. Syndromes of severe insulin resistance. J Clin Endocrinol Metab 1998;83(9):3025.

75. Grunberger G, Alfonso B. Syndromes of extreme insulin resistance. In: Poretsky L, editor. Principles of diabetes mellitus. New York: Springer; 2010. p. 259–77.

76. Poretsky L. On the paradox of insulin-induced hyperandrogenism in insulin-resistant states. Endocr Rev 1991;12(1):3–13.

77. Taylor SI, Dons RF, Hernandez E, et al. Insulin resistance associated with androgen excess in women with auto-antibodies to the insulin receptor. Ann Intern Med 1982;97(6):851.

78. Barbieri RL, Smith S, Ryan KJ, et al. The role of hyperinsulinemia in the pathogenesis of ovarian hyperandrogenism. Fertil Steril 1988;50(2):197.

79. Givens JR, Kerber IJ, Wiser WL, et al. Remission of acanthosis nigricans associated with polycystic ovarian disease and a stromal luteoma. J Clin Endocrinol Metab 1973;38(3):347.

80. Shoupe D, Lobo RA. The influence of androgens on insulin resistance. Fertil Steril 1984;41(3):385.

81. Amiel SA, Sherwin RS, Simonson DC, et al. Impaired insulin action in puberty. N Engl J Med 1986;315(4):215.

82. Friedl KE, Jones RE, Hannan CJ Jr, et al. The administration of pharmacological doses of testosterone or 19-nortestosterone to normal men is not associated with increased insulin secretion or impaired glucose tolerance. J Clin Endocrinol Metab 1989;68(5):971.

83. Billiar RB, Richardson D, Schwartz R, et al. Effect of chronically elevated androgen or estrogen on the glucose tolerance test and insulin response in female rhesus monkeys. Am J Obstet Gynecol 1987;157(5):1297.

84. Vestergaard H, Rossen M, Urhammer SA, et al. Short and long-term metabolic effects of recombinant human IGF-1 treatment in patients with severe insulin resistance and diabetes mellitus. Eur J Endocrinol 1997;136(5):475–82.

85. Stein IF, Leventhal MC. Amenorrhea associated with bilateral polycystic ovaries. Am J Obstet Gynecol 1935;29:181.

86. Okoron EM, Hooper WC, Atrash HK, et al. Prevalence of polycystic ovary syndrome among the privately insured, United States, 2003-2008. Am J Obstet Gynecol 2012;207(4):299.e1.

87. Zweig SB, Tolentino MC, Strizhevsky M, et al. Polycystic ovary syndrome. In: Poretsky L, editor. Principals of diabetes mellitus. New York: Springer; 2010. p. 515–30.

88. Azziz R, Dumesic DA, Goodarzi MO, et al. Polycystic ovary syndrome: an ancient disorder. Fertil Steril 2011;95(5):1544.

89. Ehrmann DA. Polycystic ovary syndrome. N Engl J Med 2005;352(12):1223.

90. Salehi M, Bravo-Vera R, Sheikh A, et al. Pathogenesis of polycystic ovary syndrome: what is the role of obesity? Metabolism 2004;53(3):358.

91. Dunaif A, Segal KR, Futterweit W, et al. Profound peripheral insulin resistance, independent of obesity, in polycystic ovary syndrome. Diabetes 1989;38(9):1165.

92. Paradisi G, Steinberg HO, Shepard MK, et al. Polycystic ovary syndrome is associated with endothelial dysfunction. Circulation 2001;103(10):1410.
93. Paradisi G, Steinberg HO, Shepard MK, et al. Troglitazone therapy improves endothelaial function to near normal levels in women with polcystic ovary syndrome. J Clin Endocrinol Metab 2003;88(2):576.
94. Balen A. Polycystic ovary syndrome and cancer. Hum Reprod Update 2001; 7(6):522.
95. Taylor AE, McCourt B, Martin KA, et al. Determinants of abnormal gonadotropin secretion in clinically defined women with polycystic ovary syndrome. J Clin Endocrinol Metab 1997;82(7):2248.
96. Solorzano CM, Beller JP, Abshire MY, et al. Neuroendocrine dysfunction in polycystic ovary syndrome. Steroids 2012;77(4):332.
97. Poretsky L, Clemens J, Bogovich K, et al. Hyperinsulunemia and human chorionic gonadotropin synergistically promote the growth of ovarian follicular cysts in rats. Metabolism 1992;41(8):903.
98. Repaci A, Gambineri A, Pasquali R, et al. The role of low grade inflammation in the polycystic ovary syndrome. Mol Cell Endocrinol 2011;335(1):30.
99. Lumeng CN, Bodzin JL, Saltiel AR, et al. Obesity induces a phenotype switch in adipose tissue macrophage polarization. J Clin Invest 2007;117(1):178.
100. Orio F, Manguso F, Di Biase S, et al. Metformin administration improves leukocyte count in women with polycystic ovary syndrome: a 6-month prospective study. Eur J Endocrinol 2007;157(1):69.
101. Roby KF, Terranova PF. Effects of TNFα in vitro on steroidogenesis in healthy and atretic follicles of the rat theca as a target. Endocrinology 1990;126(5): 2711.
102. Spaczynski RZ, Arici A, Duleba AJ, et al. TNFα stimulates proliferation of rat ovarian theca-interstitial cells. Biol Reprod 1999;61(4):993.
103. Path G, Bornstein SR, Ehrhart-Bornstein M, et al. IL-6 and the IL-6 receptor in the human adrenal gland: expression and effects on steroidogenesis. J Clin Endocrinol Metab 1997;82(7):2343.
104. Croton M, Botella-Carretero JI, Benguria A, et al. Differential gene expression profile in omental adipose tissue in women with PCOS. J Clin Endocrinol Metab 2007;92(1):328.
105. Xu XF, De Pergola G, Bjorntorp P, et al. Testosterone increases lipolysis and the number of beta-adrenoreceptors in male rat adipocytes. Endocrinology 1991; 128(1):379.
106. Adashi EY, Hsueh AJ, Yen SS, et al. Insulin enhancement of luteinizing hormone and follicle-stimulating hormone release by cultured pituitary cells. Endocrinology 1981;108(4):1441.
107. Soldani R, Cagnacci A, Yen SS, et al. Insulin, insulin-like growth factor I (IGF-I) and IGF-II enhance basal and gonadotropin-releasing hormone-stimulated luteinizing hormone release from rat anterior pituitary cells in vitro. Eur J Endocrinol 1994;131(6):641.
108. Samoto T, Maruo T, Matsuo H, et al. Altered expression of insulin and insulin-like growth factor-1 receptors in follicular and stromal compartments of polycystic ovaries. Endocr J 1993;40(4):413.
109. Nagamani M, Stuart CA. Specific binding sites for insulin-like growth factor-1 in the ovarian stroma of women with polycystic ovarian disease and stromal hyperthecosis. Am J Obstet Gynecol 1990;163(6 pt 1):1992.
110. Badawy A, Elnashar A. Treatment options for polycystic ovary syndrome. Int J Womens Health 2011;201(3):25.

111. Dinger JC, Heinemann LA, Kuhl-Habich D, et al. The safety of a drospirenone-containing oral contraceptive: final results from the European Active Surveillance Study on oral contraceptives based on 142,475 women-years of observation. Contraception 2007;75(5):344.

112. Seejer JD, Laughlin J, Eng PM, et al. Risk of thromboembolism in women taking ethinyl estradiol/drospirenone and other oral contraceptives. Obstet Gynecol 2007;110(3):587.

113. Parkin L, Sharples K, Hernandez RK, et al. Risk of venous thromboembolism in users of oral contraceptives containing drospirenone or levonorgestrel: nested case-control study based on UK General Practice Research Database. BMJ 2011;342:d2139.

114. Jick SS. Risk of non-fatal venous thromboembolism in women using oral contraceptives containing drospirenone compared with women using oral contraceptives containing levonogestrel: case-control study using United States claims data. BMJ 2011;342:d2151.

115. Boyle JG, Salt IP, McKay GA, et al. Metformin action on AMP-activated protein kinase: a translational research approach to understanding a potential therapeutic target. Diabet Med 2010;27(10):1097.

116. Scarpello JH, Howlett HC. Metformin therapy and clinical uses. Diab Vasc Dis Res 2008;5(3):157.

117. Patel SM, Nestler JE. Fertility in polycystic ovary syndrome. Endocrinol Metab Clin North Am 2006;35(1):137.

118. Araki T, Elias R, Rosenwaks Z, et al. Achieving a successful pregnancy in women with polycystic ovary syndrome. Endocrinol Metab Clin North Am 2011;40(4):865.

119. Escobar-Morreale HF, Botella-Carretero JI, Alvarez-Blasco F, et al. The polycystic ovary syndrome associated with morbid obesity may resolve after weight loss induced by bariatric surgery. J Clin Endocrinol Metab 2005;90(12):6364.

120. Sam S, Dunaif A. Polycystic ovary syndrome: syndrome XX? Trends Endocrinol Metab 2003;14(8):365.

121. Katsiki N, Hatzitolios AI. Insulin-sensitizing agents in the treatment of polycystic ovary syndrome: an update. Curr Opin Obstet Gynecol 2010;22(6):466.

122. Quinn CE, Hamilton PK, Lockhart CJ, et al. Thiazolidinediones: effects on insulin resistance and the cardiovascular system. Br J Pharmacol 2008;153(4):636.

123. Seto-Young D, Avtanski D, Parikh G, et al. Rosiglitazone and pioglitazone inhibit estrogen synthesis in human granulosa cells by interfering with androgen binding to aromatase. Horm Metab Res 2011;43(4):250.

124. Araki T, Varadinova M, Goldman M, et al. Rosiglitazone and pioglitazone alter aromatase kinetic porperties in human granulosa cells. PPAR Res 2011;2011: 926438.

125. Nissen SE, Wolski K. Effect of rosiglitazone on the risk of myocardial infarction and death from cardiovascular causes. N Engl J Med 2007;356(24):2457.

126. Colmers IN, Bower SL, Majumdar SR, et al. Use of thiazolidinediones and the risk of bladder cancer among people with type 2 diabetes: a meta-analysis. CMAJ 2012;184(12):E675.

127. Kahn SE, Zinman B, Lachin JM, et al. Rosiglitazone-associated fractures in type 2 diabetes: an analysis from A Diabetes Outcome Progression Trial (ADOPT). Diabetes Care 2008;31(5):845.

128. Seth A, Sy V, Pareek A, et al. Thiazolidinediones (TZDs) affect osteoblast viability and biomarkers independently of the TZD effects on aromatase. Horm Metab Res 2013;45(1):1.

129. Elkind-Hirsch K, Marrioneaux O, Bushan M, et al. Comparison of single and combined treatment with exenatide and metformin on menstrual cyclicity in overweight women with polycystic ovary syndrome. J Clin Endocrinol Metab 2008;93(7):2670.
130. Elter K, Imir G, Dumusoglu F, et al. Clinical, endocrine and metabolic effects of metformin added to ethinyl estradiol-cyproterone acetate in non-obese women with polycystic ovary syndrome: a randomized controlled study. Hum Reprod 2002;17(7):1729.
131. Lemay A, Dodin S, Turcot L, et al. Rosiglitazone and ethinyl estradiol/cyproterone acetate as single and combined treatment of overweight women with polycystic ovary syndrome and insulin resistance. Hum Reprod 2006;21(1):121.
132. Usaadi RS, Legro RS. Reproductive impact of polycystic ovary syndrome. Curr Opin Endocrinol Diabetes Obes 2012;19(6):505.
133. Legro RS, Barnhart HX, Schlaff WD, et al. Clomiphene, metformin, or both for infertility in the polycystic ovary syndrome. N Engl J Med 2007;356(6):551.
134. Qublan HS, Al-Khaderei S, Abu-Saleem AN, et al. Metformin in the treatment of clomiphene citrate-resistant women with polycystic ovary syndrome undergoing in vitro fertilization treatment: a randomized controlled trial. J Obstet Gynaecol 2009;29(7):651.
135. Badawy A, Shokeir T, Allam AF, et al. Pregnancy outcome after ovulation induction with aromatase inhibitors or clomiphene citrate in unexplained infertility. Acta Obstet Gynecol Scand 2009;88(2):187.
136. Figuerido JB, Nastri CO, Vieira AD, et al. Clomiphene combined with gonadotropins and GnRH antagonist versus conventional controlled ovarian hyperstimulation without clomiphene in women undergoing assisted reproductive techniques: systematic review and meta-analysis. Arch Gynecol Obstet 2013; 287(4):779.
137. Badawy A, Abdel Aal I, Abulatta M, et al. Clomiphene citrate or anastrozole for ovulation induction in women with polycystic ovary syndrome? A prospective randomized trial. Fertil Steril 2009;92(3):860.
138. Legro RS, Kunselman AR, Brzyski RG, et al. The Pregnancy in Polycystic Ovary Syndrome II(PPCOS II) Trial: rationale and design of a double-blind randomized trial of clomiphene citrate and letrozole for the treatment of infertility in women with polycystic ovary syndrome. Contemp Clin Trials 2012;33(3):470.
139. Heijnem EM, Eijkemans MJ, Hughes EG, et al. A meta-analysis of outcomes of conventional IVF in women with polycystic ovary syndrome. Hum Reprod Update 2006;12(1):13.
140. Lin YH, Seow KM, Hsieh BC, et al. Application of GnRH antagonist in combination with clomiphene citrate and hMG for patients with exaggerated ovarian response in previous IVF/ICSI cycles. J Assist Reprod Genet 2007;24(8):331.
141. Parasanezhad ME, Alborzi S, Motazedian S, et al. Use of dexamethasone and clomiphene citrate in the treatment of clomiphene citrate-resistant patients with polycystic ovary syndrome and normal dehydroepiandrostene sulfate levels: a prospective, double-blind, placebo-controlled trial. Fertil Steril 2002; 78(5):1001.
142. Boomsma CM, Fauser BC, Macklon NS, et al. Pregnancy complications in women with polycystic ovary syndrome. Semin Reprod Med 2008;26(1):72.
143. Iavazzo C, Vitoratos N. Polycystic ovarian syndrome and pregnancy outcome. Arch Gynecol Obstet 2010;282(3):235.
144. Dumesic DA, Padmanabhan V, Abbott DH, et al. Polycystic ovary syndrome and oocyte developmental competence. Obstet Gynecol Surv 2007;63(1):39.

145. Dumesic DA, Abbott DH. Implications of polycystic ovary syndrome on oocyte development. Semin Reprod Med 2008;26(1):53.

146. Jakubowicz DJ, Iuorno MJ, Jacubowicz S, et al. Effects of metformin on early pregnancy loss in the polycystic ovary syndrome. J Clin Endocrinol Metab 2002;87(2):524.

147. Glueck CJ, Wang P, Goldenberg N, et al. Pregnancy outcomes among women with polycystic ovary syndrome treated with metformin. Hum Reprod 2002; 17(11):2858–64.

148. Glueck CJ, Wang P, Kobayashi S, et al. Metformin therapy throughout pregnancy reduces the development of gestational diabetes in women with polycystic ovary syndrome. Fertil Steril 2002;77(3):520.

149. Glueck CJ, Phillips H, Cameron D, et al. Continuing metformin throughout pregnancy in women with polycystic ovary syndrome appears to safely reduce first trimester spontaneous abortion: a pilot study. Fertil Steril 2001; 75(1):46.

150. Schneider AE, Rayfield E, Busta A, et al. Diabetes in pregnancy. In: Poretsky L, editor. Principles of diabetes mellitus. New York: Springer; 2010. p. 233–44.

151. Landon MB, Gabbe SG. Gestational diabetes mellitus. Obstet Gynecol 2008; 118(6):1379.

152. Expert Committee on the Diagnosis and Classification of Diabetes Mellitus. Report on the expert committee on the diagnosis and classification if diabetes mellitus. Diabetes Care 2000;23(Suppl 1):S4.

153. Wang Q, Moley KH. Maternal diabetes and oocyte quality. Mitochondrion 2010; 10(5):403.

154. Negrato CA, Mattar R, Gomes MB, et al. Adverse pregnancy outcomes in women with diabetes. Diabetol Metab Syndr 2012;4(1):41.

155. Metzger BE, Lowe LP, Dyer AR, et al. HAPO Study Cooperative Research Group: hyperglycemia and adverse pregnancy outcomes. N Engl J Med 2008;358(19):1991.

156. Landon MB. The relationship between maternal glycemia and perinatal outcome. Obstet Gynecol 2011;117(2 pt 1):218.

157. Ornoy A. Growth and neurodevelopmental outcome of children born to mothers with pregestational and gestational diabetes. Pediatr Endocrinol Rev 2005;3(2): 104.

158. Clausen TD, Mathiesen ER, Hansen T, et al. High prevalence of type 2 diabetes and prediabetes in adult offspring of women with gestational diabetes mellitus or type 1 diabetes: the role of intrauterine hyperglycemia. Diabetes Care 2008;31(2):340.

159. Dabelea D. The predisposition to obesity and diabetes in offspring of diabetic mothers. Diabetes Care 2007;30(Suppl 2):S169–74.

160. Crowther CA, Hiller JE, Moss JR, et al. Australian Carbohydrate Intolerance Study in Pregnant Women (ACHOIS) Trial Group. Effect of treatment of gestational diabetes mellitus on pregnancy outcomes. N Engl J Med 2005;352(4): 2477.

161. Landon MB, Spong CY, Thom E, et al. A multicenter, randomized trial of treatment for mild gestational diabetes. N Engl J Med 2009;361(14):1339.

162. Mulford MI, Jovanovic-Peterson L, Peterson CM, et al. Alternative therpaies for the management of gestational diabetes. Clin Perinatol 1993;20(3):619.

163. Moses RG, Barker M, Winter M, et al. Can a low-glycemic index diet reduce the need for insulin in gestational diabetes mellitus? A randomized trial. Diabetes Care 2009;32(6):996.

164. Rasmussen KM. Weight gain during pregnancy: reexamining the recommendations. Washington, DC: The National Acedmic Press; 2009.
165. Avery MD, Leon AS, Kopher RA, et al. Effects of a partially home-based exercise program for women with gestational diabetes. Obstet Gynecol 1997; 89(1):10.
166. Jovanovic L, Pettitt DJ. Treatment with insulin and its analogs in pregnancies complicated by diabetes. Diabetes Care 2007;30(Suppl 2):s220.
167. Jovanovic L, Illic S, Pettitt DJ, et al. The metabolic and immunologic effects of insulin lispro in gestational diabetes. Diabetes Care 1999;22(9):1422.
168. Bhattacharyya A. Insulin lispro and regular insulin in pregnancy. QJM 2001; 94(5):225.
169. Wyatt JW, Frias JL, Hoyme HE, et al. Congenital anomaly rate in offspring of mothers with diabetes treated with insulin lispro during pregnancy. Diabet Med 2005;22(6):803.
170. Pettitt DJ, Ospina P, Kolaczynski JW, et al. Comparison of an insulin analog, insulin aspart, and regular human insulin with no insulin in gestational diabetes mellitus. Diabetes Care 2003;26(1):183.
171. Hod M, Damm P, Kaaja R, et al. Fetal and perinatal outcomes in type 1 diabetes pregnancy: a randomized study comparing insulin aspart with human insulin in 322 subjects. Am J Obstet Gynecol 2008;198(2):186.e1.
172. Mathiesen ER, Kinsky B, Amiel SA, et al. Maternal glycemic control and hypoglycemia in type 1 diabetic pregnancy: a randomized trial of insulin aspart versus human insulin in 322 pregnant women. Diabetes Care 2007;30(4):771.
173. Lepercq J, Lin J, Hall GC, et al. Meta-analysis of maternal and neonatal outcomes associated with the use of insulin glargine versus NPH insulin during pregnancy. Obstet Gynecol Int 2012;2012:649070.
174. Mathiesen ER, Hod M, Ivanisevic M, et al. Maternal efficacy and safety outcomes in a randomized controlled trial comparing insulin detemir with NPH insulin in 310 pregnant women with type 1 diabetes mellitus. Diabetes Care 2012;35(10):2012.
175. Mukhopadhyay A, Farrell T, Fraser RB, et al. Continuous subcutaneous insulin infusion vs. intensive conventional insulin therapy in pregnant diabetic women: a systematic review and metaanalysis of randomized, controlled trials. Am J Obstet Gynecol 2007;197(5):447.
176. Steel JM, Johnstone FD, Hepburn DA, et al. Can prepregnancy care of diabetic women reduce the risk of abnormal babies? BMJ 1990;301:1070.
177. Steel JM, Johnstone FD, Hume R, et al. Insulin requirements during pregnancy in women with type I diabetes. Obstet Gynecol 1994;83(2):253.
178. Dhulkotia JS, Ola B, Fraser R, et al. Oral hypoglycemic agents vs insulin in management of gestational diabetes: a systematic review and metaanalysis. Am J Obstet Gynecol 2010;203(5):457.e1.
179. Nicholson W, Bolen S, Witkop CT, et al. Benefits and risks of oral diabetic agents compared with insulin in women with gestational diabetes: a systematic review. Obstet Gynecol 2009;113(1):193.
180. Langer O, Conway DL, Berkus MD, et al. A comparison of glyburide and insulin in women with gestaional diabetes mellitus. N Engl J Med 2000;343(16):1134.
181. Rowan JA, Hague WM, Gao W, et al. Metformin versus insulin for the treatment of gestational diabetes. N Engl J Med 2008;358(19):2003.
182. Moore LE, Clokey D, Rappaport VJ, et al. Metformin compared with glyburide in gestational diabetes: a randomized controlled trial. Obstet Gynecol 2010; 115(1):55.

183. Getahun D, Fassett MJ, Jacobsen SJ, et al. Gestational diabetes: risk of recurrence in subsequent pregnancies. Am J Obstet Gynecol 2010;203(5):467.e1.

184. Bellamy L, Casas JP, Hingorani AD, et al. Type 2 diabetes mellitus after gestational diabetes: a systematic review and meta-analysis. Lancet 2009;373(9677): 1773.

185. Ferber KM, Keller E, Albert ED, et al. Predictive value of human leukocyte antigen class II typing for the development of islet autoantibodies and insulin-dependent diabetes postpartum in women with gestational diabetes. J Clin Endocrinol Metab 1999;84(7):2342.

186. Mauricio D, Balsells M, Morales J, et al. Islet cell autoimmunity in women with gestational diabetes and risk of progression to insulin-dependent diabetes mellitus. Diabetes Metab Rev 1996;12(4):275.

Complications of Diabetes Therapy

Sarah D. Corathers, MD[a,b,*], Shawn Peavie, DO[b],
Marzieh Salehi, MD, MS[b]

KEYWORDS

- Diabetes • Treatment complications • Cardiovascular outcomes • β-cell function

KEY POINTS

- The increasing incidence of diabetes over the last few decades, along with the increased pace of new antidiabetic drug development, calls for a better understanding of the efficacy, mechanism of action, and safety of these drugs.
- Current strategies for the treatment of type 2 diabetes mellitus promote the achievement of target glucose levels to minimize microvascular and macrovascular complications.
- Maintaining the glycemic control over time is a significant challenge, owing to the progressive nature of diabetes as a result of declining β-cell function.
- Given the chronic nature of diabetes management, efficacy must be balanced against side effects to achieve a tolerable long-term regimen.
- Individualized therapy started at an earlier stage of disease guided by the principle of "do not harm" seems to be essential in the patient-centric, shared decision-making model of diabetes care.

INTRODUCTION AND BACKGROUND

Type 2 diabetes mellitus (T2DM) is increasingly prevalent in the United States population and is associated with significant morbidity, mortality, and rising health care costs. Microvascular[1,2] and, to a lesser extent, macrovascular[3,4] complications are recognized to result from uncontrolled hyperglycemia. However, intensive therapy to achieve normal glucose levels is not without risk, as demonstrated by increased rates of hypoglycemia, weight gain, and all-cause mortality rates in the intensive treatment arm of the ACCORD (Action to Control Cardiovascular Risk in Diabetes)

Conflict of Interest: The authors do not have any conflict of interest to disclose.
[a] Division of Endocrinology, Cincinnati Children's Hospital Medical Center, 3333 Burnet Avenue, MLC 7012, Cincinnati, OH 45229, USA; [b] Division of Endocrinology, University of Cincinnati Medical Center, 260 Stetson, Suite 4200, Cincinnati, OH 45229, USA
* Corresponding author. Division of Endocrinology, Cincinnati Children's Hospital Medical Center, 3333 Burnet Avenue, MLC 7012, Cincinnati, OH 45229.
E-mail address: Sarah.corathers@cchmc.org

Endocrinol Metab Clin N Am 42 (2013) 947–970
http://dx.doi.org/10.1016/j.ecl.2013.06.005
0889-8529/13/$ – see front matter © 2013 Elsevier Inc. All rights reserved.

endo.theclinics.com

trial.[5] In addition, observational studies indicate that the presence of diabetes increases the risk of other comorbidities such as fracture[6] and certain cancers,[7,8] and treatment choice may affect risk. Thus, in an effort to maintain glucose control, the clinician encounters a complex interplay of primary disease management while simultaneously seeking to avoid complications associated with glucose lowering. Given the chronic nature of diabetes management, efficacy must be balanced against side effects to achieve a tolerable long-term regimen. The goal of this review is to identify complications of non-insulin treatment of diabetes. The major classes of medication are reviewed with special attention given to patient considerations, mechanism of action, effect on weight, and cardiovascular outcomes, and additional class-specific side effects including effects on bone. In addition, effects on β-cell function are highlighted. Hypoglycemia is a recognized feature of many diabetes treatment modalities, and is not covered in depth in this article.

INSULIN SENSITIZERS

The 2 classes of drugs categorized as insulin sensitizers are biguanides (metformin) and thiazolidinediones (rosiglitazone and pioglitazone).

Biguanides

Indications and patient considerations
Metformin remains the primary drug within the class of biguanides in current use, and remains the preferred initial agent for T2DM based on a recent joint statement by the American Diabetes Association (ADA) and the European Association for the Study of Diabetes (EASD) as well as the American Association of Clinical Endocrinologists (AACE).[9–11] Metformin was approved by the Food and Drug Administration (FDA) for use in the United States in 1994 for the treatment of T2DM in adults, with a pediatric indication for children older than 10 years. Concern about risk for lactic acidosis potentiated by decreased clearance of drug led to a black-box warning for use within specific populations including those with renal or hepatic impairment, acute congestive heart failure, sepsis, dehydration, and excessive alcohol intake. In addition, it is recommended that therapy be temporarily discontinued before the administration of intravascular radiocontrast agents or surgical procedures, because of the potential for dehydration and/or kidney injury.

Mechanism of action, efficacy, and kinetics
Metformin (Glucophage) reduces fasting plasma glucose and decreases hemoglobin A_{1c} (HbA1c) by approximately 1.0%.[12,13] Although the precise mechanism of action remains uncertain, the glycemic reducing effect of metformin is primarily attributed to inhibition of hepatic glucose production and, possibly, to improved peripheral insulin sensitivity.[12,14,15] Theories for the antihyperglycemic action of metformin include inhibition of key enzymes in gluconeogenesis,[15–18] direct action on the insulin receptor,[19] or modulation of components of the incretin axis.[20] The mean $t_{1/2}$ of the standard formulation is 5 hours; a sustained-release once-daily formulation is also available. Metformin is excreted unchanged in the urine, and renal clearance is the primary form of elimination of the drug.[21]

Effects on weight, cardiovascular outcomes, and risk of lactic acidosis
In the DPP (Diabetes Prevention Program) study, 3234 participants from 27 clinics in the United States were enrolled between 1996 and 1999 and randomly assigned to metformin (n = 1073) or placebo (n = 1082) treatment. Participants randomized to metformin experienced an average weight loss of 2 kg[22] that was maintained following

a 7- to 8-year open-label extension.[23] Among patients with established T2DM, reported weight benefits of metformin monotherapy ranged from a 0.6- to 2.9-kg reduction in treatment-naïve patients followed for up to 5 years.[24] Combination treatment with metformin has been also observed to mitigate weight gain associated with other agents such as sulfonylurea or thiazolidinediones.[12,24,25]

In the 1970s phenformin, an older member of the biguanide class, was removed from the market after 306 case reports of severe lactic acidosis in patients with congestive heart failure (CHF).[26] Subsequently, CHF was labeled as a contraindication to biguanide therapy in general, although the reported incidence with metformin therapy remained extremely low.[27,28] In fact, among a nested case-control series of more than 50,000 patients with T2DM, overall incidence of lactic acidosis was rare, but occurred more often in those treated with sulfonylurea (4.8 cases per 100,000 patient-years of treatment) than those in the metformin group (3.3 cases per 100,000 patient-years of treatment).[29] In several large observational studies in the United States and United Kingdom of patients with CHF, treatment with metformin had no documented events of lactic acidosis.[26,28,30] A recent meta-analysis of more than 30 clinical trials confirmed the reduction of cardiovascular mortality by metformin in comparison with any other oral diabetes agent or placebo,[31,32] suggesting that not only is metformin safe in this population, it is likely beneficial. In 2005, the FDA removed the CHF contraindication from the product labeling, although a cautionary black-box warning remains for the increased risk of lactic acidosis among patients with concurrent CHF.[26] Following the recent benefit-risk analysis there are calls for urgent reassessment of the relative contraindications of metformin use, given the paucity of data supporting the incidence of lactic acidosis and the likelihood of benefit on glucose control and mortality.[33]

Effects on bone and other side effects

Animal studies indicate that metformin may have a positive effect on osteoblast differentiation and a negative effect on osteoclast differentiation and bone loss.[6] Studies of the safety and efficacy of metformin monotherapy versus a rosiglitazone/metformin combination demonstrated improved glycemic control in the combination group but a significant reduction in lumbar bone mineral density (BMD) in comparison with the metformin monotherapy group.[34] Moreover, studies in rodent models have shown that coadministration of metformin and rosiglitazone mitigates the adverse effects of rosiglitazone on bone.[35] However, data on reduction of fracture risk in patients with T2DM treated with metformin have been inconsistent.[6]

In United States clinical trials approximately 4% of patients were unable to continue metformin because of adverse effects. The most common side effect of metformin is gastrointestinal (GI), which may be transient in nature and can often be avoided with gradual dose titration and taking the drug with meals.[14] In the DPP trial, through year 4 of analysis GI symptoms were significantly more common among the metformin-treated than the placebo participants (28% vs 16%). Nonserious adverse events during the DPP were uncommon and similar in the treatment and placebo groups. There were no reported serious adverse events of lactic acidosis during the nearly 18,000 patient-years of follow-up.[36] Additional documented side effects of metformin are rare, but include taste disturbance, decreased absorption of vitamin B_{12} (<1 in 10,000) and rashes.[14,26] A favorable association between metformin and a lower risk of cancer among patients with T2DM has been observed. Investigation into the anticancer properties and underlying mechanism of this effect is an area of active ongoing research.[37–40]

Thiazolidinediones

Indications and patient considerations

Pioglitazone (Actos) and rosiglitazone (Avandia) are thiazolidinedione (TZD) drugs approved by the FDA for the treatment of T2DM. Caution is advised for use with CHF (New York Heart Association [NYHA] class I or II), and both drugs are contraindicated in advanced CHF (NYHA class III or IV). Despite demonstrated glycemic efficacy and improved insulin sensitivity, because of troublesome side effects including weight gain and fluid retention, the ADA consensus statement favors metformin over TZD for first-line treatment of impaired glucose tolerance (IGT) or impaired fasting glucose (IFG).[41]

Mechanism of action, efficacy, and kinetics

The TZDs are synthetic ligands for peroxisome proliferative-activated receptor gamma (PPARγ), and are potent insulin sensitizers in muscle, liver, and adipocytes.[42–44] Rosiglitazone and pioglitazone bind to PPARγ, modulate the transcription of insulin-sensitive genes involved in the control of glucose and lipid metabolism,[26] and may have important effects on β cells. Because TZDs both improve insulin sensitivity and preserve β-cell function, they are very effective at preventing progression of IGT to T2DM and maintaining durable HbA1c reduction.[45] TZDs are extensively metabolized in the liver by the cytochrome P450 enzyme CYP2C8 and are eliminated through the feces.[46,47] Dose adjustment of TZDs is not required for geriatric patients, or those with renal or mild hepatic impairment. However, monitoring is recommended for patients with known hepatic toxicity (alanine aminotransferase 3 time the upper limit of the reference range) or those taking concurrent strong CYP2C8 inhibitors such as gemfibrozil.

Effects on weight and cardiovascular outcomes

Weight gain and fluid retention with associated edema are well-recognized side effects of TZDs.[24,26,48–50] Initiation of TZD in the intensive treatment arm of the ACCORD trial has been described as a predominant medication-related determinant of weight gain. Patients who received combination therapy of TZD with insulin had a weight gain of 4.6 to 5.3 kg at 2 years.[51] TZD-associated weight gain has been attributed to increased uptake of fatty acids and enhanced adipogenic capacity elicited by PPARγ activation of white adipose tissue.[48]

Within 2 years of approval by the FDA, reports of increased risk of heart failure associated with rosiglitazone began surfacing[52] and by 2002, the FDA added a precaution regarding rosiglitazone-induced heart failure followed by a more stringent "restricted access program" designation in 2011 after a meta-analysis of 42 clinical trials that compared rosiglitazone with placebo, which found a statistically significant increased risk of myocardial infarction in the rosiglitazone-treated group.[53,54] The FDA is scheduled to review a readjudication of the RECORD (Rosiglitazone Evaluated for Cardiovascular Outcomes and Regulation of Diabetes) trial findings in June 2013.

Evidence for a strong association with heart failure appears to be a class effect of TZDs.[55–57] However, in contrast to rosiglitazone, meta-analyses of pioglitazone suggest the possibility of ischemic cardiovascular benefit and overall reduction in mortality despite an increase in serious heart failure.[57] Systemic review and meta-analysis of 16 observational studies representing more than 800,000 TZD users reports that compared with pioglitazone, rosiglitazone is associated with a significantly increased risk of myocardial infarction (pooled odds ratio 1.2, 95% confidence interval [CI] 1.07–1.24), CHF (odds ratio 1.2, 95% CI 1.14–1.31) and overall mortality (odds ratio 1.1, 95% CI 1.09–1.20). The investigators calculate that the use of rosiglitazone would result in an annual number needed to harm (NNH) of 587 or an excess of 170 myocardial infarctions for every 100,000 patients who received rosiglitazone over pioglitazone. Use of rosiglitazone would result in an NNH of 154 for CHF, which equates to 649 excess cases for every 100,000 patients.[55]

Effects on bone and other side effects

PPARγ expression and the mechanism by which TZDs affect bone are complex and include antiosteoblastic, proadipocytic, and proosteoclastic activities. Multiple clinical studies in patients with T2DM and polycystic ovarian syndrome, and in postmenopausal nondiabetic women indicate that both rosiglitazone and pioglitazone decrease BMD and change bone markers.[6] Increased risk of fracture was demonstrated in posttrial analysis from ADOPT (A Diabetes Outcome Progression Trial).[58] The study was a randomized, double-blind controlled trial of 4600 individuals, designed to compare time to failure of monotherapy (defined as fasting plasma glucose >180 mg/dL) in prediabetic individuals randomly assigned to treatment with either rosiglitazone, metformin, or glyburide. Posttrial analysis of fracture rates, time to first fracture, and fracture location were analyzed after a median of 4 years of treatment. In men, there was no increased risk of fracture. However, among both premenopausal and postmenopausal women treated with rosiglitazone, the cumulative incidence of fractures was 15.1% (95% CI 11.2–19.1), whereas it was only 7.3% (95% CI 4.4–10.1) in the metformin group and 7.7% (95% CI 3.7–11.7) in the glyburide group, representing a hazard ratio of 1.8 versus 2.1 for rosiglitazone versus other therapies.[59] Subsequent meta-analysis of 10 randomized controlled trials and 2 observational studies, reflecting more than 40,000 participants, confirmed a 2-fold increased risk of fractures in women exposed to long-term TZD use, but not in men.[60] Other large-scale studies conducted in Canada, the United Kingdom, and the United States support that fracture risk is strongly associated with age and duration of TZD treatment, independent of gender. In summary, there is evidence that TZDs exert a negative effect on bone with increased risk of fracture in the following subpopulations: those with a history of prior fracture, longer duration of TZD treatment, older age, and, possibly, female predominance.[6]

Following conflicting reports, in 2012 a systematic review and meta-analysis was performed on the available studies that reported bladder cancer among adults taking either pioglitazone or rosiglitazone. In sum, a total of 3643 patients had newly diagnosed bladder cancer, for an overall incidence of 53.1 per 100,000 patient-years. All 5 studies assessing pioglitazone demonstrated an elevated risk of bladder cancer associated with pioglitazone use, whereas in the 3 studies reporting incidence of bladder cancer among rosiglitazone users, no association was found. The investigators concluded that based on a pooled estimate of 1.7 million individuals there is evidence of an increased risk of bladder cancer with pioglitazone but not with rosiglitazone.[61]

SECRETAGOGUES

Sulfonylureas and meglitinides, lower glucose levels by stimulating insulin secretion.

Sulfonylureas

Indications and patient considerations

Sulfonylureas are approved by the FDA for the treatment of T2DM in adults. In addition, clinical efficacy has been demonstrated in single-gene diabetes (HNF1A MODY) and permanent neonatal diabetes associated with the KCNJ11 and ABCC9 genes.[62] Because of the risk for hypoglycemia, sulfonylureas should be used with caution in elderly, debilitated, or malnourished patients, or in patients with renal or hepatic insufficiency. In these patients the initial dosing, dose increments, and maintenance dosage should be conservative.

Mechanism of action, efficacy, and kinetics

Sulfonylureas stimulate the release of insulin secretion by binding to the sulfonylurea receptor (SUR-1), a component of the adenosine triphosphate (ATP)-sensitive potassium channel (K_{ATP}) expressed in the pancreatic β cells,[63] leading to calcium influx and increased responsiveness of β cells to glucose and nonglucose stimuli. These drugs lower HbA1c levels by 1% to 2%,[64] and their glycemic effect is dependent on residual β-cell function. Although the therapeutic mechanism of all sulfonylureas is similar, first-generation sulfonylureas, for example, tolbutamide (Oranase) and chlorpropamide (Diabinase), have significantly lower affinity for the SUR receptor than do second-generation sulfonylureas such as glyburide (Micronase), glipizide (Glucotrol), and glimepiride (Amaryl). This difference accounts for the greater potency and efficacy of the second-generation drugs. Most sulfonylureas are transformed by cytochrome P450 in the liver to inactive metabolites; thus, their circulatory levels can be affected by any factors modifying the cytochrome P450 system.[65] Renal excretion is important for 2 drugs in this category, glyburide and chlorpropamide, therefore they should be used with caution in patients with renal impairment.[66]

Effects on weight and cardiovascular outcomes

Weight gain of 1.5 to 2.0 kg is common in the first year following initiation of sulfonylurea therapy, and typically levels off thereafter.[2,67,68] At present, all sulfonylureas carry an FDA-required warning about the increased risk of cardiovascular death. This decision was based in part on findings from the UGDP (University Group Diabetes Program) trial, in which diabetic patients treated with tolbutamide, a first-generation sulfonylurea, experienced higher cardiovascular mortality compared with insulin or placebo.[69] However, findings from the UKPDS (United Kingdom Prospective Diabetes Study) did not reveal an increased risk of cardiovascular complications over 10 years of follow-up in patients with T2DM treated with sulfonylurea.[2,70,71] Experimentally, sulfonylureas that bind to myocardial K_{ATP} channels have been shown to block the beneficial effects of ischemic preconditioning, which refers to a cardioprotective phenomenon recognized to reduce infarct size, augment postischemic function, and prevent arrhythmias.[71,72] Newer sulfonylureas, such as gliclazide (Diamicron) or glimepiride, are exclusively pancreatic β-cell specific and might offer advantages over older agents. Among sulfonylurea-treated patients in a French registry of acute myocardial infarction, in-hospital mortality was significantly lower in patients receiving pancreatic cell–specific sulfonylureas (gliclazide or glimepiride) (2.7%), compared with glyburide (7.5%). Arrhythmias and ischemic complications were also markedly less frequent in patients receiving gliclazide/glimepiride (11% vs 18%).[73] Thus, tissue-specific effects of sulfonylureas may account for the apparent conflict of beneficial and deleterious cardiovascular outcomes reported in previous studies.

Effects on bone and other adverse effects

Results from ADOPT did not indicate adverse effects of these compounds on bone mass or fracture risk.[59] Beyond the most common side effects of hypoglycemia, other adverse effects include nausea, abdominal discomfort, headache, hypersensitivity, skin reactions (including photosensitivity), and abnormal liver function tests. Differential tissue specificity of particular sulfonylureas outside the pancreas could account for variability in complications related to these drugs. Unique to chlorpropamide is water retention and potential for hyponatremia mediated through secretion of antidiuretic hormone.[66,74] In addition, chlorpropamide can cause an unpleasant flushing reaction after alcohol ingestion by inhibiting the metabolism of acetaldehyde.[75]

Meglitinides

Indications and patient considerations

Meglitinide analogues, nateglinide (Starlix) and repaglinide (Prandin), are approved for the treatment of T2DM in adults. Caution is recommended for moderate to severe hepatic impairment, and dose adjustment is indicated for creatinine clearance of less than 20 to 40 mL/min for repaglinide.

Mechanism of action, efficacy, and kinetics

Similar to sulfonylureas, meglitinides stimulate insulin release by inhibiting K_{ATP} channels, causing membrane depolarization, increased intracellular calcium, and insulin exocytosis. However, meglitinides have a distinct binding site of the β-cell membrane.[76] Although both drugs are rapid acting,[77] nateglinide dissociates from the receptor 90 times faster than repaglinide, indicating a very short on-and-off effect on insulin release. Nateglinide is hepatically cleared, with approximately 65% excreted in the bile and feces and 35% in the urine.[78] Repaglinide is metabolized by cytochrome P450 CYP3A4, with 90% excreted in bile and less than 10% in urine. Substances that inhibit CYP3A4 (eg, ketoconazole, steroids) may reduce repaglinide clearance, whereas drugs that induce CYP3A4 (eg, rifampin, carbamazepine) may accelerate repaglinide metabolism.[76] The efficacy of meglitinide monotherapy is similar to that of the sulfonylureas.[79–81] Repaglinide reduces HbA1c values by 0.1% to 2.1%, and nateglinide reduces HbA1c values by 0.2% to 0.6%.[82]

Effects on weight and cardiovascular outcomes

A Cochrane review of meglitinide analogues reports a range of weight gain from 0.7 to 2.1 kg across several trials.[82] To date, there have been no reported significant differences in blood pressure or lipid profiles among patients treated with meglitinide.[83] Because the mechanism of action of meglitinides affects the ATP-dependent potassium channels, it is possible that meglitinide analogues may have an association with poorer outcomes following a myocardial infarction, similar to sulfonylureas[73]; however, studies of long-term cardiovascular outcomes of meglitinides are lacking.

Other side effects or known complications of treatment

Similar to sulfonylureas, the most common side effect of meglitinides is mild hypoglycemia. Meglitinides have been associated with several other nonspecific side effects including dizziness, diarrhea, constipation, arthralgias, headache, and cough.[82,84,85]

α-GLUCOSIDASE INHIBITORS

Indications and Patient Considerations

The α-glucosidase inhibitors (AGI), acarbose (Precose), miglitol (Glyset), and voglibose (Voglib), are indicated for treatment of adults with T2DM. The class is contraindicated in patients with cirrhosis, inflammatory bowel disease, colonic ulceration, intestinal obstruction, or predisposition to obstruction and diabetic ketoacidosis.

Mechanism of Action, Efficacy, and Kinetics

Relative to placebo, both acarbose and miglitol have demonstrated reduction of HbA1c to 0.5% to 0.8%.[86] AGIs lower glucose levels through reversible, competitive inhibition of pancreatic α-amylase and membrane-bound intestinal α-glucoside hydrolyases. These enzymes inhibit the conversion of complex polysaccharide carbohydrates into monosaccharides, which slows the absorption of glucose and improves postprandial glucose levels.[87] In addition, following treatment with voglibose there is a measureable increase of endogenous glucagon-like peptide[88] that may further facilitate glucose-lowering effects. Acarbose has a short $t_{1/2}$ of 2 hours; thus, to be effective it must be dosed at least 3 times daily with meals. Acarbose is metabolized within the GI tract by digestive enzymes and intestinal bacteria. The fraction that is absorbed intact is excreted by the kidneys. Therefore, use with renal impairment (creatinine clearance <25 mL/min) is not recommended for acarbose or miglitol because of the risk for increased plasma concentrations of the drug; however, voglibose is minimally excreted in the urine and therefore dose adjustment is not required. Elevated liver transaminases have been reported, and the package insert recommends reduced doses or withdrawal of treatment if abnormalities of liver enzymes develop.

Effects on Body Weight and Cardiovascular Outcomes

Meta-analysis of 41 randomized controlled trials and systematic review confirm that acarbose and miglitol are weight neutral.[24] The mode of action of acarbose is to diminish glucose and insulin response to meal ingestion; and lower insulin levels are proposed to explain weight neutrality.[89]

Acarbose therapy has been shown to have a beneficial effect in comparison with placebo in preventing progression of an increase in carotid intimal wall thickness in patients with established coronary artery disease and either IGT or established T2DM,[90] as well as favorable effect on the level of low-density lipoprotein (LDL) and triglyceride.[91] Cardiovascular outcomes were the primary end point of the multicenter, international, double-blind, randomized controlled STOP-NIDDM (Study to Prevent Non Insulin Dependent Diabetes Mellitus) trial, in which 1429 patients with IGT were randomized to either placebo or acarbose 100 mg 3 times daily, and followed for a mean of 3.3 years. At the end of the study, acarbose use was associated with 49% relative risk reduction in combined cardiovascular events (coronary heart disease, cardiovascular death, CHF, cerebrovascular event, peripheral vascular disease, and hypertension >140/90 mm Hg; hazard ratio [HR] 0.51, 95% CI 0.28%–0.95%; 2.5% absolute risk reduction). The major reduction was in the risk of myocardial infarction and development of hypertension.[92]

Other Side Effects

Fermentation of an increased amount of undigested carbohydrate by bacteria in the colon accounts for the common observed side effects of abdominal pain, diarrhea, and flatulence.[91] Incidence of GI side effects varies widely across international trials. In a surveillance study of 6142 patients in the United States, intolerance was 37%, compared with 13.4% of 27,803 patients from Germany and just 2% of 14,418 patients in China and other Asian countries enrolled in postmarketing studies. The difference may in part be due to dose and titration schedules; however, given the mechanism of action it is likely that nutritional factors contribute as well. Diets higher in fiber are associated with a lower incidence of side effects. Incidence of side effects has been shown to be dose dependent, and slow titration of dose is recommended to limit the onset of unpleasant side effects.[89] Elevation of hepatic enzymes has been reported, as has one case of fulminant hepatitis with a fatal outcome. It is recommended to monitor patients with liver disease and to adjust dose or discontinue the dosing if necessary.

GLUCAGON-LIKE PEPTIDE 1–BASED DRUGS

Glucagon-like peptide 1 (GLP-1) is a gut hormone secreted in response to nutrient ingestion, which regulates postprandial glucose homeostasis. Once secreted into the circulation, GLP-1 is metabolized rapidly to inactive compounds by the action of ubiquitous enzyme dipeptidyl-peptidase 4 (DPP-4), leading to a plasma $t_{1/2}$ of 1 to 2 minutes.[93] Two classes of drugs in this category, GLP-1 receptor (GLP-1r) agonists and DPP-4 inhibitors, have been developed using strategies to bypass or block DPP-4 action, leading to compounds with half-lives longer than native GLP-1 or causing higher concentrations of native GLP-1 levels, respectively.

Indications and Patient Considerations

Exenatide (Byetta) was the first GLP-1r agonist to be approved in the United States in 2005, and sitagliptin (Januvia) the first DPP-4 inhibitor approved a year later. To date, liraglutide (Victoza) and exenatide long-acting release (LAR; Bydureon) from the class of GLP-1r agonists, and saxagliptin (Onglyza), linagliptin (Tradjenta), and alogliptin (Nesina) from the class of DPP-4 inhibitors, have been approved for the treatment of T2DM as an add-on to metformin, thiazolidinediones, sulfonylureas, and basal insulin, or a combination of these drugs. These drugs were recommended as second-line agents after metformin in the recent joint statement by the ADA/ESD[9] because of the weight neutrality with DPP-4 inhibitors or weight loss with GLP-1r agonist therapy, as well as the lack of hypoglycemia with both classes of drugs. DPP-4 inhibitors, unlike the injectable GLP-1r agonists, are administered orally, which might be preferred by patients. Caution is advised for use with concurrent renal or hepatic impairment. GLP-1r agonists are contraindicated in patients with prior history of or current pancreatitis, and individual or family history of medullary thyroid cancer.

Mechanism of Action, Efficacy, and Kinetics

GLP-1 actions are mediated by binding to a specific GLP-1 receptor that is expressed on β cells, along with many other cells such as gastric and small intestinal mucosal cells, cardiac myocytes, neurons in some brain regions, and the vagus nerve.[94,95] Administration of GLP-1 or GLP-1r agonists improves glycemia by enhancing insulin response,[96,97] inhibiting glucagon release from pancreatic α cells,[96] delaying gastric emptying,[98–100] inducing satiety,[101] and lowering hepatic glucose production.[102] The noninsulin effects of GLP-1 are equally essential in glycemic control, as GLP-1 infusion has been shown to normalize hyperglycemia in patients with type 1 diabetes mellitus (T1DM) and no residual β-cell function,[103,104] even though the use of these compounds in T1DM has not been approved. Although DPP-4 inhibitors share the insulin and glucagon effect of GLP-1r agonists, they have a trivial effect on gastric emptying.[105]

Treatment with GLP-1r agonists leads to HbA1c reduction of 1.1% to 1.6% compared with 0.6% to 1.1% with DPP-4 inhibitors; the greatest efficacy on HbA1c and fasting plasma glucose among GLP-1r agonists was reported with long-acting agents, liraglutide (once a day) and exenatide LAR once weekly, in comparison with short-acting drugs (twice a day). Available GLP-1r agonists are excreted by the kidney; therefore, their use is not recommended in the setting of severe renal impairment. In patients with moderate renal impairment, short-acting exenatide can be used with careful optimization of the dose, but there are not enough data to support the use of long-acting GLP-1r agonists. In hepatic impairment, lack of data for the use of liraglutide limits its utility, but dose adjustment is not necessary for exenatide therapy. DPP-4 inhibitors and their metabolites have distinctive pharmacokinetic properties leading to drug-specific adverse effects in this class of drugs. Saxagliptin is excreted through renal and hepatic clearance mechanisms, whereas sitagliptin is excreted mainly through renal excretion. Therefore, dose adjustment is necessary in the setting of both moderate and severe renal impairment.[106,107] By contrast, linagliptin is excreted mostly in feces through enterohepatic circulation, and requires no dose adjustment for renal impairment.[106,108] Evidence regarding the use of DPP-4 inhibitors in severe hepatic failure is lacking.

Effects of Treatment on Weight and Cardiovascular Outcomes

GLP-1r agonist therapy results in a weight reduction of greater than 2 kg, whereas DPP-4 inhibitors are weight neutral.[109] Data on long-term effects of GLP-1 based drugs on cardiovascular outcomes are lacking, although these drugs may have beneficial effects on surrogate markers of cardiovascular disease. The evidence suggests that GLP-1r agonists improve systolic blood pressure[110–112] as early as 2 weeks from initiation of treatment,[113] indicating the weight-loss independence of this effect. Moreover, comparative studies of sitagliptin versus liraglutide or exenatide LAR therapy for 26 weeks have shown a greater effect on systolic and diastolic blood pressure as a result of sitagliptin treatment, whereas the effect on weight loss was trivial in comparison with GLP-1r agonist therapy.[114] GLP-1r agonists also improve the levels of triglyceride and free fatty acid,[115] although it is not clear whether this effect is weight independent. The evidence for antilipid effects of DPP-4 inhibitors is mixed, with neutral[116] to favorable effects[117] being reported on lipid profile with sitagliptin therapy.

Other Side Effects or Known Complications of Treatment

Because of glucose dependence of GLP-1 action on insulin secretion and glucagon suppression,[118] hypoglycemia is not associated with treatment of GLP-1r agonists or DPP-4 inhibitors, unless these drugs are administered in combination with other insulin secretagogues or insulin without proper dose adjustment.[117,119–123]

GI side effects, mainly nausea and vomiting, are the most common adverse effects associated with GLP-1r agonist therapy (30%–60%) and are the main cause for early termination of treatment with these drugs. However, nausea is mostly mild and dose dependent, and wanes over time.[119,120,124] Whereas nausea is less frequently reported with long-acting GLP-1r agonists compared with short-acting exenatide,[115,125] diarrhea seems to be more frequent with long-acting agents.[125] DPP-4 inhibitors do not cause GI side effects seen with GLP-1r agonists.[117,121–123]

The FDA has issued a warning about the potential risk of acute pancreatitis with the use of GLP-1–based drugs, given early postmarketing reports[126,127] and findings from a recent population database study.[127] Although the causal relationship between pancreatitis and GLP-1–based drugs has not yet been established[128] and the number of cases reported with this condition is small, patients should be informed about the symptoms of acute pancreatitis, and therapy should be discontinued if these develop.

Long-acting GLP-1r agonists should also not be used in patients with any personal or family history of medullary thyroid cancer or multiple endocrine neoplasia type 2. Animal studies have suggested that liraglutide could increase the risk of C-cell hyperplasia and medullary thyroid cancer via activation of functional GLP-1rs that are expressed on thyroid C cells.[129,130] It is noteworthy that these results were not replicated in the studies of nonhuman primates,[131] nor did 2 years of treatment with liraglutide result in increased calcitonin levels.[131]

The wide expression of DPP-4 in different tissue cells, including T cells, has raised concerns about the potential adverse effects of DPP-4 inhibitors on immunomodulation and T-cell signaling, which need to be addressed in future studies.

AMYLIN ANALOGUES
Indications and Patient Considerations

Pramlintide (Symlin) is indicated for adjunctive use in both T1DM and T2DM in patients already taking prandial insulin. It is contraindicated in patients with a confirmed diagnosis of gastroparesis and hypoglycemia unawareness, owing to the increased risk of hypoglycemia. Dose titration is recommended, and prandial insulin doses should be reduced by 50% at the onset of therapy to limit the risk of hypoglycemia.

Mechanism of Action, Efficacy, and Kinetics

Amylin, also called islet amyloid polypeptide or diabetes-associated peptide, is produced by pancreatic β cells and is cosecreted with insulin in a 1:100 amylin/insulin ratio. Soluble amylin analogue, pramlintide acetate, is synergistic with insulin; that is, when given subcutaneously at mealtimes in combination with prandial insulin, pramlintide provides further reduction in postprandial hyperglycemia and concomitant reduction of glucagon levels in comparison with insulin monotherapy.[132] Multiple daily dosing is required, as the $t_{1/2}$ is 48 minutes; metabolism is primarily via the kidneys. Amylin may further contribute to improved glucose levels via central anorectic effects, inhibition of ghrelin release, delayed gastric emptying, and reduced insulin dose requirements.[133,134] A 1-year randomized controlled trial of pramlintide as adjunct to insulin therapy among patients with T1DM demonstrated reduction of HbA1c by 0.3% in the treated group compared with no change of HbA1c in the placebo group.[135]

Effects of Treatment on Weight and Cardiovascular Outcomes

When pramlintide is added to basal insulin, no weight gain is observed.[24] In a dose-finding study with pramlintide added to a variety of insulin regimens, weight loss (−1.4 kg) was observed across the active treatment groups.[136] Pramlintide decreases the insulin requirement, thus the weight-neutral or weight-beneficial effects may be a result of the decreased weight-promoting effects of insulin. A modest and dose-dependent beneficial effect on lipid profiles has been observed in short-term studies.[137] There are no data on long-term cardiovascular outcome.

Other Side Effects

When compared with placebo, frequently reported side effects (>10% of patients) include mild to moderate hypoglycemia, nausea, vomiting, and anorexia during the first month of therapy.[138]

SODIUM-GLUCOSE TRANSPORTER INHIBITORS
Indications and Patient Considerations

Sodium-glucose transporter 2 (SGLT2) inhibitors are a novel class of antidiabetes agents that exert glucose lowering primarily through effects on renal glucose handling. Several drugs in this class are in various stages of clinical development; canagliflozin (Invokana) is the first agent in this class to achieve a recent FDA approval for the treatment of T2DM. Use is contraindicated in severe renal impairment (glomerular filtration rate [GFR] <30 mL/min) or severe liver disease, and dose adjustment is advised for moderate renal impairment (GFR <45 mL/min). Monitoring for hypotension is recommended, particularly for elderly patients.

Mechanism of Action, Efficacy, and Kinetics

Under normal conditions, filtered glucose is actively reabsorbed by the sodium-glucose transporters SGLT1 and SGLT2 in the proximal tubule.[139] SGLT2 inhibitors

Table 1
Comparison of diabetes treatment complications and therapeutic considerations

Medication Class Drug Examples	Dose-Adjustment Considerations	Weight Effect	CV Effects	Bone Effect	Association with Cancer	Pregnancy Category
Biguanide Metformin	Renal insufficiency Hepatic insufficiency	Neutral or loss	Neutral or possible benefit on lipid profile and CV outcomes	Neutral or possible benefit	Possible beneficial effects	B
Thiazolidinedione Rosiglitazone Pioglitazone	Caution: CHF (class I and II) Contraindication: CHF (class III and IV); concurrent use of CYP2C8 inhibitors	Gain and edema	Increased risk of CHF; rosiglitazone associated with higher risk of ischemia and CV mortality	Negative impact on BMD; increased fracture risk in select populations	Pioglitazone associated with increased risk of bladder cancer	C
Sulfonylurea Chlorpropamide, tolbutamide Glyburide, glipizide, glimepiride	Renal insufficiency (chlorpropamide, glyburide) Hepatic insufficiency Elderly or malnourished	Neutral or gain	Increased risk of CV death following myocardial infarction	No effect	Unknown	C (glyburide, class B)
Meglitinide analogues Nateglinide Repaglinide	Renal insufficiency Hepatic insufficiency Concomitant use with gemfibrozil (repaglinide) Monitor with concurrent CYP3A4 metabolized medications	Neutral or gain	No change in lipids or blood pressure	Unknown	Unknown	C

α-Glucosidase inhibitors Acarbose Miglitol Voglibose	Renal insufficiency (acarbose, miglitol) Hepatic insufficiency Contraindication: cirrhosis, inflammatory bowel disease, colonic ulceration or obstruction	Neutral	Risk reduction for myocardial infarction and hypertension	Unknown	Unknown	B
GLP-1r agonist Exenatide Liraglutide	Renal insufficiency (long-acting exenatide) Hepatic insufficiency (liraglutide) Contraindicated with prior pancreatitis	Loss or neutral	Beneficial, improves blood pressure and lipid profiles	No effect	Black-box warning for personal or family history of medullary thyroid cancer or MEN 2	C
DPP-4 analogues Saxagliptin Linagliptin Alogliptin	Renal insufficiency (saxagliptin, alogliptin) Hepatic insufficiency	Neutral	Neutral, possible beneficial effects on lipid profiles	Decreased fractures	Unknown	B
Amylin analogues Pramlintide	Reduce prandial insulin	Neutral or loss	Possible beneficial effect on lipid profiles	Unknown	Unknown	C
SGLT2 inhibitors Canagliflozin	Renal insufficiency Hepatic insufficiency	Loss or neutral	Beneficial effects on systolic blood pressure	Unknown	Unknown	C

Abbreviations: BMD, bone mineral density; CHF, congestive heart failure; CV, cardiovascular; MEN 2, multiple endocrine neoplasia type 2.

reduce renal glucose reabsorption, resulting in increased excretion of urinary glucose and corresponding osmotic diuresis.[140] Completed trials of canagliflozin, dapagliflozin, and empagliflozin have demonstrated a mean reduction in HbA1c ranging from 0.6% to 0.9%.[141] Patients treated for 26 weeks with canagliflozin demonstrated decreases in proinsulin/insulin and proinsulin/C-peptide ratios compared with placebo,[139] suggestive of some improvement in β-cell function. Canagliflozin is converted to inactive metabolites via O-glucuronidation in the liver, and excreted via feces and urine.

Effects of Treatment on Weight and Cardiovascular Outcomes

SGLT2 inhibitors have demonstrated a 2- to 3-kg weight loss in short-term (12 weeks' duration) trials.[140–142] Fluid loss secondary to osmotic diuresis may account for early weight reduction; however, the glucose excreted in the urine as a result of SGLT2 inhibition equates to a loss of 200 to 300 calories daily,[140] which may provide ongoing beneficial effects on weight. A trial of dapagliflozin demonstrated a reduction in waist circumference[143] and sustained weight loss over 102 weeks when used in combination with metformin.[144] Reductions in systolic blood pressure up to 5 mm Hg have been described in trials of canagliflozin[139] and dapagliflozin,[140] likely attributable to glycosuria-induced diuresis. A statistically significant dose-related decrease in high-density lipoprotein cholesterol was observed in the 26-week randomized controlled trial of canagliflozin,[139] with a trend toward lower triglycerides and LDL cholesterol. Data regarding cardiovascular outcomes for SGLT2 inhibitors are limited; however, a series of ongoing safety trials and the CANVAS (Canagliflozin Cardiovascular Assessment Study) are anticipated to provide additional evidence in the upcoming years.[141]

Other Side Effects

The predominant reported side effect of SGLT2 inhibitors to date are increased rates of mycotic infections (vulvovaginitis, balanitis) and, less commonly, urinary tract infections,[139,141,144] presumably as a result of elevated urinary glucose levels.

EFFECTS ON β-CELL OUTCOMES

Once fasting hyperglycemia is detectable, β-cell function deteriorates progressively and contributes to further decline in the ability to maintain normal glycemic levels.[145,146] Thus, preservation of β-cell function in the prediabetes state (IGT, IFG) and prevention of further loss of β-cell function once diabetes occurs is a critical aim of therapy and is an important factor for selection of antidiabetic treatment.

Despite initial beneficial therapeutic effects, metformin may not have long-term beneficial effects on β-cell function based on disease progression (failure of monotherapy to maintain goal HbA1c).[45] Sulfonylureas may have a negative effect on β-cell function, based on some in vitro studies showing that the closure of the ATP-dependent potassium channels by tolbutamide and glibenclamide may induce calcium-dependent β-cell apoptosis in rodent and human islets.[79,81] TZDs and GLP-1–based drugs, on the other hand, may have a beneficial effect on β-cell function and may promote β-cell survival based on in vitro and animal studies.[44,147,148] However, it is not known how much of these preclinical data could be translated to clinical outcomes given the current ability to measure β-cell mass directly in humans.

Comparative studies on the durability of glycemic reduction effects of various drugs have been used to provide information about the chronic effects of these agents on islet preservation, considering that the progressive nature of β-cell dysfunction requires a continuous intensification of treatment to maintain target glycemia. ADOPT[149] is the first randomized trial to compare the long-term effect of 3 conventional oral agents, glyburide, metformin, and rosiglitazone, on glucose control for a 4-year follow-up. The findings from this trial indicated that patients with early-stage T2DM receiving glyburide had the fastest decline in glycemic control and those assigned to rosiglitazone the slowest, with patients treated with metformin being somewhere in between.

Recently, findings from a randomized trial comparing the long-term effect on glucose control of adding short-acting exenatide or glimepiride to metformin therapy in approximately 10,000 patients with uncontrolled T2DM (average basal HbA1c 7.5%) showed that more patients in the glimepiride group than in the exenatide group (54% vs 41%) experienced treatment failure. In this study, the median time to inadequate glucose control and the need for alternative treatment was markedly shorter in those treated with sulfonylurea than in patients treated with a GLP-1r agonist (140 vs 180 weeks).[150] However, the largest risk reduction as a result of GLP-1r agonist therapy was observed in patients with higher baseline HbA1c level (>7.3%), who had the highest risk of treatment failure in general. Moreover, patients in the exenatide group had an average weight loss of 3 kg, which could contribute to treatment outcome.

Although these studies are not able to prove the beneficial effects of GLP-1–based drugs or TZDs on β-cell survival and β-cell expansion based on preclinical data, they raise the question as to whether treatment with these agents should be considered for prevention purposes, or should be initiated at an earlier stage of diabetes.

SUMMARY

T2DM is a progressive disease characterized by the need for additional antidiabetic treatments over time to maintain glycemic control at the target. A large body of evidence now supports the maintenance of glycemic control as a means of eliminating the microvascular complications of diabetes. Therefore, individualized therapy started at an earlier stage of disease, guided by the principle of "do not harm," seems to be essential in the patient-centric, shared decision-making model of diabetes care. Long-term clinical outcome data are needed to address the differential disease-modifying effects of various antidiabetic drugs (**Table 1**).

REFERENCES

1. The effect of intensive treatment of diabetes on the development and progression of long-term complications in insulin-dependent diabetes mellitus. The Diabetes Control and Complications Trial Research Group. N Engl J Med 1993; 329(14):977–86.
2. Intensive blood-glucose control with sulphonylureas or insulin compared with conventional treatment and risk of complications in patients with type 2 diabetes (UKPDS 33). UK Prospective Diabetes Study (UKPDS) Group. Lancet 1998; 352(9131):837–53.
3. Stratton IM, Adler AI, Neil HA, et al. Association of glycaemia with macrovascular and microvascular complications of type 2 diabetes (UKPDS 35): prospective observational study. BMJ 2000;321(7258):405–12.
4. Holman RR, Paul SK, Bethel MA, et al. 10-year follow-up of intensive glucose control in type 2 diabetes. N Engl J Med 2008;359(15):1577–89.
5. Gerstein HC, Miller ME, Byington RP, et al. Effects of intensive glucose lowering in type 2 diabetes. N Engl J Med 2008;358(24):2545–59.

6. Lecka-Czernik B. Safety of anti-diabetic therapies on bone. Clin Rev Bone Miner Metab 2013;11(1):49–58.

7. Giovannucci E, Harlan DM, Archer MC, et al. Diabetes and cancer: a consensus report. Diabetes Care 2010;33(7):1674–85.

8. Larsson SC, Orsini N, Brismar K, et al. Diabetes mellitus and risk of bladder cancer: a meta-analysis. Diabetologia 2006;49(12):2819–23.

9. Nathan DM, Buse JB, Davidson MB, et al. Medical management of hyperglycemia in type 2 diabetes: a consensus algorithm for the initiation and adjustment of therapy: a consensus statement of the American Diabetes Association and the European Association for the Study of Diabetes. Diabetes Care 2009;32(1): 193–203.

10. Inzucchi SE, Bergenstal RM, Buse JB, et al. Management of hyperglycaemia in type 2 diabetes: a patient-centered approach. Position statement of the American Diabetes Association (ADA) and the European Association for the Study of Diabetes (EASD). Diabetologia 2012;55(6):1577–96.

11. Garber AJ, Abrahamson MJ, Barzilay JI, et al. AACE comprehensive diabetes management algorithm 2013. Endocr Pract 2013;19(2):327–36.

12. DeFronzo RA, Goodman AM. Efficacy of metformin in patients with non-insulin-dependent diabetes mellitus. The Multicenter Metformin Study Group. N Engl J Med 1995;333(9):541–9.

13. DeFronzo RA, Stonehouse AH, Han J, et al. Relationship of baseline HbA1c and efficacy of current glucose-lowering therapies: a meta-analysis of randomized clinical trials. Diabet Med 2010;27(3):309–17.

14. Kirpichnikov D, McFarlane SI, Sowers JR. Metformin: an update. Ann Intern Med 2002;137(1):25–33.

15. Cusi K, Consoli A, DeFronzo RA. Metabolic effects of metformin on glucose and lactate metabolism in noninsulin-dependent diabetes mellitus. J Clin Endocrinol Metab 1996;81(11):4059–67.

16. Dorella M, Giusto M, Da Tos V, et al. Improvement of insulin sensitivity by metformin treatment does not lower blood pressure of nonobese insulin-resistant hypertensive patients with normal glucose tolerance. J Clin Endocrinol Metab 1996;81(4):1568–74.

17. Hundal RS, Krssak M, Dufour S, et al. Mechanism by which metformin reduces glucose production in type 2 diabetes. Diabetes 2000;49(12):2063–9.

18. Natali A, Ferrannini E. Effects of metformin and thiazolidinediones on suppression of hepatic glucose production and stimulation of glucose uptake in type 2 diabetes: a systematic review. Diabetologia 2006;49(3):434–41.

19. Gunton JE, Delhanty PJ, Takahashi S, et al. Metformin rapidly increases insulin receptor activation in human liver and signals preferentially through insulin-receptor substrate-2. J Clin Endocrinol Metab 2003;88(3):1323–32.

20. Maida A, Lamont BJ, Cao X, et al. Metformin regulates the incretin receptor axis via a pathway dependent on peroxisome proliferator-activated receptor-alpha in mice. Diabetologia 2011;54(2):339–49.

21. Graham GG, Punt J, Arora M, et al. Clinical pharmacokinetics of metformin. Clin Pharmacokinet 2011;50(2):81–98.

22. Knowler WC, Barrett-Connor E, Fowler SE, et al. Reduction in the incidence of type 2 diabetes with lifestyle intervention or metformin. N Engl J Med 2002; 346(6):393–403.

23. Knowler WC, Fowler SE, Hamman RF, et al. 10-year follow-up of diabetes incidence and weight loss in the Diabetes Prevention Program Outcomes Study. Lancet 2009;374(9702):1677–86.

24. Meneghini LF, Orozco-Beltran D, Khunti K, et al. Weight beneficial treatments for type 2 diabetes. J Clin Endocrinol Metab 2011;96(11):3337–53.
25. Phung OJ, Scholle JM, Talwar M, et al. Effect of noninsulin antidiabetic drugs added to metformin therapy on glycemic control, weight gain, and hypoglycemia in type 2 diabetes. JAMA 2010;303(14):1410–8.
26. Wong AK, Struthers AD, Choy AM, et al. Insulin sensitization therapy and the heart: focus on metformin and thiazolidinediones. Heart Fail Clin 2012;8(4):539–50.
27. Salpeter SR, Greyber E, Pasternak GA, et al. Risk of fatal and nonfatal lactic acidosis with metformin use in type 2 diabetes mellitus: systematic review and meta-analysis. Arch Intern Med 2003;163(21):2594–602.
28. Masoudi FA, Inzucchi SE, Wang Y, et al. Thiazolidinediones, metformin, and outcomes in older patients with diabetes and heart failure: an observational study. Circulation 2005;111(5):583–90.
29. Bodmer M, Meier C, Krahenbuhl S, et al. Metformin, sulfonylureas, or other antidiabetes drugs and the risk of lactic acidosis or hypoglycemia: a nested case-control analysis. Diabetes Care 2008;31(11):2086–91.
30. Eurich DT, McAlister FA, Blackburn DF, et al. Benefits and harms of antidiabetic agents in patients with diabetes and heart failure: systematic review. BMJ 2007;335(7618):497.
31. Selvin E, Bolen S, Yeh HC, et al. Cardiovascular outcomes in trials of oral diabetes medications: a systematic review. Arch Intern Med 2008;168(19):2070–80.
32. Lamanna C, Monami M, Marchionni N, et al. Effect of metformin on cardiovascular events and mortality: a meta-analysis of randomized clinical trials. Diabetes Obes Metab 2011;13(3):221–8.
33. Scheen AJ, Paquot N. Metformin revisited: a critical review of the benefit-risk balance in at-risk patients with type 2 diabetes. Diabetes Metab 2013;39(3):179–90.
34. Borges JL, Bilezikian JP, Jones-Leone AR, et al. A randomized, parallel group, double-blind, multicentre study comparing the efficacy and safety of Avandamet (rosiglitazone/metformin) and metformin on long-term glycaemic control and bone mineral density after 80 weeks of treatment in drug-naive type 2 diabetes mellitus patients. Diabetes Obes Metab 2011;13(11):1036–46.
35. Sedlinsky C, Molinuevo MS, Cortizo AM, et al. Metformin prevents anti-osteogenic in vivo and ex vivo effects of rosiglitazone in rats. Eur J Pharmacol 2011;668(3):477–85.
36. Diabetes Prevention Program Research Group. Long-term safety, tolerability, and weight loss associated with metformin in the Diabetes Prevention Program Outcomes Study. Diabetes Care 2012;35(4):731–7.
37. Chung HH, Moon JS, Yoon JS, et al. The relationship between metformin and cancer in patients with Type 2 diabetes. Diabetes Metab J 2013;37(2):125–31.
38. Bost F, Sahra IB, Le Marchand-Brustel Y, et al. Metformin and cancer therapy. Curr Opin Oncol 2012;24(1):103–8.
39. Ben Sahra I, Le Marchand-Brustel Y, Tanti JF, et al. Metformin in cancer therapy: a new perspective for an old antidiabetic drug? Mol Cancer Ther 2010;9(5):1092–9.
40. Loubiere C, Dirat B, Tanti JF, et al. New perspectives for metformin in cancer therapy. Ann Endocrinol (Paris) 2013;74(2):130–6 [in French].
41. Nathan DM, Davidson MB, DeFronzo RA, et al. Impaired fasting glucose and impaired glucose tolerance: implications for care. Diabetes Care 2007;30(3):753–9.

42. Molavi B, Rassouli N, Bagwe S, et al. A review of thiazolidinediones and metformin in the treatment of type 2 diabetes with focus on cardiovascular complications. Vasc Health Risk Manag 2007;3(6):967–73.

43. Yki-Jarvinen H. Thiazolidinediones. N Engl J Med 2004;351(11):1106–18.

44. Gastaldelli A, Ferrannini E, Miyazaki Y, et al. Thiazolidinediones improve beta-cell function in type 2 diabetic patients. Am J Physiol Endocrinol Metab 2007; 292(3):E871–83.

45. DeFronzo RA, Abdul-Ghani MA. Preservation of beta-cell function: the key to diabetes prevention. J Clin Endocrinol Metab 2011;96(8):2354–66.

46. Budde K, Neumayer HH, Fritsche L, et al. The pharmacokinetics of pioglitazone in patients with impaired renal function. Br J Clin Pharmacol 2003; 55(4):368–74.

47. Kirchheiner J, Thomas S, Bauer S, et al. Pharmacokinetics and pharmacodynamics of rosiglitazone in relation to CYP2C8 genotype. Clin Pharmacol Ther 2006;80(6):657–67.

48. Ahmadian M, Suh JM, Hah N, et al. PPARgamma signaling and metabolism: the good, the bad and the future. Nat Med 2013;19(5):557–66.

49. Tschope D, Hanefeld M, Meier JJ, et al. The role of co-morbidity in the selection of antidiabetic pharmacotherapy in type-2 diabetes. Cardiovasc Diabetol 2013; 12(1):62.

50. Kung J, Henry RR. Thiazolidinedione safety. Expert Opin Drug Saf 2012;11(4): 565–79.

51. Fonseca V, McDuffie R, Calles J, et al. Determinants of weight gain in the action to control cardiovascular risk in diabetes trial. Diabetes Care 2013. [Epub ahead of print].

52. Benbow A, Stewart M, Yeoman G. Thiazolidinediones for type 2 diabetes. All glitazones may exacerbate heart failure. BMJ 2001;322(7280):236.

53. Nissen SE, Wolski K. Effect of rosiglitazone on the risk of myocardial infarction and death from cardiovascular causes. N Engl J Med 2007;356(24):2457–71.

54. Khalaf KI, Taegtmeyer H. After avandia: the use of antidiabetic drugs in patients with heart failure. Tex Heart Inst J 2012;39(2):174–8.

55. Loke YK, Kwok CS, Singh S. Comparative cardiovascular effects of thiazolidinediones: systematic review and meta-analysis of observational studies. BMJ 2011;342:d1309.

56. Singh S, Loke YK, Furberg CD. Thiazolidinediones and heart failure: a teleo-analysis. Diabetes Care 2007;30(8):2148–53.

57. Lincoff AM, Wolski K, Nicholls SJ, et al. Pioglitazone and risk of cardiovascular events in patients with type 2 diabetes mellitus: a meta-analysis of randomized trials. JAMA 2007;298(10):1180–8.

58. Kahn SE, Haffner SM, Heise MA, et al. Glycemic durability of rosiglitazone, metformin, or glyburide monotherapy. N Engl J Med 2006;355(23):2427–43.

59. Kahn SE, Zinman B, Lachin JM, et al. Rosiglitazone-associated fractures in type 2 diabetes: an analysis from A Diabetes Outcome Progression Trial (ADOPT). Diabetes Care 2008;31(5):845–51.

60. Loke YK, Singh S, Furberg CD. Long-term use of thiazolidinediones and fractures in type 2 diabetes: a meta-analysis. CMAJ 2009;180(1):32–9.

61. Colmers IN, Bowker SL, Majumdar SR, et al. Use of thiazolidinediones and the risk of bladder cancer among people with type 2 diabetes: a meta-analysis. CMAJ 2012;184(12):E675–83.

62. Klupa T, Skupien J, Malecki MT. Monogenic models: what have the single gene disorders taught us? Curr Diab Rep 2012;12(6):659–66.

63. Aguilar-Bryan L, Nichols CG, Wechsler SW, et al. Cloning of the beta cell high-affinity sulfonylurea receptor: a regulator of insulin secretion. Science 1995; 268(5209):423–6.
64. Hermann LS, Schersten B, Bitzen PO, et al. Therapeutic comparison of metformin and sulfonylurea, alone and in various combinations. A double-blind controlled study. Diabetes Care 1994;17(10):1100–9.
65. Xu H, Murray M, McLachlan AJ. Influence of genetic polymorphisms on the pharmacokinetics and pharmaco-dynamics of sulfonylurea drugs. Curr Drug Metab 2009;10(6):643–58.
66. Melander A. Kinetics-effect relations of insulin-releasing drugs in patients with type 2 diabetes: brief overview. Diabetes 2004;53(Suppl 3):S151–5.
67. Nathan DM, Buse JB, Davidson MB, et al. Management of hyperglycemia in type 2 diabetes: a consensus algorithm for the initiation and adjustment of therapy: a consensus statement from the American Diabetes Association and the European Association for the Study of Diabetes. Diabetes Care 2006;29(8):1963–72.
68. Nichols GA, Gomez-Caminero A. Weight changes following the initiation of new anti-hyperglycaemic therapies. Diabetes Obes Metab 2007;9(1):96–102.
69. Feinglos MN, Bethel MA. Therapy of type 2 diabetes, cardiovascular death, and the UGDP. Am Heart J 1999;138(5 Pt 1):S346–52.
70. UKPDS 28: a randomized trial of efficacy of early addition of metformin in sulfonylurea-treated type 2 diabetes. U.K. Prospective Diabetes Study Group. Diabetes Care 1998;21(1):87–92.
71. Zarich SW. Does choice of antidiabetes therapy influence macrovascular outcomes? Curr Diab Rep 2010;10(1):24–31.
72. Cleveland JC Jr, Meldrum DR, Cain BS, et al. Oral sulfonylurea hypoglycemic agents prevent ischemic preconditioning in human myocardium. Two paradoxes revisited. Circulation 1997;96(1):29–32.
73. Zeller M, Danchin N, Simon D, et al. Impact of type of preadmission sulfonylureas on mortality and cardiovascular outcomes in diabetic patients with acute myocardial infarction. J Clin Endocrinol Metab 2010;95(11):4993–5002.
74. Kadowaki T, Hagura R, Kajinuma H, et al. Chlorpropamide-induced hyponatremia: incidence and risk factors. Diabetes Care 1983;6(5):468–71.
75. Groop L, Eriksson CJ, Huupponen R, et al. Roles of chlorpropamide, alcohol and acetaldehyde in determining the chlorpropamide-alcohol flush. Diabetologia 1984;26(1):34–8.
76. Landgraf R. Meglitinide analogues in the treatment of type 2 diabetes mellitus. Drugs Aging 2000;17(5):411–25.
77. Dunning BE. New non-sulfonylurea insulin secretagogues. Expert Opin Investig Drugs 1997;6(8):1041–8.
78. Karara AH, Dunning BE, McLeod JF. The effect of food on the oral bioavailability and the pharmacodynamic actions of the insulinotropic agent nateglinide in healthy subjects. J Clin Pharmacol 1999;39(2):172–9.
79. Wolffenbuttel BH, Landgraf R. A 1-year multicenter randomized double-blind comparison of repaglinide and glyburide for the treatment of type 2 diabetes. Dutch and German Repaglinide Study Group. Diabetes Care 1999;22(3):463–7.
80. Hollander PA, Schwartz SL, Gatlin MR, et al. Importance of early insulin secretion: comparison of nateglinide and glyburide in previously diet-treated patients with type 2 diabetes. Diabetes Care 2001;24(6):983–8.
81. Moses R, Slobodniuk R, Boyages S, et al. Effect of repaglinide addition to metformin monotherapy on glycemic control in patients with type 2 diabetes. Diabetes Care 1999;22(1):119–24.

82. Black C, Donnelly P, McIntyre L, et al. Meglitinide analogues for type 2 diabetes mellitus. Cochrane Database Syst Rev 2007;(2):CD004654.

83. Eleftheriadou I, Grigoropoulou P, Katsilambros N, et al. The effects of medications used for the management of diabetes and obesity on postprandial lipid metabolism. Curr Diabetes Rev 2008;4(4):340–56.

84. Horton ES, Foley JE, Shen SG, et al. Efficacy and tolerability of initial combination therapy with nateglinide and metformin in treatment-naive patients with type 2 diabetes. Curr Med Res Opin 2004;20(6):883–9.

85. Horton ES, Clinkingbeard C, Gatlin M, et al. Nateglinide alone and in combination with metformin improves glycemic control by reducing mealtime glucose levels in type 2 diabetes. Diabetes Care 2000;23(11):1660–5.

86. van de Laar FA, Lucassen PL, Akkermans RP, et al. Alpha-glucosidase inhibitors for patients with type 2 diabetes: results from a Cochrane systematic review and meta-analysis. Diabetes Care 2005;28(1):154–63.

87. Chiasson JL, Josse RG, Hunt JA, et al. The efficacy of acarbose in the treatment of patients with non-insulin-dependent diabetes mellitus. A multicenter controlled clinical trial. Ann Intern Med 1994;121(12):928–35.

88. Goke B, Fuder H, Wieckhorst G, et al. Voglibose (AO-128) is an efficient alpha-glucosidase inhibitor and mobilizes the endogenous GLP-1 reserve. Digestion 1995;56(6):493–501.

89. Rosak C, Mertes G. Critical evaluation of the role of acarbose in the treatment of diabetes: patient considerations. Diabetes Metab Syndr Obes 2012;5:357–67.

90. Koyasu M, Ishii H, Watarai M, et al. Impact of acarbose on carotid intima-media thickness in patients with newly diagnosed impaired glucose tolerance or mild type 2 diabetes mellitus: a one-year, prospective, randomized, open-label, parallel-group study in Japanese adults with established coronary artery disease. Clin Ther 2010;32(9):1610–7.

91. Derosa G, Maffioli P. Efficacy and safety profile evaluation of acarbose alone and in association with other antidiabetic drugs: a systematic review. Clin Ther 2012;34(6):1221–36.

92. Chiasson JL, Josse RG, Gomis R, et al. Acarbose treatment and the risk of cardiovascular disease and hypertension in patients with impaired glucose tolerance: the STOP-NIDDM trial. JAMA 2003;290(4):486–94.

93. Hansen L, Deacon CF, Orskov C, et al. Glucagon-like peptide-1-(7-36)amide is transformed to glucagon-like peptide-1-(9-36)amide by dipeptidyl peptidase IV in the capillaries supplying the L cells of the porcine intestine. Endocrinology 1999;140(11):5356–63.

94. Bullock BP, Heller RS, Habener JF. Tissue distribution of messenger ribonucleic acid encoding the rat glucagon-like peptide-1 receptor. Endocrinology 1996;137(7):2968–78.

95. Nakagawa A, Satake H, Nakabayashi H, et al. Receptor gene expression of glucagon-like peptide-1, but not glucose-dependent insulinotropic polypeptide, in rat nodose ganglion cells. Auton Neurosci 2004;110(1):36–43.

96. Schirra J, Nicolaus M, Roggel R, et al. Endogenous glucagon-like peptide 1 controls endocrine pancreatic secretion and antro-pyloro-duodenal motility in humans. Gut 2006;55(2):243–51.

97. Salehi M, Vahl TP, D'Alessio DA. Regulation of islet hormone release and gastric emptying by endogenous glucagon-like peptide 1 after glucose ingestion. J Clin Endocrinol Metab 2008;93(12):4909–16.

98. Nauck MA, Niedereichholz U, Ettler R, et al. Glucagon-like peptide 1 inhibition of gastric emptying outweighs its insulinotropic effects in healthy humans. Am J

Physiol 1997;273(5 Pt 1): E981–8.

99. Wettergren A, Schjoldager B, Mortensen PE, et al. Truncated GLP-1 (proglucagon 78-107-amide) inhibits gastric and pancreatic functions in man. Dig Dis Sci 1993;38(4):665–73.

100. Meier JJ, Gallwitz B, Salmen S, et al. Normalization of glucose concentrations and deceleration of gastric emptying after solid meals during intravenous glucagon-like peptide 1 in patients with type 2 diabetes. J Clin Endocrinol Metab 2003;88(6):2719–25.

101. Flint A, Raben A, Astrup A, et al. Glucagon-like peptide 1 promotes satiety and suppresses energy intake in humans. J Clin Invest 1998;101(3):515–20.

102. Prigeon RL, Quddusi S, Paty B, et al. Suppression of glucose production by GLP-1 independent of islet hormones: a novel extrapancreatic effect. Am J Physiol Endocrinol Metab 2003;285(4):E701–7.

103. Kielgast U, Holst JJ, Madsbad S. Antidiabetic actions of endogenous and exogenous GLP-1 in type 1 diabetic patients with and without residual beta-cell function. Diabetes 2011;60(5):1599–607.

104. Creutzfeldt WO, Kleine N, Willms B, et al. Glucagonostatic actions and reduction of fasting hyperglycemia by exogenous glucagon-like peptide I(7-36) amide in type I diabetic patients. Diabetes Care 1996;19(6):580–6.

105. Vella A, Bock G, Giesler PD, et al. Effects of dipeptidyl peptidase-4 inhibition on gastrointestinal function, meal appearance, and glucose metabolism in type 2 diabetes. Diabetes 2007;56(5):1475–80.

106. Russell S. Incretin-based therapies for type 2 diabetes mellitus: a review of direct comparisons of efficacy, safety and patient satisfaction. Int J Clin Pharm 2013;35(2):159–72.

107. Bergman AJ, Cote J, Yi B, et al. Effect of renal insufficiency on the pharmacokinetics of sitagliptin, a dipeptidyl peptidase-4 inhibitor. Diabetes Care 2007; 30(7):1862–4.

108. Baetta R, Corsini A. Pharmacology of dipeptidyl peptidase-4 inhibitors: similarities and differences. Drugs 2011;71(11):1441–67.

109. Aroda VR, Henry RR, Han J, et al. Efficacy of GLP-1 receptor agonists and DPP-4 inhibitors: meta-analysis and systematic review. Clin Ther 2012;34(6): 1247–1258.e22.

110. Nauck MA, Duran S, Kim D, et al. A comparison of twice-daily exenatide and biphasic insulin aspart in patients with type 2 diabetes who were suboptimally controlled with sulfonylurea and metformin: a non-inferiority study. Diabetologia 2007;50(2):259–67.

111. Diamant M, Van Gaal L, Stranks S, et al. Safety and efficacy of once-weekly exenatide compared with insulin glargine titrated to target in patients with type 2 diabetes over 84 weeks. Diabetes Care 2012;35(4):683–9.

112. Bergenstal RM, Wysham C, Macconell L, et al. Efficacy and safety of exenatide once weekly versus sitagliptin or pioglitazone as an adjunct to metformin for treatment of type 2 diabetes (DURATION-2): a randomised trial. Lancet 2010; 376(9739):431–9.

113. Gallwitz B, Vaag A, Falahati A, et al. Adding liraglutide to oral antidiabetic drug therapy: onset of treatment effects over time. Int J Clin Pract 2010;64(2):267–76.

114. Pratley RE, Nauck M, Bailey T, et al. Liraglutide versus sitagliptin for patients with type 2 diabetes who did not have adequate glycaemic control with metformin: a 26-week, randomised, parallel-group, open-label trial. Lancet 2010; 375(9724):1447–56.

115. Buse JB, Rosenstock J, Sesti G, et al. Liraglutide once a day versus exenatide twice a day for type 2 diabetes: a 26-week randomised, parallel-group, multinational, open-label trial (LEAD-6). Lancet 2009;374(9683):39–47.

116. Aschner P, Kipnes MS, Lunceford JK, et al. Effect of the dipeptidyl peptidase-4 inhibitor sitagliptin as monotherapy on glycemic control in patients with type 2 diabetes. Diabetes Care 2006;29(12):2632–7.

117. Charbonnel B, Karasik A, Liu J, et al. Efficacy and safety of the dipeptidyl peptidase-4 inhibitor sitagliptin added to ongoing metformin therapy in patients with type 2 diabetes inadequately controlled with metformin alone. Diabetes Care 2006;29(12):2638–43.

118. Nauck MA, Heimesaat MM, Behle K, et al. Effects of glucagon-like peptide 1 on counterregulatory hormone responses, cognitive functions, and insulin secretion during hyperinsulinemic, stepped hypoglycemic clamp experiments in healthy volunteers. J Clin Endocrinol Metab 2002;87(3):1239–46.

119. Buse JB, Henry RR, Han J, et al. Effects of exenatide (exendin-4) on glycemic control over 30 weeks in sulfonylurea-treated patients with type 2 diabetes. Diabetes Care 2004;27(11):2628–35.

120. Kendall DM, Riddle MC, Rosenstock J, et al. Effects of exenatide (exendin-4) on glycemic control over 30 weeks in patients with type 2 diabetes treated with metformin and a sulfonylurea. Diabetes Care 2005;28(5):1083–91.

121. Raz I, Hanefeld M, Xu L, et al. Efficacy and safety of the dipeptidyl peptidase-4 inhibitor sitagliptin as monotherapy in patients with type 2 diabetes mellitus. Diabetologia 2006;49(11):2564–71.

122. DeFronzo RA, Hissa MN, Garber AJ, et al. The efficacy and safety of saxagliptin when added to metformin therapy in patients with inadequately controlled type 2 diabetes with metformin alone. Diabetes Care 2009;32(9):1649–55.

123. Del Prato S, Barnett AH, Huisman H, et al. Effect of linagliptin monotherapy on glycaemic control and markers of beta-cell function in patients with inadequately controlled type 2 diabetes: a randomized controlled trial. Diabetes Obes Metab 2011;13(3):258–67.

124. DeFronzo RA, Ratner RE, Han J, et al. Effects of exenatide (exendin-4) on glycemic control and weight over 30 weeks in metformin-treated patients with type 2 diabetes. Diabetes Care 2005;28(5):1092–100.

125. Drucker DJ, Buse JB, Taylor K, et al. Exenatide once weekly versus twice daily for the treatment of type 2 diabetes: a randomised, open-label, non-inferiority study. Lancet 2008;372(9645):1240–50.

126. Elashoff M, Matveyenko AV, Gier B, et al. Pancreatitis, pancreatic, and thyroid cancer with glucagon-like peptide-1-based therapies. Gastroenterology 2011;141(1):150–6.

127. Singh S, Chang HY, Richards TM, et al. Glucagonlike peptide 1-based therapies and risk of hospitalization for acute pancreatitis in type 2 diabetes mellitus: a population-based matched case-control study. JAMA Intern Med 2013;173(7):534–9.

128. Garg R, Chen W, Pendergrass M. Acute pancreatitis in type 2 diabetes treated with exenatide or sitagliptin: a retrospective observational pharmacy claims analysis. Diabetes Care 2010;33(11):2349–54.

129. Crespel A, De Boisvilliers F, Gros L, et al. Effects of glucagon and glucagon-like peptide-1-(7-36) amide on C cells from rat thyroid and medullary thyroid carcinoma CA-77 cell line. Endocrinology 1996;137(9):3674–80.

130. Butler PC, Elashoff M, Elashoff R, et al. A critical analysis of the clinical use of incretin-based therapies: are the GLP-1 therapies safe? Diabetes Care 2013;36(7):2118–25.

131. Bjerre Knudsen L, Madsen LW, Andersen S, et al. Glucagon-like peptide-1 receptor agonists activate rodent thyroid C-cells causing calcitonin release and C-cell proliferation. Endocrinology 2010;151(4):1473–86.
132. Adeghate E, Kalasz H. Amylin analogues in the treatment of diabetes mellitus: medicinal chemistry and structural basis of its function. Open Med Chem J 2011;5(Suppl 2):78–81.
133. Young A. Inhibition of food intake. Adv Pharmacol 2005;52:79–98.
134. Fineman M, Weyer C, Maggs DG, et al. The human amylin analog, pramlintide, reduces postprandial hyperglucagonemia in patients with type 2 diabetes mellitus. Horm Metab Res 2002;34(9):504–8.
135. Ratner RE, Dickey R, Fineman M, et al. Amylin replacement with pramlintide as an adjunct to insulin therapy improves long-term glycaemic and weight control in type 1 diabetes mellitus: a 1-year, randomized controlled trial. Diabet Med 2004;21(11):1204–12.
136. Hollander PA, Levy P, Fineman MS, et al. Pramlintide as an adjunct to insulin therapy improves long-term glycemic and weight control in patients with type 2 diabetes: a 1-year randomized controlled trial. Diabetes Care 2003;26(3): 784–90.
137. Thompson RG, Pearson L, Schoenfeld SL, et al. Pramlintide, a synthetic analog of human amylin, improves the metabolic profile of patients with type 2 diabetes using insulin. The Pramlintide in Type 2 Diabetes Group. Diabetes Care 1998; 21(6):987–93.
138. Singh-Franco D, Robles G, Gazze D. Pramlintide acetate injection for the treatment of type 1 and type 2 diabetes mellitus. Clin Ther 2007;29(4):535–62.
139. Stenlof K, Cefalu WT, Kim KA, et al. Efficacy and safety of canagliflozin monotherapy in subjects with type 2 diabetes mellitus inadequately controlled with diet and exercise. Diabetes Obes Metab 2013;15(4):372–82.
140. List JF, Woo V, Morales E, et al. Sodium-glucose cotransport inhibition with dapagliflozin in type 2 diabetes. Diabetes Care 2009;32(4):650–7.
141. Foote C, Perkovic V, Neal B. Effects of SGLT2 inhibitors on cardiovascular outcomes. Diab Vasc Dis Res 2012;9(2):117–23.
142. Ferrannini E, Seman LJ, Seewaldt-Becker L, et al. The potent and highly selective sodium-glucose co-transporter (SGLT-2) inhibitor BI 10773 is safe and efficacious as monotherapy in patients with type 2 diabetes mellitus [abstract]. Diabetologia 2010;53(Suppl 2):877.
143. Bailey CJ, Gross JL, Pieters A, et al. Effect of dapagliflozin in patients with type 2 diabetes who have inadequate glycaemic control with metformin: a randomised, double-blind, placebo-controlled trial. Lancet 2010;375(9733):2223–33.
144. Bailey CJ, Gross JL, Hennicken D, et al. Dapagliflozin add-on to metformin in type 2 diabetes inadequately controlled with metformin: a randomized, double-blind, placebo-controlled 102-week trial. BMC Med 2013;11:43.
145. Turner RC, Cull CA, Frighi V, et al. Glycemic control with diet, sulfonylurea, metformin, or insulin in patients with type 2 diabetes mellitus: progressive requirement for multiple therapies (UKPDS 49). UK Prospective Diabetes Study (UKPDS) Group. JAMA 1999;281(21):2005–12.
146. Levy J, Atkinson AB, Bell PM, et al. Beta-cell deterioration determines the onset and rate of progression of secondary dietary failure in type 2 diabetes mellitus: the 10-year follow-up of the Belfast Diet Study. Diabet Med 1998;15(4):290–6.
147. Farilla L, Bulotta A, Hirshberg B, et al. Glucagon-like peptide 1 inhibits cell apoptosis and improves glucose responsiveness of freshly isolated human islets. Endocrinology 2003;144(12):5149–58.

148. Farilla L, Hui H, Bertolotto C, et al. Glucagon-like peptide-1 promotes islet cell growth and inhibits apoptosis in Zucker diabetic rats. Endocrinology 2002; 143(11):4397–408.

149. Viberti G, Kahn SE, Greene DA, et al. A diabetes outcome progression trial (ADOPT): an international multicenter study of the comparative efficacy of rosiglitazone, glyburide, and metformin in recently diagnosed type 2 diabetes. Diabetes Care 2002;25(10):1737–43.

150. Gallwitz B, Guzman J, Dotta F, et al. Exenatide twice daily versus glimepiride for prevention of glycaemic deterioration in patients with type 2 diabetes with metformin failure (EUREXA): an open-label, randomised controlled trial. Lancet 2012;379(9833):2270–8.

Index

Note: Page numbers of article titles are in **boldface** type.

Endocrinol Metab Clin N Am 42 (2013) 971–1014
http://dx.doi.org/10.1016/S0889-8529(13)00103-5
0889-8529/13/$ – see front matter © 2013 Elsevier Inc. All rights reserved.

Printed and bound by CPI Group (UK) Ltd, Croydon, CR0 4YY

03/10/2024

01040409-0014